Social Isolation and Loneliness in Older Adults

OPPORTUNITIES FOR THE HEALTH CARE SYSTEM

Committee on the Health and Medical Dimensions of Social Isolation and Loneliness in Older Adults

Board on Health Sciences Policy

Health and Medicine Division

Board on Behavioral, Cognitive, and Sensory Sciences

Division of Behavioral and Social Sciences and Education

A Consensus Study Report of

The National Academies of
SCIENCES · ENGINEERING · MEDICINE

AF622502

THE NATIONAL ACADEMIES PRESS
Washington, DC
www.nap.edu

THE NATIONAL ACADEMIES PRESS 500 Fifth Street, NW Washington, DC 20001

This activity was supported by a contract between the National Academy of Sciences and the AARP Foundation. Any opinions, findings, conclusions, or recommendations expressed in this publication do not necessarily reflect the views of any organization or agency that provided support for the project.

International Standard Book Number-13: 978–0-309-67100-2
International Standard Book Number-10: 0-309-67100-0
Digital Object Identifier: https://doi.org/10.17226/25663
Library of Congress Control Number: 2020934003

Additional copies of this publication are available from the National Academies Press, 500 Fifth Street, NW, Keck 360, Washington, DC 20001; (800) 624-6242 or (202) 334-3313; http://www.nap.edu.

Copyright 2020 by the National Academy of Sciences. All rights reserved.

Printed in the United States of America

Suggested citation: National Academies of Sciences, Engineering, and Medicine. 2020. *Social isolation and loneliness in older adults: Opportunities for the health care system.* Washington, DC: The National Academies Press. https://doi.org/10.17226/25663.

The National Academies of

SCIENCES · ENGINEERING · MEDICINE

The **National Academy of Sciences** was established in 1863 by an Act of Congress, signed by President Lincoln, as a private, nongovernmental institution to advise the nation on issues related to science and technology. Members are elected by their peers for outstanding contributions to research. Dr. Marcia McNutt is president.

The **National Academy of Engineering** was established in 1964 under the charter of the National Academy of Sciences to bring the practices of engineering to advising the nation. Members are elected by their peers for extraordinary contributions to engineering. Dr. John L. Anderson is president.

The **National Academy of Medicine** (formerly the Institute of Medicine) was established in 1970 under the charter of the National Academy of Sciences to advise the nation on medical and health issues. Members are elected by their peers for distinguished contributions to medicine and health. Dr. Victor J. Dzau is president.

The three Academies work together as the **National Academies of Sciences, Engineering, and Medicine** to provide independent, objective analysis and advice to the nation and conduct other activities to solve complex problems and inform public policy decisions. The National Academies also encourage education and research, recognize outstanding contributions to knowledge, and increase public understanding in matters of science, engineering, and medicine.

Learn more about the National Academies of Sciences, Engineering, and Medicine at **www.nationalacademies.org.**

The National Academies of
SCIENCES · ENGINEERING · MEDICINE

Consensus Study Reports published by the National Academies of Sciences, Engineering, and Medicine document the evidence-based consensus on the study's statement of task by an authoring committee of experts. Reports typically include findings, conclusions, and recommendations based on information gathered by the committee and the committee's deliberations. Each report has been subjected to a rigorous and independent peer-review process and it represents the position of the National Academies on the statement of task.

Proceedings published by the National Academies of Sciences, Engineering, and Medicine chronicle the presentations and discussions at a workshop, symposium, or other event convened by the National Academies. The statements and opinions contained in proceedings are those of the participants and are not endorsed by other participants, the planning committee, or the National Academies.

For information about other products and activities of the National Academies, please visit www.nationalacademies.org/about/whatwedo.

COMMITTEE ON THE HEALTH AND MEDICAL DIMENSIONS OF SOCIAL ISOLATION AND LONELINESS IN OLDER ADULTS

DAN G. BLAZER II (*Chair*), J.P. Gibbons Professor Emeritus of Psychiatry, Duke University School of Medicine
SUSAN BEANE, Vice President and Medical Director, Healthfirst, Inc.
CYNTHIA M. BOYD, Professor, Johns Hopkins Bloomberg School of Public Health
LINDA BURNES BOLTON, Senior Vice President and Chief Health Equity Officer, Cedars-Sinai Medical Center
GEORGE DEMIRIS, Penn Integrates Knowledge University Professor, University of Pennsylvania
NANCY J. DONOVAN, Director, Division of Geriatric Psychiatry, Brigham and Women's Hospital, Harvard Medical School
ROBERT ESPINOZA, Vice President of Policy, PHI
COLLEEN GALAMBOS, Professor and Helen Bader Endowed Chair in Applied Gerontology, University of Wisconsin–Milwaukee Helen Bader School of Social Welfare
JULIANNE HOLT-LUNSTAD, Professor, Brigham Young University
JAMES S. HOUSE, Angus Campbell Distinguished University Professor Emeritus, Survey Research University of Michigan Institute for Social Research
KATHLEEN McGARRY, Professor and Vice Chair, Department of Economics, University of California, Los Angeles
JEANNE MIRANDA, Professor, Department of Psychiatry and Biobehavioral Sciences, University of California, Los Angeles
LAURIE LOVETT NOVAK, Assistant Professor, Department of Biomedical Informatics, Vanderbilt University School of Medicine
CARLA M. PERISSINOTTO, Associate Professor of Medicine and Associate Chief of Clinical Programs in Geriatrics, University of California, San Francisco
JULIANN G. SEBASTIAN, Dean and Professor, College of Nursing, University of Nebraska Medical Center

Study Staff

TRACY A. LUSTIG, Study Director
JENNIFER A. COHEN, Program Officer
CAROLINE M. CILIO, Associate Program Officer (*through October 2019*)
KENDALL LOGAN, Senior Program Assistant
ANDREW M. POPE, Senior Director, Board on Health Sciences Policy

Consultant

MARITA G. TITLER, University of Michigan School of Nursing

Reviewers

This Consensus Study Report was reviewed in draft form by individuals chosen for their diverse perspectives and technical expertise. The purpose of this independent review is to provide candid and critical comments that will assist the National Academies of Sciences, Engineering, and Medicine in making each published report as sound as possible and to ensure that it meets the institutional standards for quality, objectivity, evidence, and responsiveness to the study charge. The review comments and draft manuscript remain confidential to protect the integrity of the deliberative process.

We thank the following individuals for their review of this report:

LINDA FRIED, Columbia University Mailman School of Public Health
TERRY T. FULMER, The John A. Hartford Foundation
CARMEN GARCIA-PENA, National Institute of Geriatrics
LOUISE HAWKLEY, NORC at the University of Chicago
MITCHELL H. KATZ, Health + Hospitals
JAMES LUBBEN, University of California, Los Angeles
JOSÉ A. PAGÁN, New York University School of Global Public Health
MICHELLE PUTNAM, Simmons University School of Social Work
NIRAV R. SHAH, Stanford University
ROBYN STONE, LeadingAge
PAUL C. TANG, Stanford University
WINSTON WONG, Kaiser Permanente

Although the reviewers listed above provided many constructive comments and suggestions, they were not asked to endorse the conclusions or recommendations of this report nor did they see the final draft before its release. The review of this report was overseen by **BOBBIE A. BERKOWITZ,** Columbia University School of Nursing and University of Washington, and **NANCY FUGATE WOODS,** University of Washington. They were responsible for making certain that an independent examination of this report was carried out in accordance with the standards of the National Academies and that all review comments were carefully considered. Responsibility for the final content rests entirely with the authoring committee and the National Academies.

Acknowledgments

The study committee and the Health and Medicine Division (HMD) project staff take this opportunity to recognize and thank the many individuals who shared their time and expertise to support the committee's work and to inform deliberations.

This study was sponsored by the AARP Foundation. We thank the AARP Foundation president, Lisa Marsh Ryerson, for her guidance and support. We also wish to recognize the important contributions of Emily Allen and Eliza Heppner, who were instrumental in helping to launch this effort.

The committee benefitted greatly from discussions with individuals who made presentations during the committee's open sessions: Martha Bruce, James Coen, Sara Czaja, Steve Ewell, Maureen Feldman, Linda Fried, Jeanne-Marie Guise, Sachin Jain, Michael Monson, Jessica Retrum, Lucy Savitz, Bert Uchino, and Colin Walsh. The committee is very grateful to these presenters for volunteering to share their knowledge, data, and expert opinions with the committee and members of the public who attended the committee's open sessions. Special thanks are also extended to Sara Czaja for her early interest in this effort and her ongoing support of the National Academies' work. The staff also recognize Martha Coven, Robin Mockenhaupt, Sheila Shapiro, and Bob Wallace for providing expertise and replying to staff inquiries.

The committee is grateful for the many staff within HMD who provided support at various times throughout this project. Special thanks are extended to Rebecca Morgan, senior librarian, who compiled literature searches; Bardia Massoudkhan, the financial associate for this project; and Robert Pool, for his editorial assistance provided in preparing the final report.

Preface

Human beings are social by nature, and high-quality social relationships are vital for health and well-being. Like many other social determinants of health, however, social isolation (an objective lack of social contact with others) and loneliness (the subjective feeling of being isolated) are significant yet underappreciated public health risks. Social isolation and loneliness are associated with poor physical and mental health outcomes, including higher rates of mortality, depression, and cognitive decline. Recent research documents the high prevalence of social isolation and loneliness among older adults. For example, data from the National Health and Aging Trends Study found that 24 percent of community-dwelling older adults are considered socially isolated, and a 2018 survey by the AARP Foundation found that more than one-third (35 percent) of adults aged 45 and older are lonely. Additionally, a 2018 study by the Kaiser Family Foundation found that 22 percent of adults in the United States say they "often or always feel lonely, feel that they lack companionship, feel left out, or feel isolated from others."

While the science of social relationships and their consequences on health and well-being has been documented for decades, the topics of social isolation and loneliness have recently garnered increased attention in the mass media. For example, in the past few years, articles in *The New York Times* featured headlines such as "How Social Isolation Is Killing Us" and "The Surprising Effects of Loneliness on Health."

In particular, the AARP Foundation has played a key role in bringing attention to the health and medical impacts of social isolation and loneliness. In this context, the AARP Foundation came to the National Academies of Sciences, Engineering, and Medicine for an examination of the health and medical dimensions of social isolation and loneliness and for recommendations on the role of the health care system in helping to reduce the incidence and adverse health impacts of social isolation and loneliness among older adults in clinical settings. This exploration is notable in that relatively few stakeholders have paid attention to the particular role that health care professionals and providers can play.

During this broad-based review of the issues of social isolation and loneliness, the committee identified several overarching challenges. Most prominently is the multiplicity of terms for different aspects of social relationships (such as social isolation, social support, loneliness, and social networks, among others). Furthermore, the terms social isolation and loneliness are often conflated, but they represent distinct concepts, each with their own measures. As a result, the literature base on the health and medical impacts of social isolation and loneliness, as well as potential interventions, are confounded by this confusion of terminology. In the report, the committee sought to carefully report the evidence accurately in terms of the specific aspects of social isolation and loneliness that were actually targeted and measured.

This report presents a comprehensive review of the impacts of social isolation and loneliness on mortality and morbidity, the risk factors for social isolation and loneliness, the mechanisms by which social isolation and loneliness impact health, the factors that affect those mechanisms, and the ways in which researchers measure social isolation and loneliness and their resultant impacts on health. Furthermore, the committee discusses the role of the health care system in addressing these issues, the ways in which we can better educate and train our health care workforce, and which interventions (particularly for the clinical setting) show the most promise. Finally, the committee discusses general principles of dissemination and implementation that will be important for translating research into practice, especially as the evidence base for effective interventions continues to flourish.

Overall, this committee comes to the firm conclusion that the health care system is well poised to develop and evaluate methods and processes to identify social isolation and loneliness among older adults in clinical settings. In fact, the committee notes that a single interaction with the health care system may represent the only opportunity to identify those individuals who are the most isolated and lonely. However, we emphasize that the health care system cannot solve the problems of social isolation and loneliness alone; rather, the goals and recommendations presented in this report represent a vision for how the health care system can help as part of a larger global effort to combat the adverse health impacts of social isolation and loneliness among adults aged 50 and older in the United States.

As chair of the committee I would like to recognize and thank each committee member for his/her contributions to the report. Our committee was most engaged with, even passionate, about the topic yet throughout our discussions and drafting of the report the committee maintained the highest level of critical thinking and reliance on the evidence available to us. The entire committee owes a special thanks to Tracy Lustig, Jennifer Cohen, Caroline Cilio, and Kendall Logan. We could not have asked for a more dedicated and thoughtful staff from the National Academies. Finally I offer thanks to Andy Pope, the senior director of the Board on Health Sciences Policy at the National Academies and to the AARP Foundation for supporting this exciting and meaningful exploration.

Dan G. Blazer II, *Chair*
Committee on the Health and Medical Dimensions of
Social Isolation and Loneliness in Older Adults

Contents

Summary

Social isolation (the objective state of having few social relationships or infrequent social contact with others) and loneliness (a subjective feeling of being isolated) are serious yet underappreciated public health risks that affect a significant portion of the older adult population. Approximately one-quarter (24 percent) of community-dwelling Americans aged 65 and older are considered to be socially isolated, and a significant proportion of adults in the United States report feeling lonely (35 percent of adults aged 45 and older and 43 percent of adults aged 60 and older). While there are challenges in measuring social isolation and loneliness precisely, there is strong evidence that many older adults are socially isolated or lonely in ways that puts their health at risk. For example:

- Social isolation has been associated with a significantly increased risk of premature mortality from all causes;
- Social isolation has been associated with an approximately 50 percent increased risk of developing dementia;
- Loneliness among heart failure patients has been associated with a nearly four times increased risk of death, 68 percent increased risk of hospitalization, and 57 percent increased risk of emergency department visits; and
- Poor social relationships (characterized by social isolation or loneliness) have been associated with a 29 percent increased risk of incident coronary heart disease and a 32 percent increased risk of stroke.

Understanding the full scope and complexity of the influence of social relationships on health is challenging. In addition to the absolute number or extent of social relationships, the quality of such relationships is also an important factor in their impact on health. Two aspects of social relationships, social isolation and loneliness, have become increasingly prominent in the scientific literature. While both social isolation and loneliness can affect health throughout the life course, this report focuses on the health impacts of social isolation and loneliness among adults aged 50 and older. Of note, it is incorrect to assume that all older adults are isolated or lonely or that aging, independent of other factors, causes social isolation and loneliness. Rather, older adults are at increased risk for social isolation and loneliness because they are more likely to face predisposing factors such as living alone, the loss of family or friends, chronic illness, and sensory impairments. Over a life course, social isolation and loneliness may be episodic or chronic, depending on an individual's circumstances and perceptions.

Many approaches have been taken to improve social connections for individuals who are socially isolated or lonely, but opportunities to intervene may be most challenging for those who are at highest risk. For example, people who do not have consistent interactions with others (e.g., have unstable housing, do not belong to any social or religious groups, or do not have significant personal relationships) may never be identified in their own communities. However, nearly all persons 50 years of age or older interact with the health care system in some way. Therefore, this report focuses on the role of the health care system as a key and relatively untapped partner in efforts to identify, prevent, and mitigate the adverse health impacts of social isolation and loneliness in older adults.

STUDY CONTEXT AND CHARGE

A systematic and rigorous science of social relationships and their consequences, especially in terms of health, emerged in the latter part of the 20th century as part of a broader recognition of the role of social determinants of health. By the beginning of the 21st century, several aspects of social relationships were being studied systematically in research and had been identified as potential influences on human health. Only recently have the adverse health effects of social isolation and loneliness received public attention nationally and internationally. For example, in January 2018, Theresa May, the prime minister of the United Kingdom, established and appointed a Minister of Loneliness to develop policies for both measuring and reducing loneliness.

With support from the AARP Foundation, the National Academies of Sciences, Engineering, and Medicine (the National Academies) formed the Committee on the Health and Medical Dimensions of Social Isolation and Loneliness in Older Adults in fall 2018. The committee's charge essentially consisted of two parts. First, the committee was charged with summarizing the evidence for how social isolation and loneliness affect health and quality of life in adults aged 50 and older, particularly among low-income, underserved, and vulnerable subpopulations (groups the committee refer to as "at-risk" populations). Second, the committee was charged with identifying and recommending opportunities specifically for clinical settings of health care to help reduce the incidence and adverse health impacts of social isolation and loneliness (such as clinical tools and methodologies, professional education, and public awareness) and to examine avenues for the dissemination of information targeted to health care practitioners.[1]

While this report focuses on the role of the health care system, the committee emphasizes that the health care system alone cannot solve all of the challenges of social isolation and loneliness; rather, the health care system needs to connect with the broader public health and social care communities. Furthermore, the committee recognizes that in the larger context of addressing social isolation and loneliness, the most effective interventions may not require the participation of the health care system. However, this does not mean that the health care system should not strive to help improve the health and well-being of those who suffer the adverse health impacts of social isolation and loneliness. In fact, health care providers may be in the best position to identify individuals who are at highest risk for social isolation or loneliness—individuals for whom the health care system may be their only point of contact with their broader community. In this way, the health care system can help those individuals to connect with the most appropriate care, either inside or outside the health care system. Therefore, the health care system has the potential to be a critical component of a much larger solution.

DEFINING ASPECTS OF SOCIAL RELATIONSHIPS

The broad, interdisciplinary scientific fields that together form the modern science of social relationships have used a variety of terms—social isolation, social connection, social networks, social support, social relationships, loneliness, and so forth—to refer to related situations. There are important distinctions among these terms in what they describe or measure, but they are often erroneously used interchangeably. An individual can be isolated and not feel lonely, or can feel lonely even if he or she is not isolated. Social isolation and loneliness represent distinct phenomena. *Social isolation* typically refers to the objective lack of (or limited) social contact with others and is marked by a person having few social network ties, having infrequent social contact, or, potentially, living alone.

[1] The complete Statement of Task is presented in Chapter 1 of this report.

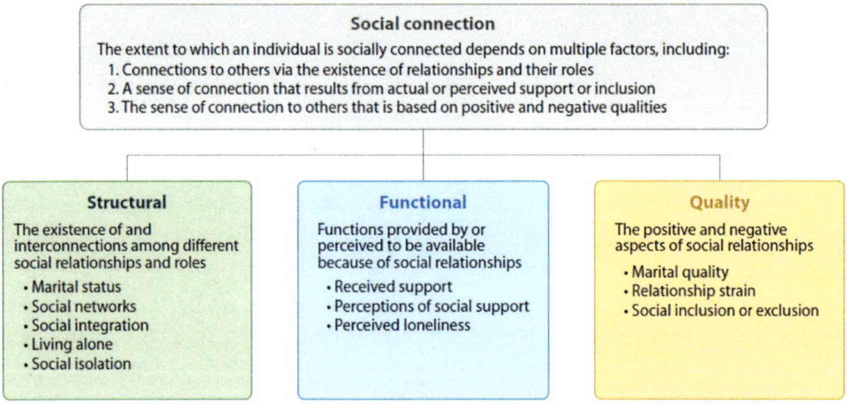

FIGURE S-1 Social connection as a multifactorial construct including structural, functional, and quality components.
SOURCE: Holt-Lunstad, 2018a. Reproduced with permission from the *Annual Review of Psychology*, Volume 69 © 2018 by Annual Reviews, http://www.annualreviews.org (accessed March 13, 2020).

Loneliness, by contrast, refers to the perception of social isolation or the subjective feeling of being lonely. Although those who lack social contact may feel lonely, social isolation and loneliness often are not significantly correlated. Thus, it is important to distinguish between the two states.

The term "social relationships" is arguably the most common way of referring to the connections and intersections among human beings, and it derives from and is employed in broader common usage. In 1979 Berkman and Syme documented the strong association between social relationships and all-cause mortality and, hence, life expectancy, using the terms "social networks" and "social integration" to denote a broad pattern of social relationships (with both individuals and groups). Additionally, there has been much research on the concept of *social support*, the actual or perceived availability of resources from others. Over the past several decades there has been a new focus on loneliness as a risk factor for health. While each of these terms have been linked to important health outcomes, they are not highly correlated, suggesting that they may influence health through different mechanisms. Thus, the term "social connection" has been proposed to encompass the different conceptual and measurement approaches (see Figure S-1). Social isolation is reflected in Figure S-1 as a structural indicator of social connection while loneliness is functional indicator.

The literature concerning social isolation and loneliness uses all of these terms. To describe the evidence base as accurately as possible, when the evidence does not differentiate among or combines several related terms, this report uses

> **BOX S-1**
> **Goals for Enhancing the Role of the Health Care Sector in Addressing the Impacts of Social Isolation and Loneliness in Older Adults**
>
> 1. ***Develop a more robust evidence base*** for effective assessment, prevention, and intervention strategies for social isolation and loneliness;
> 2. ***Translate current research into health care practices*** in order to reduce the negative health impacts of social isolation and loneliness;
> 3. ***Improve awareness*** of the health and medical impacts of social isolation and loneliness across the health care workforce and among members of the public;
> 4. ***Strengthen ongoing education and training*** related to social isolation and loneliness in older adults for the health care workforce; and
> 5. ***Strengthen ties between the health care system and community-based networks and resources*** that address social isolation and loneliness in older adults.

the term "social connection" to refer to the various structural, functional, and quality aspects of social relationships. This report uses the specific terms "social isolation," "loneliness," or other terms when the data are specific to these terms.[2]

GOALS AND RECOMMENDATIONS

The committee formulated its recommendations in accordance with five goals, each of which addresses an aspect of enhancing the role of the health care system in addressing the health impacts of social isolation and loneliness in older adults (see Box S-1). While not all of the recommendations are explicitly directed to clinicians or clinical settings of care, the committee identified recommendations that would be most helpful to reach the ultimate goal of developing and improving clinical interventions to mitigate the negative health impacts of social isolation and loneliness. Furthermore, the committee emphasizes that the preservation of an individual's own decisions regarding his or her life is essential as a guiding principle for all interventions. The following sections discuss the overall goals and recommendations of this report, all of which apply to interventions in health care settings for adults aged 50 and older.

[2] While social integration can describe high social connection, low scores on measures of social integration (e.g., on the Berkman–Syme Social Network Index) are frequently used as an indication of social isolation. Thus, the term "social isolation" will also be used to represent these data.

Goal 1: Develop a More Robust Evidence Base

While a substantial and growing body of evidence demonstrates the health impacts of social isolation and loneliness, the evidence base for interventions for specific populations or settings is less robust. Recommendations are provided for meeting the goal of developing a more robust evidence base on effective assessment, prevention, and intervention strategies.

Social Isolation, Loneliness, and Mortality

Social isolation and loneliness are as prevalent and play as large a role in today's society as many other well-established risk factors for health, yet limited resources and attention have been committed to better understanding social isolation and loneliness and their individual and collective impacts on health. More than four decades of research has produced robust evidence that lacking social connection—and, particularly, scoring high on measures of social isolation—is associated with a significantly increased risk for premature mortality from all causes. Furthermore, there is some evidence that the magnitude of the effect of social connection on risk for mortality may be comparable to or greater than other well-established risk factors that are widely recognized and acted on by the public health and health care systems.

While there is evidence that loneliness is associated with mortality, the existing evidence does not yet approach the cumulative weight of evidence for the association between social isolation and mortality. More research is needed to establish the strength and robustness of the predictive association of loneliness with mortality in relation to social isolation and to clarify how social isolation and loneliness relate to and operate with each other.

> **RECOMMENDATION 2-1: Major funders of health research, including the government (e.g., the National Institutes of Health, the Center for Medicare & Medicaid Innovation, and the Patient-Centered Outcomes Research Institute), foundations, and large health plans should fund research on social isolation and loneliness at levels that reflect their associations with mortality.[3]**

Risk Factors and Health Impacts

The relationships among risk factors, social isolation or loneliness, and health impacts can be reciprocal in that not only can being socially isolated or lonely have an impact on health, but the resultant health conditions can increase an

---

[3] The committee's recommendations are numbered according to the chapter of the main report in which they appear. Thus, Recommendation 2-1 is the first recommendation in Chapter 2.

individual's likelihood of experiencing social isolation or loneliness. Furthermore, some factors may increase the risk for social isolation and loneliness (and ultimately, result in negative health impacts) while other factors may provide protective benefits. Substantial evidence indicates that social isolation, loneliness, and other indicators of social connection have associations with major forms of physical, cognitive, and psychological morbidity; health-related behaviors; and health-related quality of life. However, the evidence for specific impacts in the at-risk populations is sparse.

Beyond these associations, the mechanisms by which social connection, or lack thereof, affects the development and course of disease have been elucidated by a growing evidence base. Strong evidence links social isolation, loneliness, and other indicators of social connection to changes in biological and behavioral responses which may in turn influence health risk. Thus, current evidence supports plausible biological and behavioral mechanisms that explain how social isolation and loneliness ultimately influence health outcomes.

The committee identified the increased funding of basic research as key to developing a more robust evidence base on effective assessment, prevention, and intervention strategies for social isolation and loneliness (Goal 1). Specifically, the committee concluded that identifying, prioritizing, and developing ways to translate scientific knowledge about the impacts of social isolation and loneliness on health into effective and efficient clinical and public health interventions first requires a better understanding of how social isolation and loneliness are connected with each other and how they impact health. This includes understanding the mechanisms through which social isolation and loneliness affect health, the risk factors for social isolation and loneliness, and the factors that affect those relationships.

RECOMMENDATION 3-1: Major funders of health research, including the government (e.g., the National Institutes of Health, the Center for Medicare & Medicaid Innovation, and the Patient-Centered Outcomes Research Institute), foundations, and large health plans should fund research to improve the basic scientific understanding of the links between social connection and health, including the study of risk factors and mechanisms.

The Current Evidence Base for Interventions

The overall quality of the evidence for specific clinical and public health interventions for social isolation and loneliness in older adults is mixed. In part, this is due to the heterogeneity of older people themselves and the underlying causes of their isolation or loneliness. While there is some evidence for promising approaches, the committee concludes that researchers are only beginning to understand which specific approaches work best for which populations and which risk factors. In particular, the committee emphasizes that different intervention approaches may be needed for social isolation versus loneliness. Furthermore, in the case of technological interventions, many gaps in understanding remain, particularly related to possible unintended harms and ethical concerns as well as the impact of current trends, such as the use of social media on future generations of older adults.

The committee identified three major aspects of the evidence base for effective clinical and public health interventions that need to be addressed in order to determine best practices and approaches: quality, funding, and research gaps. That is, the overall quality of the evidence base needs to be improved, adequate funding of research will be required, and research on major gaps in the current evidence base needs to be prioritized. Therefore, the committee makes the following recommendations:

RECOMMENDATION 9-3: Funders should prioritize research that builds a scientific foundation for clinical and public health interventions that reduce the health and medical impacts of social isolation and loneliness based on standard theoretical frameworks. Researchers and health care providers and systems that study interventions for social isolation or loneliness should consider the following key elements in the design and evaluation of any intervention in order to enhance the ability to compare across studies:

- **A theoretical framework that drives particular approaches**
- **Appropriate choice of measure**
- **A specific target population**
- **Scalability**
- **Sustainability**
- **Ways to encourage data sharing**

RECOMMENDATION 9-4: Major funders of health research, including the government (e.g., the National Institutes of Health, the Center for Medicare & Medicaid Innovation, and the Patient-Centered Outcomes Research Institute), foundations, and large health plans should fund research on interventions in clinical settings to identify, prevent, and mitigate the effects of social isolation and loneliness in older adults.

RECOMMENDATION 9-5: Those who fund, develop, and operate programs to assess, prevent, and intervene in social isolation and loneliness should prioritize research on the following major gaps in the evidence base:

- **Tailored interventions based on a public health framework of primary, secondary, and tertiary prevention. In particular, researchers should examine improved measures to identify individuals who may be at**

high risk for social isolation or loneliness and primary interventions in order to target such individuals.

- **Trends among current younger adults as they age (e.g., use of technology, economic trends) to gain knowledge that informs future approaches to addressing social isolation and loneliness.**
- **Flexibility in funding to allow for the pilot testing and evaluation of innovative funding mechanisms for interventions.**
- **Approaches for assessments of and interventions among understudied groups of older adults (e.g., low income, lesbian, gay, bisexual, and transgender) and those who face unique barriers to health.**

RECOMMENDATION 9-6: System designers as well as those who are developing and deploying technology in interventions should ensure that technological innovations related to social isolation and loneliness are properly assessed and tested so as to understand their full range of benefits and potential adverse consequences in order to prevent harm, and they should work to understand and take into account contextual issues, such as broadband access and having sufficient knowledge and support for using the technology.

Goal 2: Translate Current Research into Health Care Practices

Older adults are high-volume and high-frequency users of the health care system. Targeting the major social and behavioral risk factors for health offers a way to improve population health and even reduce health disparities. Health care delivery systems are exploring the feasibility and impact of using practice-based strategies to identify and address the social determinants of health, including social isolation and loneliness. Many intervention efforts for social isolation and loneliness focus only on community-based organizations, but given the evidence for the broad-reaching impacts of social isolation and loneliness on the health of older adults and the emerging evidence for their impacts on health care utilization, the committee concluded that the health care system is well poised to develop methods for beginning to identify social isolation and loneliness in health care settings. By first identifying those at highest risk, clinicians and health care researchers may be able to use these findings to better target meaningful clinical and public health interventions to individual patients as well as to high-need populations served by a practice or health care system. Furthermore, this will support a step-wise approach to care that includes the identification of individuals at risk, the provision of education, and ultimately, intervention.

RECOMMENDATION 7-1: Health care providers and practices should periodically perform an assessment using one or more validated tools to identify older adults experiencing social isolation and loneliness in order to

initiate potential preventive interventions after having identified individuals who are at an elevated risk due to life events (e.g., loss of a significant relationship, geographic move, relevant health conditions).

- **In the case of older adults who are currently socially isolated or lonely (or at an elevated risk for social isolation or loneliness), health care providers should discuss the adverse health outcomes associated with social isolation and loneliness with these older adults and their legally appointed representatives. Providers should make appropriate efforts to connect isolated or lonely older adults with needed social care.**
- **For older adults who are currently socially isolated or lonely, health care providers should attempt to determine the underlying causes and use evidence-based practices tailored to appropriately address those causes (e.g., hearing loss, mobility limitations).**

A variety of established research tools can be used to measure social isolation and loneliness, each with its own strengths and weaknesses. Despite the limits of the evidence base concerning how best to implement these tools in clinical settings, the committee concluded that an important aspect of selecting a tool for use in clinical settings is standardization. This means that within a specific health care system or organization, all clinicians should use the same tool or set of tools; they should use only validated tools and refrain from using only parts of existing tools or creating new, unvalidated tools. While the committee recognizes that some variation in choice of appropriate tools may be necessary for assessing certain specific populations or health conditions, it emphasizes that the chosen measurement tool needs to match the research question. (That is, if assessing for loneliness, for instance, the tool needs to be validated specifically for the measurement of loneliness, as opposed to other indicators of social connection.) In spite of limitations to existing tools, their use is necessary to address social isolation and loneliness more fully in clinical settings. More effort is needed to update existing tools and to develop and validate better tools that can fully capture the experience of social isolation and loneliness among today's older adults.

Additional research is needed to evaluate the ethical implications and unintended consequences of clinical assessments and also to determine specific implementation details, including

- who should receive the assessment,
- who should conduct the assessment,
- the ideal frequency of assessment for different subpopulations, and
- the appropriate interventions, referrals, and follow-up care.

Many initiatives to address social isolation and loneliness in clinical settings are being undertaken by individuals without formal research training.

Linking clinicians and others who are implementing new interventions with formally trained researchers early on in the design of the intervention can help to ensure robust research design, and thereby improve the evidence concerning the use of validated tools in clinical settings.

RECOMMENDATION 7-2: Health care systems should create opportunities for clinicians to partner with researchers to evaluate the application of currently available evidence-based tools to assess social isolation and loneliness in clinical settings, including testing and applications for specific populations.

Finally, the committee concludes that assessment data need to be included in clear locations in the electronic health record.

RECOMMENDATION 7-3: The committee endorses the recommendation of previous National Academies reports that social isolation should be included in the electronic health record or medical record.

Research will be needed to determine how to best integrate information from a patient's assessments into his or her health record in order to make determinations about future care and the identification of risk.

Goals 3 and 4: Improve Awareness and Strengthen Ongoing Education and Training

Educating and training the health care workforce about addressing social isolation and loneliness will require a broad approach similar to educating the workforce to address the social determinants of health. Workforce development is needed within formal degree and postgraduate programs for health professionals, in training programs for direct care workers and community members, and in lifelong learning opportunities. It will be necessary to educate and train all members of the health care workforce, including professionals, direct care workers, community health workers, volunteers, family caregivers, and members of the larger community, such as police officers and mail carriers, who provide a broad array of services to or regularly interact with older adults.[4]

Improving Overall Awareness

Based on the significant evidence base concerning the health and medical impacts of social isolation and loneliness, the committee concluded that, as with

[4] This report focuses on the education and training of health care workers, particularly health care professionals and direct care workers.

other public health issues of the same magnitude, a critical step toward preventing, mitigating, or eliminating negative health impacts will be to improve awareness among the general public and, specifically for this report, among the health care workforce itself.

RECOMMENDATION 8-1: The U.S. Department of Health and Human Services should advocate for including measures of social isolation and loneliness in major large-scale health strategies (e.g., Healthy People) and surveys (e.g., National Health Interview Survey).

RECOMMENDATION 8-2: Health and aging organizations, relevant government agencies, and consumer-facing organizations should create public awareness and education campaigns that highlight the health impacts of social isolation and loneliness in adults.

- **Health care systems, associations representing all types of health care workers (e.g., American Medical Association, American Nurses Association, American Psychological Association, National Association of Social Workers, American Geriatrics Society, American Association for Geriatric Psychiatry, organizations representing direct care workers); health-related organizations (e.g., American Heart Association); consumer-facing, health-related organizations (e.g., AARP); aging professional associations (e.g., American Society on Aging, Gerontological Society of America); aging services organizations (e.g., area agencies on aging, state departments on aging); and organizations working with at-risk older adults (e.g., National Hispanic Council on Aging) should actively communicate information about the health impacts of social isolation and loneliness through print and digital media.**
- **Organizations representing health plans and providers should include consumer-friendly information about the health impacts of social isolation and loneliness in their repository of patient resources (e.g., where the organization provides information about the self-management of various chronic diseases).**

Strengthening Education and Training

While research-based evidence is not yet available to support curricular content on specific interventions for social isolation and loneliness in older adults, enough is known about the health impacts to warrant broad curricular recommendations for all health professions and careers. Education is needed about the prevalence of social isolation and loneliness in older adults, the health outcomes and risk factors for social isolation and loneliness, and how to assess for these problems. Health professionals also need to learn how to work directly with older adults and their significant others to support and encourage ways to prevent or reduce social isolation and loneliness, including how to make and follow-up on referrals to appropriate community-based services. This will include learning to work with direct care workers, community health workers, family caregivers, and other community members as part of a team-based approach to helping older adults. Health care professionals also need to learn how to work with community partners to develop, implement, and evaluate programs for preventing or mitigating social isolation and loneliness in older adults. Competency in each of these areas will become increasingly important as systems of care are developed for preventing, assessing, and treating the negative health impacts of social isolation and loneliness in older adults. Therefore, as a first step, the committee makes the following recommendations:

RECOMMENDATION 8-3: Health professions schools and colleges as well as direct care worker training programs should include education and training related to social isolation and loneliness in their curricula, optimally as interprofessional team-based learning experiences.

- **Health education and training programs should include information on clinical approaches to assessing and intervening when an older adult is at risk for social isolation and loneliness.**
- **As evidence on effective interventions develops, health education and training programs should provide education on integrating care related to social isolation and loneliness into clinical practice and as part of discharge planning, care coordination, and transitional care planning with community organizations.**

RECOMMENDATION 8-4: Health professional associations should incorporate information about the health and medical impacts of social isolation and loneliness on older adults in their advocacy, practice, and education initiatives.

- **Health professional associations should include social isolation and loneliness in conference programming, webinars, toolkits, clinical guidelines, and advocacy priorities.**

RECOMMENDATION 8-5: Health professional associations, membership organizations, academic institutions, health insurers, researchers, developers of education and training programs, and other actors in the public and private sectors should support, develop, and test different educational and training approaches related to the health and medical impacts of social isolation and loneliness in older adults across different segments of the

health care workforce (including health care professionals and direct care workers) in order to determine the most effective ways to enhance competencies. In addition to initial clinical education, these approaches should apply to professional education, continuing education modules, online learning, and other forms of lifelong learning.

Depending on the complexity of the knowledge to be disseminated or the evidence-based practices to be implemented, a variety of teaching strategies can be considered. As the evidence for interventions evolves, the educational and training opportunities need to expand to include new and updated evidence-based practices for preventing, assessing, and treating the negative health impacts of social isolation and loneliness.

Goal 5: Strengthen Ties Between the Health Care System and Community-Based Networks and Resources

Like other social determinants of health, social isolation and loneliness are community-wide problems and some solutions will require coordinated solutions between the health care system and community-based social care providers. National, state, and local coalitions of public and private health care leaders, including minority-based community organizations, need to work collectively to develop strategies to address social isolation and loneliness in older adults.

RECOMMENDATION 9-1: Health care providers, organizations, and systems should partner with social service providers, including those serving vulnerable communities, in order to create effective team-based care (which includes services such as transportation and housing support) and to promote the use of tailored community-based services to address social isolation and loneliness in older adults.

Many health care organizations (e.g., hospitals) are required under federal law to submit community benefit reports. Efforts by such entities to partner with social service providers could be used as an example of their community benefit. The 2019 National Academies consensus study report *Integrating Social Care into the Delivery of Health Care* cites the provision of transportation vouchers and the investment in community ride-sharing programs as examples of activities that can improve the integration of care. Such services could allow individuals to travel to health care appointments and to overcome individual transportation-related barriers to being more integrated into local community events, both of which could help to reduce social isolation and loneliness.

A variety of stakeholders, both within and outside of the formal health care system, are testing new approaches to preventing, identifying, and intervening in social isolation or loneliness for older adults. The committee concluded that as new evidence develops, a centralized sharing of resources and best practices would benefit all stakeholders.

> **RECOMMENDATION 9-2: Given the public health impact of social isolation and loneliness, the U.S. Department of Health and Human Services should establish and fund a national resource center to centralize evidence, resources, training, and best practices on social isolation and loneliness, including those for older adults and for diverse and at-risk populations.**

DISSEMINATION AND IMPLEMENTATION

The dissemination and implementation of evidence into regular and effective use is complex because of the multiplicity and varying capacities of health care systems and providers and the diversity of the target audiences. However, such efforts are imperative in order to improve quality of care, outcomes, and population health. Two main challenges exist for the dissemination and implementation of evidence related to the social isolation and loneliness of older adults. First, better dissemination is needed of the evidence of the health impacts. Second, the best practices of implementation science need to be used in order to ensure that health care systems and providers are able to more quickly adopt evidence-based practices. This will be particularly important as the evidence base on the effectiveness of specific interventions improves.

1

Introduction

A social instinct is implanted in all [people] by nature. . . .
—Aristotle, *Politics*, 350 B.C.E., Jowett (2009)

The scientific evidence is convincing. Strong social ties are good for one's health.
—Lubben (2017)

Social isolation (the objective state of having few social relationships or infrequent social contact with others) and loneliness (a subjective feeling of being isolated) are serious yet underappreciated public health risks that affect a significant portion of the population. Approximately one-quarter (24 percent) of community-dwelling Americans aged 65 and older are considered to be socially isolated, and a significant proportion of adults in the United States report feeling lonely (35 percent of adults aged 45 and older and 43 percent of adults aged 60 and older) (Anderson and Thayer, 2018; Cudjoe et al., 2020; Perissinotto et al., 2012). In spite of some challenges related to the measurement of social isolation and loneliness, current evidence suggests that many older adults are socially isolated or lonely (or both) in ways that put their health at risk. For example:

- Social isolation significantly increases a person's risk of mortality from all causes, a risk that may rival the risks of smoking, obesity, and physical activity (Holt-Lunstad et al., 2017);
- Being socially connected in a variety of ways is associated with having a 50 percent greater likelihood of survival, with some indicators of social integration being associated with a 91 percent greater likelihood of survival (Holt-Lunstad et al., 2010);

- Social isolation has been associated with a 29 percent increased all-cause risk for mortality and a 25 percent increased risk for cancer mortality (Fleisch Marcus et al., 2017; Holt-Lunstad et al., 2015);
- Loneliness has been associated with higher rates of clinically significant depression, anxiety, and suicidal ideation (Beutel et al., 2017);
- Loneliness has been associated with a 59 percent increased risk of functional decline and 45 percent increased risk of death (Perissinotto et al., 2012);
- Poor social relationships (characterized by social isolation or loneliness) have been associated with a 29 percent increased risk of incident coronary heart disease and a 32 percent increased risk of stroke (Valtorta et al., 2016a);
- Loneliness among heart failure patients has been associated with a nearly four times increased risk of death, 68 percent increased risk of hospitalization, and 57 percent increased risk of emergency department visits (Manemann et al., 2018); and
- Social isolation has been associated with an approximately 50 percent increased risk of developing dementia (Kuiper et al., 2015; Penninkilampi et al., 2018).

Understanding the full scope and complexity of the influence of social relationships on health is challenging. In addition to the absolute number or extent of social relationships, the quality of such relationships is also important for their impact on health. As such, two aspects of social relationships, social isolation and loneliness, have become most prominent in the scientific literature. While both social isolation and loneliness can affect health throughout the life course, this report focuses specifically on the health and medical impacts of social isolation and loneliness among adults aged 50 and older. Of note, it is incorrect to assume that all older people are isolated or lonely. Rather, older adults are at increased risk for social isolation and loneliness because they are more likely to face predisposing factors such as living alone, the loss of family or friends, chronic illness, and sensory impairments. Over a life course, social isolation and loneliness may be episodic or chronic, depending on an individual's circumstances and perceptions.

Many approaches have been taken to improve social connections for individuals who are socially isolated or lonely, but finding opportunities to intervene may be most challenging for those who are at highest risk. For example, people who do not have consistent interactions with others (e.g., have unstable housing, do not belong to any social or religious groups, or do not have significant personal relationships) may never be identified in their own communities. However, nearly all persons who are 50 years of age or older interact with the health care system in some way, regardless of where they fall on the social isolation or loneliness continuum, and so this interaction may serve as a touchpoint to identify those who are isolated or lonely. Therefore, this report focuses on the role of the health care system as a key and relatively untapped partner in efforts to identify, prevent, and mitigate the adverse health impacts of social isolation and loneliness in older adults.

STUDY CONTEXT

A systematic and rigorous science of social relationships and their consequences, especially in terms of health, emerged in the latter part of the 20th century as part of a broader recognition of the role of social determinants of health. By the beginning of the 21st century, several aspects of social relationships were being studied systematically in research and identified as potential influences on human health. Only recently have the adverse health effects of social isolation and loneliness received public attention nationally and internationally through governmental initiatives, the work of nonprofit organizations, and mass media coverage (Anderson and Thayer, 2018; Brody, 2017; DiJulio et al., 2018; Frank, 2018; Hafner, 2016; Khullar, 2016). For example, in January 2018, Theresa May, prime minister of the United Kingdom, established and appointed a Minister of Loneliness to develop policies for both measuring and reducing loneliness (Yeginsu, 2018).

In his keynote address for the Accreditation Council for Graduate Medical Education (ACGME) 2019 Annual Educational Conference, Vivek Murthy, the 19th Surgeon General of the United States, spoke of an "epidemic of loneliness" that he recognized during his tenure as Surgeon General, stating,

> I see [loneliness] actually as a primary concern, not just a health concern but as a concern as a society. . . . While the negative impact of loneliness cannot be denied, the treatment can be relatively simple. Part of treating loneliness is creating moments for genuine human interaction, which can be achieved on several levels. (ACGME, 2019)

Prevalence of Social Isolation and Loneliness

Understanding the prevalence of social isolation and loneliness is important in two ways. First, the population health impact of any risk factor is a function of the strength of its impact and its prevalence in a population. Second, whether a risk factor is becoming more or less prevalent is an indicator of whether its importance for population health is waxing or waning. However, it is very difficult to measure social isolation or loneliness in any population or to ascertain the degree of increase or decrease. A range of estimates have been made for the prevalence of social isolation and loneliness among different segments of the adult population in the United States. For example:

- Data from the National Health and Aging Trends Study found that 24 percent of community-dwelling adults aged 65 and older in the United States were categorized as being socially isolated and 4 percent were severely socially isolated (Cudjoe et al., 2020);
- A 2012 study by Perissinotto and colleagues found that 43 percent of adults aged 60 and older reported feeling lonely. Furthermore, among those who reported at least one symptom of loneliness, 13 percent reported the symptom as occurring "often" (Perissinotto et al., 2012);

- A survey by the AARP Foundation found that more than one-third (35 percent) of adults aged 45 and older in the United States report feeling lonely (Anderson and Thayer, 2018);
- A 2018 survey by the Kaiser Family Foundation found that "more than a fifth of adults [aged 18 and older] in the United States (22 percent) . . . say they often or always feel lonely, feel that they lack companionship, feel left out, or feel isolated from others" (DiJulio et al., 2018);
- A study by Hawkley and colleagues (2017) using data from the National Social Life, Health, and Aging Project found that 19 percent of adults aged 62–91 report frequent loneliness (with an additional 29 percent reporting occasional loneliness); and
- A study by Cigna of adults aged 18 and older found that 46 percent reported "sometimes or always feeling alone" (Cigna/Ipsos, 2018).

Depending on how social isolation or loneliness is measured, the demographic trends contributing to it may include an increase in the number of people living alone, decreased marriage rates, higher rates of childlessness, or decreased community involvement (e.g., volunteerism, religious affiliation) (Holt-Lunstad, 2018b; Putnam, 2001). Social isolation and loneliness may occur unequally across age groups, including within the group of adults 50 years of age and older who are the focus of this report. Furthermore, the oldest adults may not be the most isolated or lonely. For example, the 2018 survey by the Kaiser Family Foundation found that 59 percent of the respondents who reported feeling lonely were under age 50 (DiJulio et al., 2018); the Cigna study found that adults aged 18–22 were the loneliest, and that loneliness decreased with age (Cigna/Ipsos, 2018); and a study by Hawkley and colleagues (2019) found that "loneliness decreased with age through the early 70s, after which it increased" (p. 1144).

Aside from looking for differences among various age segments of the adult population, several studies have examined whether there are variations in the prevalence of social isolation or loneliness among subsets of adults related to demographic factors such as socioeconomic status, race and ethnicity, gender, educational status, employment status, and marital status. Several studies have found that those who report feeling lonely are more likely than others to report lower incomes and assets, having poorer health, and not being married (Anderson and Thayer, 2018; DiJulio et al., 2018; Hawkley et al., 2017). According to the study from Hawkley and colleagues (2017), "loneliness is not significantly more prevalent in the oldest old adults, nor in minority groups relative to whites, nor in women relative to men" (p. 6) and Anderson and Thayer (2018) found that individuals who identify as lesbian, gay, bisexual, transgender, and questioning (or queer) (LGBTQ) are more likely to say they are lonely. Cudjoe and colleagues (2020) found that "being unmarried, male, having low education, and low income were all independently associated with social isolation" (p. 107). They further found that "Black and Hispanic older adults had lower odds of social isolation compared with white older adults" (p. 107).

Differences in findings among many studies on the prevalence of social isolation and loneliness may be due, in part, to the challenges of defining and measuring social isolation and loneliness, including the use of different measures to assess different aspects of social isolation and loneliness in various groups that may differ by various demographic factors. Despite the variance in measurement, there are clearly a vast number of people who are socially isolated or lonely. Furthermore, the implications of these findings for physical or mental health, morbidity, and mortality underscore the urgency surrounding these issues and render them topics of highest concern to both public health and clinical health care.

CHARGE TO THE COMMITTEE

With support from the AARP Foundation, the National Academies of Sciences, Engineering, and Medicine (the National Academies) formed the Committee on the Health and Medical Dimensions of Social Isolation and Loneliness in Older Adults in fall 2018. The committee's charge essentially consisted of two parts. First, the committee was asked to examine how social isolation and loneliness affect health and quality of life in adults aged 50 and older, particularly among low-income, underserved, and vulnerable subpopulations. Second, the committee was charged to identify and recommend opportunities specifically for clinical settings of health care to help reduce the incidence and adverse health impacts of social isolation and loneliness (such as clinical tools and methodologies, professional education, and public awareness) and to examine avenues for translation and dissemination of information targeted to health care practitioners (see Box 1-1).

The committee was asked to focus on adults aged 50 and older. Social connections are considered to be a fundamental human need and thus are vital across the lifespan. The committee acknowledges the importance of social connection at all ages and recognizes that social processes at earlier ages influence the trajectory of risk as one ages. For example, there is evidence that social disruptions (e.g., adverse childhood experiences) at early ages can place individuals on a worse health trajectory (Anda et al., 2006; Uchino, 2009a). However, for the purposes of this study and the specific task, the committee did not examine the evidence base related to the health impacts on younger generations or interventions aimed at those populations. Furthermore, the committee notes that studies of both the health impacts of social isolation or loneliness and of potential interventions also often include different segments of the population over age 50, which can make comparisons across studies challenging.

While this report focuses on the specific role of the health care system (and the role of clinicians and clinical care in particular), the committee emphasizes that the health care system alone cannot solve all of the challenges related to social isolation and loneliness; rather, the health care system needs to connect with the

BOX 1-1
Statement of Task

An ad hoc committee under the auspices of the National Academies of Sciences, Engineering, and Medicine will examine how isolation and loneliness impact health outcomes in older adults aged 50 and older, particularly among low-income, underserved, and vulnerable subpopulations. The committee will:

- Summarize and examine the evidence that social isolation and loneliness predict poor health outcomes and increase a person's risk for premature morbidity, including evidence for:
    - Predictors of social isolation and loneliness;
    - Impact of social isolation and loneliness on the cognitive, emotional, medical, and quality-of-life outcomes; and
    - Factors that moderate and mediate the links between social isolation/loneliness and health outcomes.
- Explore how social isolation and loneliness affect health care access and utilization.
- Make evidence-based recommendations on translating research into practice within the clinical setting that could facilitate progress in reducing the incidence and adverse health impacts of social isolation and loneliness among the low-income 50+ population. These recommendations will focus on the following issues:
    - Opportunities for the identification of, prevention of, and interventions for social isolation and loneliness that can be incorporated into clinical environments ***that may include*** social and environmental programs; the education of health care professionals; tools and methodologies that can be used in clinical settings; and public awareness.
    - Current financing for social isolation and loneliness interventions and future opportunities.
- Examine avenues for translation and dissemination of new findings and communication of new information targeting health care practitioners.

broader public health and social care communities. Furthermore, the committee recognizes that in the larger context of addressing social isolation and loneliness, the most effective interventions may not require the participation of the health care system. However, the committee argues that this does not mean that the health care system should not strive to help improve the health and well-being of those who suffer the adverse health impacts of social isolation and loneliness. In fact, health care providers may be in the best position to identify individuals who are at highest risk for social isolation or loneliness—individuals for whom the health care system may be their only point of contact with their broader community. In this way, the health care system can help those individuals to connect with the most appropriate care, either inside or outside the health care system. Therefore, the health care system has the potential to be a critical component of a much larger solution. As noted by Lisa Marsh Ryerson, president of the AARP Foundation, in an open session of the committee's first meeting:

> We have been working in the space of social isolation and loneliness among older adults since 2010 and we have been working on advancing a variety of solutions as well as funding and examining the research. But for us this study fills an important research and recommendation gap because from our point of view we will not make measurable significant steps toward solving [social isolation and loneliness] unless we figure out the path for health care.

RELEVANT NATIONAL ACADEMIES REPORTS

The National Academies have produced many reports related to the social determinants of health, and several of them are directly relevant to this current study. The work, conclusions, and recommendations of the current committee reinforce, extend, and elaborate on the work, conclusions, and recommendations of prior National Academies committees. Box 1-2 provides some examples of previous National Academies work related to the work of this committee.

STUDY APPROACH

The Committee on the Health and Medical Dimensions of Social Isolation and Loneliness in Older Adults consisted of 15 members with expertise in bioinformatics, economics, epidemiology, geriatrics, health care, health care administration, medicine, nursing, psychiatry, psychology, public health, rural health, social work, and sociology. (See Appendix B for the biographies of the committee members.)

A variety of sources informed the committee's work. The committee met in person five times, and during three of those meetings it held public sessions to obtain input from a broad range of relevant stakeholders, including the sponsor. (See Appendix A for the public meeting agendas with topics and speakers listed.) In addition, the committee conducted extensive literature reviews, reached out to a variety of public and private stakeholders, and commissioned one paper.

To address its charge, the committee set the following parameters

- Created a guiding framework that highlighted the role of the health care system
- Addressed relevant definitions
- Defined the scope of health care providers and settings
- Identified the populations at risk and age groups to be studied
- Considered the quality of the existing evidence base

BOX 1-2
Previous Reports of the National Academies

In *The Second Fifty Years* (IOM, 1992), the committee noted "a lack of family and community supports plays an important role in the development and exacerbation of disease" (p. 8). The report further indicated that "clinicians, family, friends, and social institutions bear a responsibility for diminishing social isolation" (p. 8). The committee recommended the identification of at-risk individuals, noting "there are indications that the first opportunity for such an identification of needs is at the source of medical care" (p. 256).

In *Capturing Social and Behavioral Domains and Measures in Electronic Health Records: Phase 2* (IOM, 2014), the committee recommended social isolation as one of 10 domains best suited for inclusion in all electronic health records (EHRs). In assessing the usefulness of collecting data on social connections and social isolation, the committee noted:

> If health care providers know the social integration/isolation, social support, and loneliness of individual patients, they may better understand not only the patient's health but also his or her use of and need for health care services. . . . If the health system is aware that social integration/isolation, social support, and loneliness can be major risk and protective factors for health, it can use this information to identify patients and work to assess and intervene at a population or community level. . . . For researchers, the availability of more data on integration/isolation, social support, and loneliness can advance the knowledge of how much these determinants affect health and enable the establishment of better screening and treatment programs for loneliness and interventions within the health system. (pp. 97–98)

That committee further concluded that the updated and adapted Berkman–Syme Social Network Index (as used for the National Health and Nutrition Examination Survey III) could be adopted into EHRs. They acknowledged that specific tools exist to assess "social isolation and disconnectedness" in geriatric populations, but decided that this measure was appropriate for use in all adults (p. 197).

In *Cognitive Aging* (IOM, 2015), the committee described how social isolation and loneliness are associated with declines in global cognition, psychomotor

Guiding Framework

Pursuant to its charge, the committee focused heavily on the clinical health care setting. This focus also seemed appropriate as clinical care is itself an aspect of, or an intervention related to, social connection. Clinical settings offer major opportunities for identifying problems related to social isolation and loneliness and for advancing interventions to alleviate these problems either within the clinical care setting itself or by mobilizing broader social and policy resources that may be needed for effective intervention.

To guide its deliberations, the committee developed a conceptual framework to better understand the relationships among several aspects of social connections processing speed, and delayed visual memory; Alzheimer's disease; and other physical problems. In particular, the committee noted that "cognitive declines may lead to lower social engagement, creating a downward spiral of social isolation and loneliness" (p. 121). Overall, the committee concluded that "although evidence from some epidemiological and observational studies indicates that increases in social activity and social engagement may be associated with higher levels of cognition, evidence from RCTs [randomized controlled trials] is needed before recommendations can be made for specific social interaction interventions" (p. 123).

In *A Framework for Educating Health Professionals to Address the Social Determinants of Health* (NASEM, 2016a), the committee developed a framework to "align the education, health, and other sectors, in partnership with communities, to educate health professionals in the social determinants of health" (p. 4). The committee recommended use of the framework to "guide and support evaluation research aimed at identifying and illustrating effective approaches for learning about the social determinants of health in and with communities while improving health outcomes, thereby building the evidence base" (p. 13).

In *Accounting for Social Risk Factors in Medicare Payment* (NASEM, 2017), the committee identified social relationships as one of five domains of social risk factors "that are associated with health care outcomes independently of quality of care" (p. 2).

In *Integrating Social Care into the Delivery of Health Care* (NASEM, 2019), the committee defined social risk factors as "social determinants that may be associated with negative health outcomes, such as poor housing or unstable social relationships" (p. 28). The committee recommended that "health care organizations should take steps to integrate social care into health care" and that effective strategies for screening and assessing social risk factors "should include standardized and validated questions, as available, and should use interoperable data systems to document results" (p. 10). Furthermore, the committee noted that clinical personnel who should address social needs includes nurses, physicians, community health workers, home health aides, and geriatricians, among others.

and how they are embedded in the overarching public health focus on social determinants of health (see Figure 1-1). The framework in Figure 1-1 has a presumed causal flow (indicated by the thicker unidirectional arrows) from risk factors (for social connections and other variables in the framework) through social connections (i.e., social isolation and loneliness and other aspects of social connection such as social support, considered both independently and in relation to each other) to mediators (e.g., medical, biological, behavioral, social, and psychological pathways) through which social isolation or loneliness affect health outcomes and, potentially, mortality.

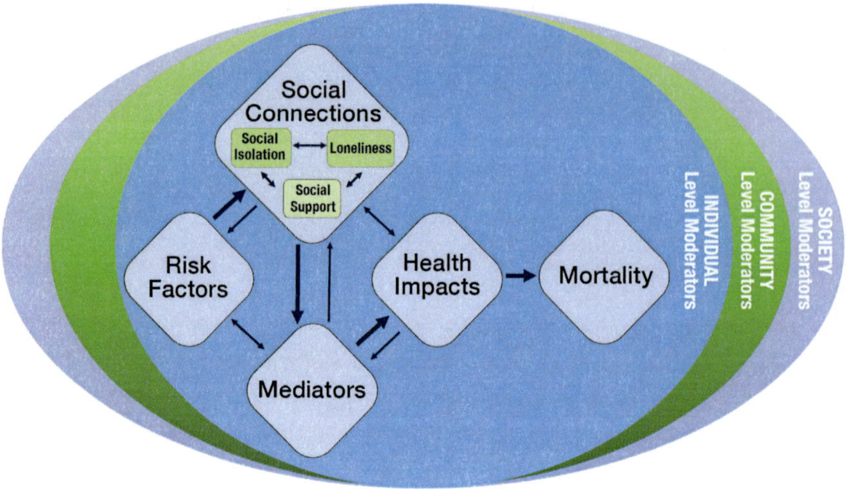

FIGURE 1-1 Guiding framework.

In this report and more generally, variables or boxes that intervene between a presumed causal factor and any subsequent variables or boxes that the cause is presumed to affect are termed mediators of that causal effect. *Mediators* (i.e., mechanisms or pathways) are the factors that help explain how social isolation or loneliness affects health outcomes. Most notably, variables in the box labeled pathways are hypothesized to mediate the effect of risk factors or social connections on health impacts, which in turn usually mediate these effects on mortality. Any of the variables in Figure 1-1, as well as other variables not specified there, may also act as moderators of any of the relationships between variables in the framework. *Moderators* are the factors that can influence the magnitude or direction of the effect of social isolation or loneliness on health. For example, the existence, nature, or strength of any empirical relationship hypothesized in Figure 1-1 may vary as a function of age, sex/gender, race/ethnicity, socioeconomic position, geographic location, or pre-existing health status.

Many of the relationships in the model are potentially bi-directional, as indicated by the thinner arrows. For example, social isolation and loneliness do causally affect health, but they, in turn, may also be affected by health status. That is, a chronic condition, for example, can be both a risk factor for or a consequence of social isolation or loneliness. The committee recognizes that separating discussions of health impacts (see Chapter 3) from risk and protective factors (see Chapter 4) can be challenging and confusing given that the same health condition is often discussed in both chapters, albeit for different reasons. Similarly, factors that mediate the relationship between social isolation/loneliness and health can also serve as moderators of those relationships. Therefore, the committee emphasizes that the conceptual framework serves in part to highlight the complexity of all of these interrelationships. Individual elements of this framework will be discussed in more detail throughout the first half of this report. Specifically, the different aspects of social connections are discussed later in this chapter, mortality is discussed in Chapter 2, health impacts are discussed in Chapter 3, and risk (and protective) factors are discussed in Chapter 4. Chapter 5 discusses the potential role of many variables as mediators or moderators of the relationships among variables in the Figure 1-1 framework. All of these concepts and pathways offer opportunities for intervention (both directly and indirectly) by the health care system as a way of improving the ultimate health outcomes.

Finally, all of these relationships fit within a typical ecological model of health wherein factors contributing to social isolation and loneliness at the individual level are also potentially affected by the broader contextual factors at the levels of the community and society. Factors that influence social isolation and loneliness at the community level may include factors such as availability of transportation, broadband access, natural disasters, gentrification, and housing displacement. Factors that influence social isolation and loneliness at the society level may, for example, include racism, ageism, changes in family structure (e.g., lower rates of intergenerational living, higher rates of divorce and childlessness), trends in use of technology, and broader laws and policies that may affect social isolation and loneliness.

These influences at the level of the community and society are key to understanding risk for social isolation and loneliness and often have a reciprocal relationship with risk and protective factors at the individual level. For example, a key lifestyle feature of Blue Zones (geographic areas characterized by populations with low levels of chronic disease and long lifespans) is social connection. This may be in part due to how the overall social norms of these communities impact individual-level factors for social isolation and loneliness; Blue Zones are often characterized by living in proximity to one's family, belonging to a faith-based community, and supporting healthy behaviors (e.g., healthy diets and exercise). These ideas are captured in the person-environment fit theory which "focuses on the interaction between the characteristics of the individual and the environment, whereby the individual not only influences his or her environment, but the environment also affects the individual" (Holmbeck et al., 2008, p. 33). This may be particularly important for individuals with disabilities for whom their social and physical environments influence participation, engagement, inclusion, and social relationships. Chapter 4 provides some insight for the contextual factors at the levels of the community and society, but an extensive discussion of all of these broader concepts and the bio-psycho-social model of health, is beyond the scope of this report.

This report focuses on social isolation, loneliness, and several related concepts, each of which contributes to health. However, because social isolation and loneliness are seldom included together in the same study as predictors of health outcomes, the evidence concerning the impact of each on health largely exists in parallel literature bases. Social isolation and loneliness need to continue to be independently examined as potential predictors of the other related aspects of social connection as well as of health outcomes. More importantly, they need to be examined together (1) to discover potential pathways by which one may be operating through, or in combination with, the other in determining health outcomes; and (2) to better estimate the relative strength of their impacts on health outcomes and mortality.

Defining Social Isolation, Loneliness, and Related Aspects of Social Relationships

The broad, interdisciplinary scientific fields that together form the modern science of social relationships have used a variety of terms (e.g., social isolation, social connection, social networks, social integration, social support, social exclusion, social deprivation, social relationships, loneliness) to refer to empirical phenomena related to social relationships. Although there are important distinctions among these terms concerning what they describe or measure, they are often, incorrectly, used interchangeably. Some of the key terms that will be used throughout this report are presented in Box 1-3.

BOX 1-3
Key Definitions

Loneliness: the perception of social isolation or the subjective feeling of being lonely.

Mediators: also known as mechanisms or pathways; the factors that help explain how social isolation or loneliness affects health outcomes.

Moderators: the factors that can influence the magnitude or direction of the effect of social isolation or loneliness on health.

Social connection: an umbrella term that encompasses the structural, functional, and quality aspects of how individuals connect to each other.

Social isolation: the objective lack of (or limited) social contact with others.

Social support: the actual or perceived availability of resources (e.g., informational, tangible, emotional) from others, typically one's social network.

Social Isolation and Loneliness

Social isolation and loneliness represent distinct phenomena. *Social isolation* typically refers to the objective lack of (or limited) social contact with others, and it is marked by an individual having few social network ties, having infrequent social contact, or, potentially, living alone. Markers of social isolation objectively and quantitatively establish a dearth of social contact and network size. *Loneliness* refers to the perception of social isolation or the subjective feeling of being lonely that "occurs when there is a significant mismatch or discrepancy between a person's actual social relations and his or her needed or desired social relations" (Perlman and Peplau, 1998, p. 571). While loneliness is subjective, there are measurement tools that can help to quantify the degree of loneliness (see Chapter 6). Although those who lack social contact may feel lonely (Yildirim and Kocabiyik, 2010), social isolation and loneliness are often not highly correlated (Coyle and Dugan, 2012; Perissinotto and Covinsky, 2014). Thus, it is important to distinguish between social isolation and loneliness.

Related Aspects of Social Relationships

"Social relationships" is arguably the most common term for the connections and intersections among human beings, and it derives from and is employed in broader common usage. The term "social networks" has been used for some time as a similarly broad rubric for the connections among human beings and also other creatures, but it is also used more specifically to refer to the structure and way of analyzing relationship data (Scott, 1988). Berkman and Syme (1979) documented the powerful impact of social relationships on all-cause mortality and hence life expectancy, using the terms "social networks" and also "social integration" to denote the broad pattern of social relationships that they were examining; these terms are now part of the concept of social isolation. Beginning before the Berkman and Syme study and continuing over the succeeding four decades, the study of social relationships and health came to focus on social support. *Social support* is defined as the actual or perceived availability of resources (e.g., informational, tangible, emotional) from others, typically one's social network (Cohen and Wills, 1985). While each of these terms used to describe social relationships have been linked to important health outcomes, they are not highly correlated, suggesting that each may influence health through different pathways (Cohen et al., 2000). Thus, the literature often refers to organizing themes—the structure, functions, and quality of our social relationships—that categorize the broader class of terms that have been termed social relationships by sociologists and epidemiologists or social connection by psychologists (Berkman et al., 2000; Holt-Lunstad, 2018b; Holt-Lunstad et al., 2017; House et al., 1988). "Social connection" is an umbrella term that some have proposed using to encompass the different conceptual and measurement approaches represented

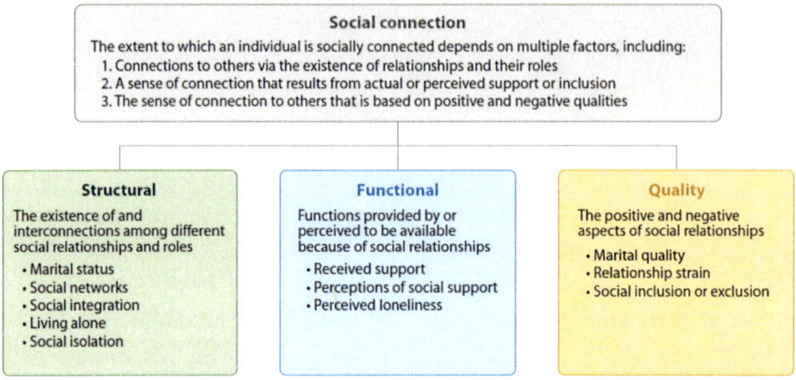

FIGURE 1-2 Social connection as a multi-factorial construct including structural, functional, and quality components.
SOURCE: Holt-Lunstad, 2018a. Reproduced with permission from the *Annual Review of Psychology,* Volume 69 © 2018 by Annual Reviews, http://www.annualreviews.org.

in the scientific literature. (Holt-Lunstad, 2018a). According to Holt-Lunstad et al. (2017), social connection encompasses the variety of ways one can connect to others socially—through physical, behavioral, social–cognitive, and emotional channels. The extent to which an individual is socially connected takes a multifactorial approach, including (1) [*structural aspects*] connections to others via the existence of relationships and their roles; (2) [*functional aspects*] a sense of connection that results from actual or perceived support or inclusion; and (3) [*qualitative aspects*] the sense of connection to others that is based on positive and negative qualities. Figure 1-2 shows the three categories of indicators of social connection (i.e., structural, functional, and quality indicators) and provides examples of such indicators.

When considering risk factors and protective factors for social isolation and loneliness, having indicators of high social connection is typically considered protective while having indicators of low social connection is typically considered detrimental. Social isolation and loneliness are examples of low social connection, with social isolation being a structural aspect and loneliness a functional aspect. Some indicators of social connection are more stable than others, and the acute or chronic nature of these indicators will influence the degree of risk or protection.

The committee recognizes that the literature on social isolation and loneliness uses all of these terms. To describe the evidence base as accurately as possible, when the evidence does not differentiate among or combines several related terms, this report uses the term "social connection" to refer to the various structural, functional, and quality aspects of social relationships. This report uses the specific terms "social isolation," "loneliness," or other terms when the data are specific to these terms.[1]

The Health Care System and Its Providers

For the purposes of this study, the committee examined the potential role of the formal health care system and settings where health care services are provided in reducing the impacts of social isolation and loneliness in older adults. The committee considered health care settings broadly to include not just hospital and professional offices, but also other community-based settings where clinical health care services are provided (e.g., homes, long-term care settings). In accordance with discussions with the sponsor in open session at the committee's first meeting, the committee agreed to consider the settings of care broadly, but to focus on the provision of clinical care by qualified clinicians and health care workers (not including family caregivers). Therefore, the committee used the lens of the health care system itself on the role of health care professionals (e.g., nurses, physicians, social workers), direct care workers (e.g., home health aides, nurse aides, personal care aides), and others involved in the delivery of health care (e.g., community health workers, health care administrators, health information technology professionals). While the committee recognizes the vital importance of family caregivers (the family, friends, and others who provide care, sometimes called informal caregivers) to the delivery of health care as well as their role in mitigating the social isolation and loneliness of their family members, the committee and sponsor agreed that the focus for this study was to gain a comprehensive understanding of how social isolation and loneliness affect the individual and then explore the role of the formal health care system as described above.

The committee also limited its examination largely to literature from the United States. The committee based this approach not only on the likely differences among different countries that can affect social isolation and loneliness (e.g., societal norms, cultural expectations, and family structures), but also on the fact that the health care systems in other countries are markedly different from the U.S. health care system, and could make comparisons of clinical approaches quite challenging. However, the committee did review and include notable examples from other countries wherever relevant.

Finally, the committee considered general public health principles, including connection to the community and other public health partners, to be considered a part of comprehensive clinical care, especially given that the Statement of Task calls for the committee to consider "opportunities that can be incorporated into health care environments" (e.g., education, tools, public awareness). While the

---

[1] While social integration can describe high social connection, low scores on measures of social integration (e.g., on the Berkman–Syme Social Network Index) are frequently used as an indication of social isolation. Thus, the term "social isolation" will also be used to represent these data.

committee's ultimate recommendations are not all explicitly directed to health care professionals and other health care workers, the committee asserts that its recommendations are the ones that would be most helpful in reaching the ultimate goal of improving the role of individuals involved in clinical care in particular to help mitigate the negative health impacts of social isolation and loneliness.

Identifying Populations at Risk

Pursuant to its charge, the committee primarily focused its efforts on addressing the health and medical dimensions of loneliness and social isolation as they pertain to adults aged 50 and older. The committee's work was necessarily limited by the available research on this population. Also in response to the charge, the committee sought to include relevant research pertaining to low-income, underserved, or vulnerable populations. To address these subpopulations of older adults, the committee included available research on specific populations as defined by race, geographic area (e.g., rural versus urban), immigration status, sexual orientation, and other characteristics. Although the research on many of these subpopulations is sparse, examinations of studies focusing on these subpopulations are included throughout the report as part of the evidentiary data for each topic area. A separate section specifically addressing particular subpopulations (i.e., gay, lesbian, and bisexual populations; minorities; immigrants; and victims of elder abuse) is included in Chapters 4 and 5. However, the committee emphasizes that the literature base specific to at-risk populations is quite sparse, and much more research is needed to determine the risks, impacts, and appropriate interventions for a variety of at-risk subpopulations.

Quality of Available Evidence

A significant and robust literature demonstrates the impact of social isolation and loneliness on health and well-being (see Chapters 2 and 3). However, the literature on effective interventions, particularly for the role of the health care system, is less robust. The existing studies of interventions vary in their terminology, measures, and measured outcomes. While this variability made comparing the studies and their overall conclusions quite challenging for the committee, the variability can also be a strength in the sense that it makes it possible to look for convergent validity (i.e., robustness of the empirical relationships among conceptual variables even in the face of some variation in measures and study designs; see Lykken, 1968) in establishing the effect of social isolation and loneliness on health and well-being.

The committee prioritized the available literature according to known principles of evidence-based health research intended to reduce the risk of bias affecting study conclusions (Podsakoff et al., 2003). Important factors include how participants are allocated to different types of interventions, the comparability of study populations, controls for confounding factors, how outcomes are assessed, how representative the study group is of the older U.S. population, and the degree to which statistical analyses help reduce bias.

OVERVIEW OF THE COMMITTEE'S REPORT

The work of the current committee reinforces, extends, and elaborates on the work of prior National Academies committees. Chapter 2 examines the history and context of how social isolation in particular (and loneliness to a lesser extent) came to be recognized as a factor influencing mortality and how social support came to be recognized as a protective factor. Chapter 3 summarizes the evidence base for the impacts of social isolation and loneliness on morbidity and quality of life, while Chapter 4 summarizes the evidence base for the factors that put people at risk for social isolation and loneliness. Chapter 5 discusses the moderators and mediators of the relationships of social isolation and loneliness with health. Chapter 6 presents a brief overview of the tools used for measurement and assessment in research settings as well as of the use of information technology to identify individuals at risk for social isolation or loneliness. Chapter 7 discusses the role of the health care system specifically in addressing social isolation and loneliness. Chapter 8 considers the importance of education and training of the general public and the health care workforce, particularly in raising awareness of the health impacts of social isolation and loneliness. Chapter 9 presents an overview of interventions for social isolation and loneliness, focusing on approaches that are most applicable to health care providers and settings. Chapter 10 reflects on the principles of dissemination and implementation in order to explore avenues for translating research into practice. The citations for all chapters have been merged into a single reference list that follows Chapter 10. Appendix A provides the agendas of the committee's open sessions, including the topics and speakers. Appendix B contains the biographical sketches of the committee members and project staff.

2

Evaluating the Evidence for the Impacts of Social Isolation, Loneliness, and Other Aspects of Social Connection on Mortality

> *Strong social relationships are essential for a good life. The consequences of neglecting this fact become especially apparent in old age. Thus it is urgent that more attention be given to social isolation as a potential killer.*
>
> —Lubben (2017)

Developing the current understanding of the health impacts of social isolation and loneliness as well as other aspects of social connection has been part of a larger development regarding the importance of social determinants of health (i.e., the recognition that biomedical treatments are actually not, on average, the most significant determinants of the health outcomes of individuals). A major endpoint of this historical trend has been the scientific identification of social isolation as a major risk factor for human mortality, morbidity, and well-being. Loneliness and other aspects of social connection are also emerging potential risk factors for mortality.

This chapter considers the evidence for social isolation, loneliness, and other aspects of social connection as potentially causal risk factors for mortality, while Chapter 3 will do the same for morbidity and well-being. (Unless otherwise specified, mortality in this chapter is defined as all-cause mortality.) Both chapters consider the current evidence for social isolation, loneliness, and other aspects of social connection being risk factors for health and well-being.

The development of any area of scientific inquiry is rarely a simple, logical linear process. Knowing how we have gotten to where we are in any area of science is essential to understanding how and why we know what we do and what we do not. It can also clarify issues such as concepts and their definitions (see Chapter 1), their empirical measurement (see Chapter 6), and the nature of the scientific

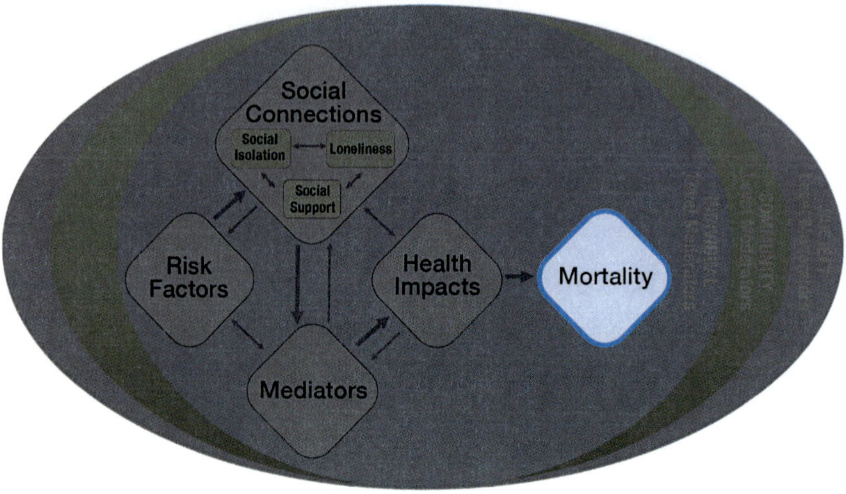

FIGURE 2-1 Committee's guiding framework with focus on mortality.

evidence regarding putatively causal relationships. Thus, this chapter begins with an overview of how social factors (e.g., the social determinants of health), including major social disparities and inequalities, have come to be recognized as major determinants of or risk factors for health and especially how and why social isolation and loneliness have come to be particularly pivotal at this point in time. This chapter represents the portion of the committee's guiding framework related to mortality (see Figure 2-1). Given the complexity of the terminology used in relation to social isolation and loneliness, a reminder of key definitions is provided in Box 2-1.

A HISTORY OF UNDERSTANDING THE CONTRIBUTORS TO HUMAN HEALTH

For most of human history human life was, in the famous words of Thomas Hobbes, "solitary, poor, nasty, brutish, and short" (Hobbes, 1965, p. 97). The life expectancy of human individuals and populations never exceeded 30–35 years of age until the beginning of the 18th century, and it was not until the end of the first half of the 20th century that life expectancy increased to about 65 years of age, after which it increased to almost 80 years by the end of the 20th century. The period since the 18th century saw the development of modern biomedical health science as well as such public health advances as the decline in infectious disease between the mid-18th and mid-20th centuries and the decline in rates of smoking in the last half of the 20th century. Thus, it seemed logical to

BOX 2-1
Key Definitions

Loneliness: the perception of social isolation or the subjective feeling of being lonely.

Mediators: also known as mechanisms or pathways; the factors that help explain how social isolation or loneliness affects health outcomes.

Moderators: the factors that can influence the magnitude or direction of the effect of social isolation or loneliness on health.

Social connection: an umbrella term that encompasses the structural, functional, and quality aspects of how individuals connect to each other.

Social isolation: the objective lack of (or limited) social contact with others.

Social support: the actual or perceived availability of resources (e.g., informational, tangible, emotional) from others, typically one's social network.

attribute the dramatic rise of human life expectancy to the application of biomedical science, clinical medicine, and biomedically based public health. Such an attribution continues to dominate much thinking about health policy even to the present day, though its validity has been increasingly challenged, and most health researchers now agree that clinical medicine, public health, and social changes all contributed to this increase in life expectancy (see House, 2015, especially Chapter 4; McGinnis et al., 2002; McKeown, 1976, 1979, 1988; Szreter, 1988, 1997, 2000). This growing appreciation for the impact of public health and social changes on health has given rise to a new appreciation of non-medical (e.g., environmental, health behavior, social and community, psychological, and socioeconomic) factors in health, most often referred to as *social determinants of health*.

The Role of Public Health

The era of the industrial revolution of the 18th, 19th, and 20th centuries saw the development of a public health approach to ensure "the conditions in which people can be healthy" (IOM, 1988, p. 1). Immunizations, improvements in drinking water and sanitation, increasing food safety, and the pharmacological treatment of infectious diseases resulted in reductions or eradication of many acute illnesses (CDC, 2001). These public health approaches led to an "epidemiological transition"—a shift from acute to chronic illnesses as the leading causes of death (Omran, 1971). As a result, "public health has shifted its primary focus from addressing infectious disease to tackling chronic disease" (IOM, 2012, p. 3). Understanding the impacts of the physical, chemical, and biological environments on health led to the recognition of a broader set of determinants of health that is beyond clinical medicine, though still largely within the biomedical framework.

The identification of cigarette smoking and other negative health behaviors as major risk factors for mortality and morbidity was pivotal to the movement toward a conception of the broader social determinants of health. The recognition of the danger of tobacco was considered one of the 10 greatest public health achievements of the 20th century (CDC, 2001). However, in spite of compelling evidence linking cigarette smoking to lung cancer and other causes of death, it took almost a quarter century to move from the strong scientific evidence to an effective comprehensive public health policy and then another quarter century to see major health improvements. The case of cigarette smoking and health gave rise to broader science, policy, and practice regarding the impacts of other health-related behaviors such as excessive consumption of alcohol, overeating, and the lack of physical activity (Berkman and Breslow, 1983). Increasingly, these behaviors joined cigarette smoking as major targets of intervention in both health care and broader public health policy (HHS, 2001, 2010).

Social Disparities in Health

As the understanding of the importance of social determinants of health grew in the last decades of the 20th century, there was also a renewed recognition of the disparities in health by socioeconomic position, race/ethnicity, gender, sexual orientation, and various combinations thereof. Most notably, in the late 1970s and early 1980s a commission in the United Kingdom found that differences in mortality by occupational status had not declined at all and perhaps had even grown in the quarter century after the National Health Service had presumably equalized access to health services (Black, 1982). Others found similar trends of differences in mortality by education and income in the United States (Pappas et al., 1993) and Canada (Wilkins et al., 1989). The World Health Organization (WHO) has focused attention on the social injustices that underlie inequities and inequalities in longevity and quality of life. A 2008 report of WHO's Commission on Social Determinants of Health stated:

> These inequities in health, avoidable health inequalities, arise because of the circumstances in which people grow, live, work, and age, and the systems put in place to deal with illness. The conditions in which people live and die are, in turn, shaped by political, social, and economic forces. (CSDH, 2008)

The identification of social disparities in the prevalence of any or all risk factors for health or in their impact became another major component of the growing science, policy, and practice regarding the social determinants of health.

DISCOVERING SOCIAL CONNECTIONS AS A DETERMINANT OF HEALTH AND LONGEVITY

Despite a long history of suggestions that social connections were integral to human health and well-being, a systematic investigation of social relationships, especially in relation to health, did not emerge until several decades after research on the social determinants of health had begun following World War II. In the mid-1970s, two physician social epidemiologists, John Cassel and Sidney Cobb, independently linked social support to health (Cassel, 1976; Cobb, 1976). Cassel and Cobb each reviewed a wide range of evidence from humans and animals showing that social connections were protective of health, especially in the face of biological and psychosocial risk factors for disease, most notably psychosocial stress, and both emphasized the ability of social support to buffer or moderate the adverse effects of such risk factors to health across a wide range of health outcomes. By the late 1970s and early 1980s, however, multiple researchers had identified various issues concerning the research on social support and health, including (1) what the causal associations between social support and health were, (2) "whether social relationships and supports [only or mainly] buffered the impact of stress on health or had more direct effects," and (3) how consequential the effects of social relationships on health really were (House et al., 1988, p. 541).

A number of researchers began to explore existing prospective longitudinal cohort studies for evidence of the long-term impacts of social connection on mortality that would be analogous to the evidence that had been used to identify other major biomedical and behavioral risk factors for mortality. Researchers focused on measures of the presence, extent, and types of social ties or relationships (e.g., marital status, contacts with friends and relatives, membership in—or at least attendance at services or meetings of—religious congregations or other formal and informal voluntary organizations or groups). These types of measures at baseline (individually and, especially, collectively) proved to be highly predictive of mortality, even after controlling for a large number of other predictors of mortality.

In the seminal study of this type, Berkman and Syme (1979) analyzed four measures collected in the Alameda County Study: (1) marital status, (2) frequency of contacts with other friends and relatives, (3) membership and frequency of participation in voluntary organizations, and (4) frequency of attendance at religious services. They found that all four of these factors predicted mortality over the succeeding 9 years in multivariate analyses that controlled for self-reports of physical health, socioeconomic status, smoking, alcohol consumption, physical activity, and the use of preventive health services. A "social network index" combining all four factors produced a relative risk ratio for all-cause mortality of about 2.0 for the socially isolated versus the more socially integrated—that is, socially isolated individuals were twice as likely to die in any given year as those who were more socially integrated (Berkman and Syme, 1979). A similar analysis in the Tecumseh Community Health Study that added biomedical baseline measures (e.g., blood pressure, cholesterol, respiratory function, electrocardiograms) to a similar set of self-reported controls at baseline obtained similar results (House et al., 1982). Further replicating studies came from the United States (Schoenbach et al., 1986) and Europe (Orth-Gomer and Johnson, 1987; Tibblin et al., 1986; Welin et al., 1985), and in 1988 House and colleagues summarized these data and other experimental and quasi-experimental evidence from animals and humans as follows:

> [S]ocial relationships, or the relative lack thereof, constitute a major risk factor for health—rivaling the effect of well established health risk factors such as cigarette smoking, blood pressure, blood lipids, obesity, and physical activity. (House et al., 1988, p. 541)

The conclusions of House et al. (1988) have remained valid over the succeeding three decades, and research on the mortality impacts of lack of social relationships or connections, increasingly called "social isolation," have continued. Furthermore, the number of studies has expanded tremendously. The remainder of this chapter summarizes the current state of the evidence in terms of overall magnitude of the effect on mortality of different aspects of social connection (e.g., social isolation, loneliness, social support) and why these may be causal effects.

THE CURRENT STATE OF THE EVIDENCE ON IMPACTS OF SOCIAL ISOLATION, LONELINESS, AND SOCIAL SUPPORT ON MORTALITY

As described in Chapter 1, the scientific evidence concerning social isolation and loneliness is based on a variety of different related conceptual and measurement approaches that all characterize related aspects of social relationships. To describe this evidence as accurately as possible, when the evidence does not differentiate among several related terms or perhaps combines them this report uses the term "social connection" (or "connectedness") as an umbrella term to refer to the structural, functional, and quality aspects of social relationships (Holt-Lunstad, 2018a,b; Holt-Lunstad et al., 2017). Social isolation and loneliness are common indicators of low social connection, while social support is a common indicator of high social connection. (See Chapter 1 for additional indicators of high and low social connection.) This report uses the specific terms "social isolation," "loneliness," and "social support" only when the data are specific to these terms.

The following sections summarize the evidence from meta-analyses and systematic reviews that synthesize the overall evidence for the mortality impacts of social isolation, loneliness, and social support across many studies as well as data from important individual studies.

Evidence Establishing Social Isolation as a Major Risk Factor for Mortality

A comprehensive meta-analysis by Holt-Lunstad and colleagues (2010) has been widely cited and influential in refocusing attention on the impacts of social connections on mortality. This analysis included 148 prospective studies that measured the structural (e.g., social integration,[1] network size, marital status, living alone), functional (e.g., perceived support, received support, perceived loneliness), or combined aspects (e.g., complex social integration) of social relationships and that followed participants over time (an average of 7.5 years) to determine the predictive association with mortality. This analysis, which examined studies with data from more than 300,000 participants, found that having a stronger social connection was associated with 50 percent greater odds of survival. Furthermore, these findings were consistent across age, gender, cause of death, and country of origin. Since this publication, several additional prospective studies and meta-analyses have replicated these findings (Holt-Lunstad et al., 2015; Luo et al., 2012; Rico-Uribe et al., 2018; Shor and Roelfs, 2015; Tanskanen and Anttila, 2016). Figure 2-2 provides their estimates, as well as more recent estimates, of the odds of decreased mortality of various indicators of social connection and other major risk factors for health.

The strongest results come from studies that used complex measures of social integration (which essentially correspond to the absence of social isolation). One example of such a measure is the Berkman–Syme Social Network Index, which is now included in several ongoing national surveys and recommended for inclusion in electronic medical records by a prior Institute of Medicine (IOM) committee (IOM, 2014). Low scores on this measure are often used as an indicator of social isolation. The measure has been and can be varied modestly across epidemiologic studies and could also be adapted slightly for clinical use. (See Chapters 6 and 7 for more on the use of the Berkman–Syme Social Network Index and other measures in clinical settings.)

In sum, more than four decades of research has produced robust evidence that lacking social connections has been associated with significantly increased risk for premature mortality—and this is strongest among measures of social isolation. Furthermore, in spite of a variety of challenges in the definitions and

[1] While social integration can describe high social connection, low scores on measures of social integration (e.g., the Berkman–Syme Social Network Index) are frequently used to measure social isolation. Thus, the term social isolation will also be used to represent these data.

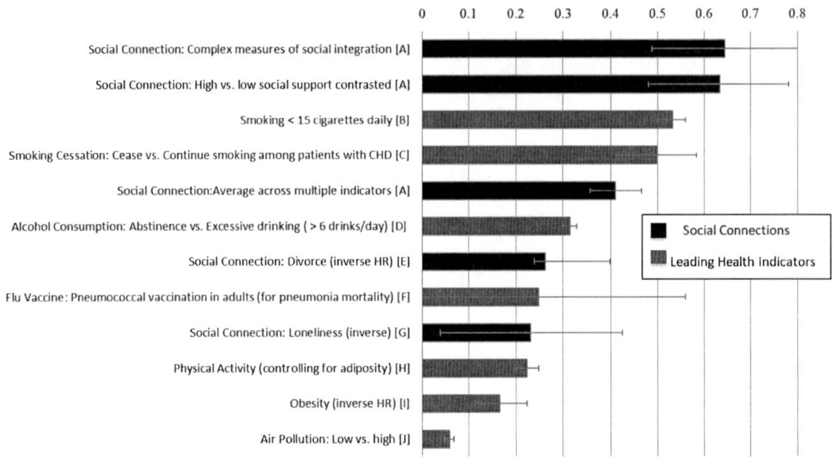

FIGURE 2-2 Odds of decreased mortality for indicators of social connection relative to leading health indicators.
NOTES: Odds (lnOR) or Hazards (lnHR). Effect size of zero indicates no effect. The effect sizes were estimated from meta-analyses: A = Holt-Lunstad et al., 2010; B = Shavelle et al., 2008; C = Critchley and Capewell, 2003; D = Holman et al., 1996; E = Shor et al., 2012; F = Fine et al., 1994; G = Holt-Lunstad et al., 2015; H = Katzmarzyk et al., 2003; I = Flegal et al., 2013; J = Schwartz, 1994.
SOURCE: Holt-Lunstad et al., 2017.

subsequent measurement of both social isolation and loneliness, there is some evidence that the magnitude of the effect on mortality risk may be comparable to or greater than other well-established risk factors such as smoking, obesity, and physical inactivity (which also have their own challenges in terms of determining causality). Importantly, this effect is independent of age and initial health status, which argues against reverse causality (Holt-Lunstad et al., 2010; Leigh-Hunt et al., 2017; Rico-Uribe et al., 2018; Shor and Roelfs, 2015). (See later in this chapter for a discussion of causality using Bradford Hill criteria.)

Evidence on Loneliness as a Risk Factor for Mortality, Considered Independently and in Relation to Social Isolation

In addition to the compelling evidence regarding social isolation as a major risk factor for mortality, evidence is emerging on the association between mortality and loneliness. Attention to loneliness grew because of two main factors: (1) the development of the concept and measurement of loneliness as a cognitive/emotional personality state or trait, and (2) the development of social neuroscience. Russell and colleagues (1980) developed the concept and the still-dominant measure of loneliness, the UCLA Loneliness Scale, while a related scale was developed in the Netherlands (de Jong Gierveld and Kamphuis, 1985). (See Chapter 6 for more on the measurement of social isolation and loneliness in research.) Many researchers have explored a causal link between loneliness and health, and, as a result, a growing number of predictive associations of loneliness with mortality have been found (e.g., Drageset et al., 2013; Luo and Waite, 2014; Perissinotto et al., 2012). In a recent meta-analysis focused exclusively on the association between loneliness and mortality, which included 35 prospective studies with 77,220 participants, the researchers concluded that loneliness significantly increases the risk for all-cause mortality—by 22 percent—independent of depression (Rico-Uribe et al., 2018). The authors did note that the variability in the instruments used to measure loneliness among the studies may be a limitation of interpreting the results. However, the finding was consistent with a previous meta-analysis that found that loneliness was associated with a 26 percent increased risk for premature mortality (Holt-Lunstad et al., 2015). Thus the predictive effect of loneliness on mortality (independent of depression) appears to be replicable, if smaller than that for social isolation.

Evidence on Social Isolation and Loneliness Considered Together

While substantial research has documented the risk of premature mortality posed by both social isolation and loneliness, most studies have examined these factors separately. And because only a handful of studies have examined both loneliness and social isolation in the same sample, there is currently limited ability to explore and compare their effects on mortality as independent or joint factors or to explore the degree to which loneliness is more a mediator of the health impacts of social isolation. Among studies that have examined both social isolation and loneliness in the same sample, most have tested which had the most important unique contribution—in essence, pitting social isolation and loneliness against each other. The strongest study that contained good measures of both social isolation and loneliness was done in a large nationally representative sample in the United Kingdom, which found that both social isolation and loneliness were associated with mortality when considered independently and with limited control variables. The effect of loneliness though was not independent of demographic factors such as age or health problems and did not increase the risk associated with social isolation. Therefore the subjective experience of loneliness, which may be the psychological manifestation of social isolation, appears not to be the primary mechanism explaining the association between social isolation and mortality in this study (Steptoe et al., 2013).

Similarly, the UK Biobank cohort study, which included 479,054 men and women, found that social isolation, but not loneliness,[2] predicted increased mortality

---

[2] In this study the authors used a two-item scale to measure loneliness (i.e., "Do you often feel lonely?" and "How often are you able to confide in someone close to you?").

in those with a history of acute myocardial infarction (Hakulinen et al., 2018). Thus, it appears that social isolation has an independent influence on the risk for mortality, which remains significant even when adjusting for loneliness, but the same is not true for loneliness.

Ong et al. (2016) reached similar conclusions in a review focused specifically on older adults that considered broader indicators of health as well as mortality:

> Although there is growing interest in studying the prevalence and detrimental effects of loneliness in later life . . . [q]uestions remain about whether the associations between loneliness and health reflect the effects of loneliness, the effects of objective social isolation, or the effects of unmeasured variables. Thus longitudinal and experimental studies addressing the direct, indirect [mediating], and moderating effects of social isolation and loneliness on health are urgently needed. (Ong et al., 2016, pp. 448–449)

A 20-year prospective study with a nationally representative sample of more than 4,800 middle-aged and older adults in Germany suggests there may be synergistic effects of social isolation and loneliness (Beller and Wagner, 2018a). The evidence indicates that the greater the social isolation, the larger the effect of loneliness on mortality and that the greater the loneliness, the larger the effect of social isolation (Beller and Wagner, 2018a,b).

To summarize, there is a large literature of studies that examine social isolation and loneliness separately as predictors of premature mortality; however, to date only five published studies have examined both social isolation and loneliness within the same sample. These five studies are all large population-based studies, but none were conducted within the United States. While these studies confirm their respective effect on risk for premature mortality, they also begin to elucidate more complex findings when considering their joint contributions. When social isolation and loneliness are considered together, social isolation has remained a robust predictor of mortality, but loneliness appears more tenuous.

Evidence Regarding Social Support and Mortality

Social support is one of the three major components of social connection, and it has been extensively studied in relation to health. Among the 148 studies included in the meta-analysis by Holt-Lunstad and colleagues (2010) on mortality risk, roughly half included measures of social support, and its role as a major independent risk factor for mortality has substantial support. However, the term "social support" has many different specific meanings and measures. For example, support may be instrumental, emotional, or informational; it may also be received, perceived[3] (as helpful or available if needed), or provided

[3] Perceived social support is conceptually similar to loneliness.

to others. When the effect of social relationships on mortality was broken down by measurement approach, perceived support and received support were found to have different effects. Perceived social support significantly predicted 35 percent increased odds of survival, which is stronger than the effect of loneliness (see Figure 2-2). However, the effect of received support, which was in the moderate range, was non-significant (Holt-Lunstad et al., 2010). Uchino (2009a,b) and Uchino et al. (2011) have discussed multiple possible reasons why received support may be less predictive than perceived support (or other indicators of social connection).

Research on social support as a construct has also been distinct from the literature on social isolation, although the two are intimately intertwined. Thus, we do not know the degree to which these may overlap (e.g., those who are isolated or lonely may perceive low social support). As with loneliness, more research in this area is needed.

Evidence of the Impact of Social Isolation and Loneliness on Specific Causes of Mortality

While all-cause mortality provides the most compelling evidence of the impact of social isolation and potentially loneliness, these two factors are also necessarily associated with the elevation of certain specific major causes of death. For example, individuals who are socially isolated or lonely and have a history of acute myocardial infarction or stroke have been shown to be at increased risk of death (Hakulinen et al., 2018). Among nearly 15,000 patients with chronic heart disease, living alone was related to a higher risk of cardiovascular death, while being married (compared to being widowed) was associated with a lower risk of cardiovascular death (Hagström et al., 2018). Among heart failure patients, those reporting high levels of loneliness had a nearly four times greater risk of death than patients who self-reported low levels of loneliness (Manemann et al., 2018). (See Chapter 3 for a discussion of suicidal ideation and suicide attempts.)

A FURTHER NOTE ON SOCIAL ISOLATION, AND SOCIAL CONNECTION MORE GENERALLY, AS A POTENTIAL CAUSAL RISK FOR MORTALITY

Substantial evidence supports an association between social connection (across varied measurement approaches) and both better health and a reduced risk for mortality; there is also substantial evidence for an association between a lack of social connection (especially social isolation) and poorer health and an increased risk of mortality. However, some may ask whether, in the absence of randomized control trials, this can truly be said to be a causal association. Causality is difficult to determine experimentally in this case because one cannot randomly assign individuals to be socially isolated. Furthermore, as discussed previously, there is uncertainty related to the different definitions of and measures for various aspects of social connection and so measurement uncertainties can make it difficult to determine causality with certainty. Table 2-1 outlines the Bradford Hill criteria, a framework for determining causality in epidemiology studies, and applies them to social isolation, including whether the criteria have been met, and

TABLE 2-1 Applying the Bradford Hill Criteria to Consider the Causal Influence of Social Isolation on Mortality

Guideline	Description of Guideline	Evidence	Evidence That the Guideline Has Been Satisfied
Experiment	Is there experimental evidence?	✓	Experimental evidence in animals shows that isolation increases mortality. Humans randomly assigned to loneliness induction, exclusion, or support conditions show different health-relevant physiological responses.
Strength	Is the effect size greater than combined effect of confounders?	✓	Overall magnitude of effect (risk ratio) is about 2.0, which is strong and comparable to or greater than other accepted risk factors.
Temporality	Does the cause occur before the effect? (temporal precedence)	✓	Prospective evidence establishes direction of effect. Poor social connection precedes mortality and poor health.
Biological gradient	Is there a dose–response effect?	✓	Animal and human evidence demonstrates a dose–response effect.
Biological plausibility	Are there plausible mechanisms of action?	✓	Established biological, behavioral, and cognitive pathways (see Chapter 5 for details).
Coherence	Is the evidence coherent with (does not contradict) other known mechanisms?	✓	Coheres with animal and human studies showing that increasing care support for children and neonates improves their health.
Replicability	Can the effect be repeated across multiple studies?	✓	Many studies in 2010 meta-analysis plus several more now have replicated these findings.
Similarity	Do similar studies show consistent results?	✓	Across the varied measurement approaches of social isolation and other aspects of social connection, there is converging evidence.

SOURCE: Adapted from Howick et al., 2019.

also provides a summary of the evidence that satisfies each criterion. By adapting the Bradford Hill criteria for social connections in general, evidence is found to support a potential causal link between social isolation and mortality.

FINDINGS AND CONCLUSIONS

- Social isolation has been associated with a significantly increased risk of premature mortality from all causes.
- There is some evidence that the magnitude of the effect of social isolation on mortality risk may be comparable to or greater than other well-established risk factors such as smoking, obesity, and physical inactivity.
- While there is evidence of a significant association between loneliness and mortality, existing evidence does not yet approach the cumulative weight of evidence of the association between social isolation and mortality. Further research is needed to establish the strength and robustness of the predictive association of loneliness with mortality in relation to social isolation and to clarify how social isolation and loneliness relate to and operate with each other (as well as other aspects of social connection, such as social support).

NEXT STEPS AND RECOMMENDATION

In today's society social isolation and loneliness are as prevalent as many other well-established risk factors for health, yet limited resources and attention have been paid to better understanding social isolation and loneliness and their individual and collective impacts on health. To enhance the role of the health care sector in addressing the impacts of social isolation and loneliness among older adults, the committee identifies the following goal:

GOAL: Develop a more robust evidence base for effective assessment, prevention, and intervention strategies for social isolation and loneliness.

Achieving this goal will require increasing funding for basic research on social isolation and loneliness. The body of evidence for the association of social connection (particularly of social isolation) with all-cause mortality is strong, and the magnitude of this association may rival that of other risk factors that are widely recognized and acted upon by the public health and health care systems (e.g., smoking, obesity, physical inactivity). However, given this evidence, current funding for social isolation and loneliness is not adequate. The committee concludes that in particular, further research is needed to establish the strength and robustness of the predictive association of loneliness with mortality in relation to social isolation and to clarify how social isolation and loneliness relate to and operate with each other in order to inform effective clinical interventions. Therefore, the committee recommends:

> **RECOMMENDATION 2-1: Major funders of health research, including the government (e.g., the National Institutes of Health, the Center for Medicare & Medicaid Innovation, and the Patient-Centered Outcomes Research Institute), foundations, and large health plans should fund research on social isolation and loneliness at levels that reflect their associations with mortality.**

3

Health Impacts of Social Isolation and Loneliness on Morbidity and Quality of Life

Feelings of social connection as well as feelings of disconnection have enormous influences on our bodies, as well as on our behaviors.

—Cacciopo and Patrick (2008)

As described in Chapter 2, studies of all-cause mortality provide compelling evidence of the health impacts of social isolation, and several aspects of social connection have been associated with specific causes of death (e.g., cardiovascular disease, cancer). But the health effects of social isolation and loneliness extend beyond mortality. Social isolation, loneliness, and other aspects of social connection can also significantly affect the risk of developing certain health conditions as well as the course of these health conditions and various measures of the quality of life. While most of the studies in this area evaluate social isolation and loneliness as risk factors and the health conditions as outcomes, the relationship between social isolation or loneliness and health is often bi-directional. (See Chapter 4 for more on health conditions as risk factors for social isolation and loneliness.) This chapter focuses on the evidence base for the impact of social isolation and loneliness on a wide range of physical, cognitive, and mental health conditions as well as on self-reported health and quality of life among adults aged 50 and older. The material presented in this chapter provides a summary of the relevant published literature. It is not intended to serve as a comprehensive review of every study published on these topics. This chapter represents the portion of the committee's guiding framework related to health impacts (see Figure 3-1). Given the complexity of the terminology used in relation to social isolation and loneliness, a reminder of key definitions is provided in Box 3-1.

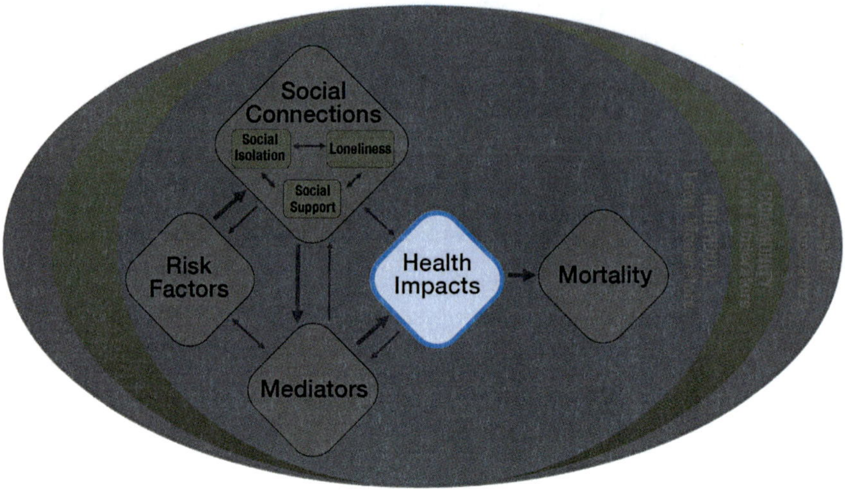

FIGURE 3-1 Committee's guiding framework with focus on health impacts.

BOX 3-1
Key Definitions

Loneliness: the perception of social isolation or the subjective feeling of being lonely.

Mediators: also known as mechanisms or pathways; the factors that help explain how social isolation or loneliness affects health outcomes.

Moderators: the factors that can influence the magnitude or direction of the effect of social isolation or loneliness on health.

Social connection: an umbrella term that encompasses the structural, functional, and quality aspects of how individuals connect to each other.

Social isolation: the objective lack of (or limited) social contact with others.

Social support: the actual or perceived availability of resources (e.g., informational, tangible, emotional) from others, typically one's social network.

IMPACT ON HEALTH OUTCOMES

In addition to the robust evidence linking social isolation and loneliness with mortality (see Chapter 2), other research has established that social isolation and loneliness are linked with specific health conditions. As described in previous chapters, the scientific literature concerning social isolation and loneliness draws on a variety of conceptual and measurement approaches that collectively characterize related aspects of social relationships. In the following sections, the committee presents evidence of the effects of different aspects of social connection on health, using the terminology and definitions as described by the individual authors of the cited studies.

Cardiovascular Disease and Stroke

Cardiovascular disorders and morbidities have been studied extensively as outcomes of social isolation and loneliness. A meta-analysis of 23 studies using 16 longitudinal datasets found that poor social relationships (e.g., social isolation, loneliness) increased the risk of developing coronary heart disease and stroke, independent of traditional cardiovascular disease risk factors (Valtorta et al., 2016a). Despite variability in the measurement of social isolation and loneliness across studies, poor social relationships were found to be associated with a 29 percent increase in risk of incident coronary heart disease and a 32 percent increase in the risk of stroke, and this was consistent across genders (Valtorta et al., 2016a). Other studies support these findings. For example, studies of patients after myocardial infarction have consistently found low social support to be a marker of poor prognosis and to be associated with increased mortality, readmission, and re-infarction rates (Barth et al., 2010; Glozier et al., 2013). An earlier review found both low social integration and loneliness to be associated with an increased risk for hypertension (Cuffee et al., 2014). A longitudinal study of nearly 5,400 adults over the age of 50 found loneliness to be associated with an increased risk for cardiovascular disease (defined by coronary heart disease and stroke), but not social isolation (Valtorta et al., 2018a). Data from the United Kingdom Biobank found that isolated and lonely persons were at increased risk of acute myocardial infarction and stroke (Hakulinen et al., 2018). One study of heart failure patients who self-reported high "perceived social isolation" (i.e., loneliness) found a 68 percent increased risk of hospitalization, a 57 percent increased risk of emergency department visits, and a 26 percent increased risk of outpatient visits compared with patients reporting low perceived social isolation (Manemann et al., 2018). (See Chapter 9 for more on the impacts of social isolation and loneliness on health care use.)

Consistent with this evidence for social isolation or loneliness as a major risk factor for cardiovascular disease, a review of currently available and widely used cardiovascular risk assessment models concluded that traditional screening for cardiovascular risk may be improved by taking social relationships into account (Ruwanpathirana et al., 2015).

Dementia and Cognition

Numerous observational studies have examined the associations of high levels of loneliness, low frequency of contact with family and friends, and low levels of participation in community groups with the risk of dementia and cognitive decline in older adults. A 2015 meta-analysis found an increased risk of dementia to be associated with high levels of loneliness, infrequent social contacts, and low-level group participation (Kuiper et al., 2015). Furthermore, this meta-analysis indicated that these social factors increased the risk of dementia by approximately 50 percent, which was comparable to such dementia risk factors as physical inactivity, low education, type 2 diabetes mellitus, and late-life depression (Diniz et al., 2013; Leoutsakos et al., 2015; Norton et al., 2014; Vagelatos and Eslick, 2013).

Similarly, another meta-analysis that included more than 2.3 million participants found that living alone, having a limited social network, having a low frequency of social contact, and having poor social support were all risk factors for dementia (Penninkilampi et al., 2018). The risk ratios for a weak social network and few social contacts were even stronger after adjusting for the presence of depression, indicating that low social connection has discrete effects on dementia risk that are distinct from the effects of depression (Penninkilampi et al., 2018). An elevated risk of dementia was also associated with low social support. Findings for an association between loneliness and risk of dementia in studies were mixed and, being based on a small number of studies, were non-significant overall. Furthermore, a reduced risk of dementia was reported to be associated with high levels of social contacts and social activity, indicating possible protective effects of high social engagement (in addition to the increased risk of dementia at low levels of social engagement) (Penninkilampi et al., 2018).

Social isolation and loneliness have also been examined in multiple cohorts for their association with cognitive decline (Bassuk et al., 1999; Crooks et al., 2008; Ertel et al., 2008; Kelly et al., 2017). The evidence indicates that less frequent social contacts and lower levels of participation in community groups are associated with declines in global cognition, processing speed, executive function, and visuospatial abilities (Braak and Del Tredici, 2012). These associations were found to be independent of many factors, including age, sex, educational attainment, wealth, levels of depression, and physical activity (Saczynski et al., 2006; Shankar et al., 2013). Greater loneliness in older adults has also been associated with worsening performance on measures of global cognition and on specific tests of immediate and delayed recall (Holwerda et al., 2014; Shankar et al., 2013; Tilvis at al., 2004; Wilson et al., 2007).

Notably, social isolation and loneliness have been found to have independent and cumulative effects on cognitive decline and dementia risk in some but not all studies, suggesting that the structural and functional aspects of social connection may influence cognitive health through both shared and distinct mechanisms (Donovan et al., 2017; Holwerda et al., 2014; Shankar et al., 2013; Wilson et al., 2007). Social interactions are thought to enhance cognitive capacity by activating and maintaining the efficiency of brain networks (Stern, 2012). This effect may point to the existence of a form of neural reserve that supports cognitive function as age-related and pathological brain changes accrue over time (Bennett et al., 2006; Yu et al., 2015). In older adults greater emotional support has been associated with both higher serum levels of brain-derived neurotropic factor and a reduced risk of dementia, suggesting that enriching relationships may also promote neurogenesis and synaptic plasticity (Salinas et al., 2017). In addition, higher loneliness in mid- to late life has been associated with elevated cardiovascular and neuroendocrine markers of stress, impaired sleep, and pro-inflammatory physiological effects, which may accelerate neurodegeneration in the hippocampus and in other brain regions vulnerable to Alzheimer's disease and vascular cognitive impairment (Cacioppo et al., 2002; Hackett et al., 2012; Hawkley and Cacioppo, 2010; Hawkley et al., 2006; Jaremka et al., 2013a; McHugh and Lawlor, 2013). In cognitively normal older adults, greater loneliness has been associated with higher levels of brain amyloid and regional accumulation of tau protein, linking loneliness with the pathological changes of early Alzheimer's disease (d'Oleire Uquillas et al., 2018; Donovan et al., 2016). Furthermore, less social engagement with friends, family, and community groups has been associated with a more rapid cognitive decline in these unimpaired older adults with high brain amyloid, indicating an adverse interactive effect of low social connection and early Alzheimer's pathology on cognitive health (Biddle et al., 2019).

A small number of observational studies have investigated the possibility of reverse causation (i.e., the possibility that low cognitive function may precede declines in social function). These studies have found inconsistent and, most often, opposing evidence that low cognitive function leads to subsequent social disengagement or loneliness in population-based cohorts; however, other research has demonstrated that older adults with declining cognitive performance experience disruptions in their larger and more diversified social networks (Aartsen et al., 2004; Ayalon et al., 2016; Donovan et al., 2017; Ellwardt et al., 2015; James et al., 2011; Wilson et al., 2007). These and other complementary findings raise the possibility that social function and cognitive abilities are reciprocally related and, in certain aging adults, may decline in tandem (Biddle et al., 2019).

Depression and Anxiety

In cross-sectional studies, social isolation and loneliness have been associated with both depression and anxiety throughout adulthood, including in older adults. In one of the largest studies to date, which included more than 15,000 German adults aged 35–74 years, greater loneliness was related to higher rates of clinically significant depression, anxiety, and suicidal ideation, independent of age, sex, partnership, and socioeconomic status (Beutel et al., 2017). A systematic review of this topic included eight cross-sectional studies of adults aged 60 and older and found loneliness to have been associated with depression in seven studies and low social engagement to have been associated with depression in one study (Choi et al., 2015). In a cross-sectional study of 314 older U.S. adults living in retirement communities, loneliness was found to be associated with both depression and anxiety, but not with perceived health, medical conditions, or functional status (Bekhet and Zauszniewski, 2012). While loneliness is commonly associated with clinically significant depression, loneliness and depression are recognized as distinct constructs that can also be experienced independently of each other. A study of more than 8,000 older adult participants from the U.S. Health and Retirement Study found that nearly 18 percent of the sample reported frequent feelings of loneliness. Within this lonely group, 53 percent reported levels of depressive symptoms above the threshold for clinically significant depression, and 47 percent reported either no depressive symptoms or depressive symptoms in a subthreshold range (Donovan et al., 2017). A systematic review by Schwarzbach and colleagues (2014) of 25 cross-sectional and 12 longitudinal studies (but not including studies of loneliness) evaluated the relationship between depression and a range of social support and social network measures for older adults. Qualitative aspects of social relations, such as social support, the quality of relations, and a confidant relationship, were most consistently associated with the presence or absence of depression in the cross-sectional studies. However, in the longitudinal studies a lower quantity of social interactions was most often associated with depression over time. Schwarzbach and colleagues (2014) interpreted this to mean that having fewer social interactions or connections may predispose adults to later having inadequate social support when it is needed during stressful events, thereby elevating the risk of incident depression. Correspondingly, close relationships and social support may be experienced as more acutely inadequate in those who are depressed because of the distress and disabilities imposed by these symptoms.

A cross-sectional study of more than 1,400 older U.S. adults also found that the qualitative aspects of social relationships were more strongly related to depression than the quantitative aspects when the depression and social relationships were measured at the same time-point, which was consistent with the pattern observed earlier (Taylor et al., 2018a). Also consistent were findings from a longitudinal study of more than 11,000 older U.S. adults, which quantified the number and types of social contacts as a potential predictor of future depression. A lower frequency of in-person social contacts was related to higher rates of depression over 2 years. Notably, the frequencies of telephone, written, or email contacts were not associated with depression at 2 years, indicating that in-person modes of contact were uniquely protective (Teo et al., 2015).

A growing number of international studies have employed validated instruments for measuring loneliness and have found positive associations of loneliness with higher depression and anxiety over time. These include analyses from the Irish Longitudinal Study of Ageing, which found both loneliness and low social network to be associated with rates of clinically significant depression and anxiety over 2 years; from the Netherlands Study of Depression in Older Persons, which found that loneliness at baseline predicted a poorer course of depression in persons with late-life depression; and from the Chicago Health, Aging, and Social Relations Study, which found greater loneliness, but not social support or social network, to be associated with higher depression scores over 5 years (Cacioppo et al., 2010; Doménech-Abella et al., 2019; Jeuring et al., 2018). One German study that sought to compare different measurement approaches found that subjective loneliness and network quality best predicted mental health, whereas network size and living alone best predicted physical and cognitive health (Beller and Wagner, 2018b).

Collectively, these studies establish that social support, social isolation, and loneliness are strongly linked to depression and anxiety. While these associations do not establish causality, the temporal associations suggest that social isolation and loneliness likely cause or worsen depression and anxiety, with in-person contacts and the perceived adequacy of relationships having the largest impacts. The relationships of social isolation and loneliness with depression and anxiety have also been shown to have reciprocal effects over time. (See Chapter 4 for research describing loneliness and social isolation as outcomes of depression and anxiety and for further discussion of loneliness and depression as distinct constructs.)

Chronic Health Conditions and Other Physical Health–Related Factors

In a cross-sectional, population-based sample of 20,007 participants from the Swiss Health Survey, individuals who self-identified as being lonely were found to be 41 percent more likely to be affected by self-reported chronic diseases, 31 percent more likely to have high cholesterol levels, 40 percent more likely to have diabetes, and 94 percent more likely to report self-perceived impaired health (Richard et al., 2017). In a Danish sample, self-reported loneliness was associated with a more than 2.5 times higher risk for poor self-rated health, 91 percent higher risk of limited physical abilities, and a 77 percent higher risk of multiple diagnoses (Jessen et al., 2017). In the United States the relationship between loneliness and functional decline or death was assessed in 1,604 subjects 60 years of age and older, who participated in a longitudinal cohort study between 2002 and 2008; the assessments were conducted every 2 years (Perissinotto et al., 2012). Participants who self-identified as lonely (as measured by the three-item UCLA Loneliness Scale) were more likely to have experienced reductions in the activities of daily living (e.g., bathing, eating), in mobility, and in stair-climbing ability, and they had more difficulty with upper extremity tasks (e.g., pushing or pulling large objects, lifting weights heavier than 10 pounds), ultimately resulting in a 59 percent increased risk of function loss. A longitudinal community-based cohort study of 985 older adults who reported loneliness and being alone examined the loss of motor function (Buchman et al., 2010). Assessed loneliness at baseline was found to correspond with the rate of motor function decline, with a higher assessed loneliness at baseline resulting in more rapid rates of motor function decline. (See Chapter 4 for information regarding risk factors associated with frailty in older adults.)

Several aspects of the structural and functional characteristics of social connection have been associated with newly and previously diagnosed type 2 diabetes mellitus (T2DM). One study found that individuals with a smaller social network size were more likely to have newly diagnosed and previously diagnosed T2DM; no such relationship was found for pre-diabetes (Brinkhues et al., 2017). On the other hand, pre-diabetes was found to be associated with a lack of social participation, and living alone was associated with a greater likelihood of previously diagnosed T2DM in men, but not in women (Brinkhues et al., 2017).

Loneliness may also have a reciprocal relationship with diabetic outcomes. Diabetes-related complications can limit physical mobility, which may in turn limit an individual's ability to initiate social interactions or may strain relationships, thus leading to greater loneliness (Jaremka et al., 2013b; Ribu and Wahl, 2004). In a population-based study of adults without diabetes, low satisfaction with one's social network (perhaps an indirect indication of social isolation and loneliness) was associated with a significantly increased risk of developing T2DM, and the risk for incident T2DM was still significant after controlling for social isolation and living alone (Lukaschek et al., 2017).

Social connections even appear to influence susceptibility to colds. In viral challenge studies, for which all participants are infected with a cold virus, loneliness was associated with greater self-reported cold symptoms (LeRoy et al., 2017). Sociability (assessed using measures of extraversion, agreeableness, and positive relationship style) has been linearly associated with a decreased probability of developing a cold, independent of baseline, demographics, emotional styles, stress hormones, and health practices (Cohen et al., 2003). Having more diverse social networks has been associated with having a greater resistance to upper respiratory illness (Cohen et al., 1997). Furthermore, having a greater number of social roles has been associated with better pulmonary function in older adults (Crittenden et al., 2014).

IMPACT ON HEALTH-RELATED BEHAVIORS

Different aspects of social connection may affect health-related behaviors (e.g., smoking, substance use, exercise, diet, sleep patterns) both positively and negatively. Health-related behaviors have been studied for decades, and early theories held that being married or being a parent helped inhibit risk-taking behaviors such as drinking, smoking, or illicit substance use because these roles afforded a sense of importance or purpose or because having a partner helped to favorably regulate these health behaviors (Gove, 1973; Syme, 1974; Umberson, 1987).

Social connections and supports have been associated with levels of use (as well as the cessation and relapse) of tobacco and alcohol (Christakis and Fowler, 2008; Havassy et al., 1991; Rosenquist et al., 2010; Seeman and Anderson, 1983). That is, an individual's levels of alcohol and tobacco use may be affected by the degree of use of his or her social contacts or, in the case of cessation, by the strength of his or her social supports. However, these effects can be positive or negative. For example, studies have shown that smoking cessation among one's social contacts improves the likelihood that an individual will stop smoking, while living with a smoker or having smokers among one's social networks decreases the likelihood of smoking cessation (Holahan et al., 2012; Lacey et al., 1993; Moore et al., 2014).

Evidence specifically related to the connection between social isolation and health-related behaviors has shown that older people who are isolated are more likely to have less healthy behaviors such as poor diets, tobacco use, heavy alcohol use, and a lack of physical activity (Choi and DiNitto, 2015; Ho et al., 2018; Kharicha et al., 2007; Kobayashi and Steptoe, 2018; Locher et al., 2005; Schrempft et al., 2019).

While some research has found no relationship specifically between loneliness and certain health-related behaviors (Canham et al., 2016; Hawkley et al., 2009; Kobayashi and Steptoe, 2018; Schrempft et al., 2019), other studies of adults and older adults have found associations of loneliness with low physical activity, being overweight, higher levels of smoking, and greater alcohol consumption (Åkerlind and Hornquist, 1992; Barretta et al., 1995; Hawkley et al., 2009; Lauder et al., 2006a; Shankar et al., 2011; Stickley et al., 2013). Also, limited evidence links loneliness with risky sexual behaviors and psychotropic drug use among older adults (Boehlen et al., 2015; Golub et al., 2010). (See Chapter 5 for more on health-related behaviors as a mediator of the relationship between social connection and health.)

Suicidal Ideation and Suicide Attempts

Suicide is a concern for families and communities, and both social isolation and loneliness have been identified as risk factors for suicide for individuals of all ages (Calati et al., 2019; Kochanek et al., 2019). Between 1999 and 2017 suicide rates increased among adults aged 45–74 (from 6.0 to 9.7 per 100,000 adults aged 45–64 and from 4.1 to 6.2 per 100,000 adults aged 65–74), and white males over the age of 85 have been identified as being most at risk for suicide (Hedegaard et al., 2018; Steele et al., 2018). Depression has been found to be the most relevant cause of suicide attempts, but both loneliness and social isolation have also been identified as major contributing factors (Minayo and Cavalcante, 2015).

A number of studies have evaluated the relationship of social isolation with suicide in older adults. In a review of nine studies published between 2010 and 2017 that focused on suicide attempts or suicide ideation in adults 60 years of age and older, the authors found a relationship between both loneliness and social isolation and suicidal thoughts or ideation (Heuser and Howe, 2019).

Similar findings were seen in a systematic review of studies examining suicide risk in nursing homes and other long-term care facilities conducted between 1985 and 2013 (Mezuk et al., 2014). Researchers found that both loneliness and social isolation were correlated with suicidal ideation among residents in these settings.

The majority of studies examine either social isolation or loneliness when evaluating suicide risk. Several recent interview studies found a relationship between suicidal ideation or self-harm in older adults and feelings of loneliness or "aching loneliness" (Huang et al., 2017; van Wijngaarden et al., 2015; Wand et al., 2018). Self-harm in older adults was evaluated in a recent systematic review that included 40 articles published through February 2018. This study, which included a total of 62,755 older adults, found that increased loneliness was among the primary motivations reported for self-harm (Troya et al., 2019). Wiktorsson and colleagues (2010) interviewed 103 suicide attempters aged 70 or older treated at five emergency departments in Western Sweden and compared them with matched community controls. A strong relationship was found between perceived loneliness and attempted suicide, independent of depression. The association between social relationships and suicidal ideation were evaluated in a meta-analysis by Chang et al. (2017), which included findings from 31 studies published between 2000 and November 2016. In that analysis, elderly adults were found to be 57 percent more likely to experience suicide ideation if they had discordant social relationships, and perceived loneliness along with elderly mistreatment and poorly perceived social support were found to be the measures associated with the greatest effect (Chang et al., 2017). Furthermore, death wishes, which may lead to suicidal ideation or future suicide attempts, were found to be significantly associated with loneliness, depression, and poor self-reported health in a study of more than 35,000 people over 65 years of age (Cheung et al., 2017). Bernier et al. (2020) evaluated Seniors Health Survey results from 2,787 French-speaking community dwellers between the ages of 65 and 69 and found that the 5 percent of respondents who wished for death were significantly more isolated than other respondents.

Taken together, these results indicate that social isolation and loneliness are related to both suicidal ideation and suicide attempts. None of these studies were designed to determine whether social isolation or loneliness cause suicidality, but they are clearly associated with suicidal thoughts and behaviors, even apart from depression.

IMPACT ON QUALITY-OF-LIFE OUTCOMES

A growing body of research indicates that social isolation and loneliness negatively affect quality of life among older adults, although the empirical literature on these relationships remains relatively limited. The variability in the measures of social isolation and loneliness used in these studies, coupled with the small number of the studies, allows for only a limited scientific understanding of how both phenomena relate to an older adult's quality of life.

The definitions of quality of life vary across the available research on social isolation and loneliness among older adults. Many of these studies define quality of life as a health-related construct—either as health-related quality of life (HRQL), which offers a broad, multi-dimensional picture of a person's health and well-being from the individual's perspective, or as health status, which captures a person's physical and mental health in narrower terms and represents only one aspect of HRQL (Golden et al., 2009). Other studies employ a more expansive definition of quality of life, including factors such as perceived financial adequacy, satisfaction with life, and "global happiness," among others (Chappell and Badger, 1989). Holmén et al. (1999) commented that while the common definitions of quality of life at the time focused on health and illness, emerging definitions were generally more expansive in that they allowed for subjective dimensions such as overall life satisfaction.

Current evidence indicates that social isolation negatively affects the quality of life of older adults. Hawton et al. (2011) found that social isolation—defined by a person's level of contact with others—has a significant, independent, and negative effect on HRQL among older adults, even when accounting for factors such as depression, physical comorbidity, age, gender, living alone, employment status, and accommodation type. In the Hawton et al. (2011) study, older adults who were severely socially isolated were found to have particularly low HRQL scores when compared to peers of similar age in the general population. Other work done in the context of older people's social networks has found social isolation to be associated with decreased satisfaction with one's life, hopelessness, increased risk of depressed mood, and decreased happiness (Golden et al., 2009). Additionally, research has illustrated how certain dimensions of social isolation might have a greater effect than others on an older person's quality of life. Chappell and Badger (1989) interviewed 743 older adults aged 60 years or older to examine 10 indicators of social isolation—whether an older person lives alone, is married, has children, or interacts with confidants or companions, and so on—and they observed that companionship and confidants were more related to an older person's well-being than the individual's marital status, living arrangements, or presence of children.

While few studies have documented the impact of loneliness on quality of life among older adults, the research that has been done indicates that both severe and moderate loneliness significantly reduce the physical and mental quality of life among older adults. Being lonely might also lead to reduced satisfaction with one's life and lower levels of happiness, and one study concluded that older adults who were not lonely showed fewer depressive symptoms (Ekwall et al., 2005; Lim and Kua, 2011; Musich et al., 2015). The combination of loneliness and social isolation might also have an adverse effect on the quality of life among older adults. Golden et al. (2009) discovered that the prevalence of hopelessness—an indicator for a diminished quality of life—was higher among older adults who did not have an integrated social network.

ELDERS AT RISK FOR ABUSE

Elder abuse, which can affect an older adult's physical health, mental health, and quality of life, is burgeoning globally, and isolated or lonely individuals can be more vulnerable to mistreatment. According to the World Health Organization, approximately one in six adults aged 60 years or older have experienced at least one form of abuse—financial exploitation, physical abuse, psychological (or verbal) abuse, sexual abuse, or outright neglect—during the past year (WHO, 2018). In the United States it has proved difficult to determine the precise extent of elder abuse. Efforts to evaluate the scope of abuse have been hampered by the lack of standardization in how cases of abuse are defined, prosecuted, and reported from one jurisdiction to the next as well as by the large number of abuse cases that go unreported (Acierno et al., 2010; Wang et al., 2015). However, an estimated 5 to 10 percent of older adults in the United States fall victim to some form of abuse (Lachs and Pillemer, 2015; Wang et al., 2015). Based on projections of aging, the number of older victims of abuse could grow from an estimated 2.5 million to 4.9 million in 2016 to as many as 9.8 million by 2060 (ACL, 2018; Ortman et al., 2014).

Physical or social isolation can increase a person's susceptibility to abuse. Socially isolated individuals are both more vulnerable to abuse (Acierno et al., 2010) and more likely to become abusers (Amstadter et al., 2011). In addition to any psychological anguish it may cause, elder abuse can lead to housing displacement or disruption, worse physical health, or, in extreme cases, even death (Wong and Waite, 2017). Perpetrators of elder abuse are most often family members—spouses or adult children—or unrelated caregivers and are often male and financially dependent on the abused adult; substance abuse problems or having a history of mental health issues are common in abusers (Fulmer et al., 2005; Labrum and Solomon, 2015; Lachs and Pillemer, 2015; Sibbald and Holroyd-Leduc, 2012; Wong and Waite, 2017). Many cases of abuse go unreported by both the abused individuals and the perpetrators of abuse because of other factors, such as the possibility of losing housing or a caregiver, or emotional or financial reasons that could be at stake (Wong and Waite, 2017).

FINDINGS AND CONCLUSIONS

- Substantial evidence shows that social isolation and loneliness are strongly associated with a greater incidence of major psychological, cognitive, and physical morbidities and lower perceived well-being or quality of life.
- Strong evidence indicates that social isolation and loneliness have effects on the risk of cardiovascular and cerebrovascular morbidities. A smaller amount of evidence indicates that social connection has effects on the course of other chronic health conditions, such as type 2 diabetes mellitus, or on health characteristics, such as mobility and functioning in the activities of daily living.

- Substantial evidence links social isolation and loneliness with accelerated cognitive decline in older adults and an increased risk of incident dementia.
- Social connection is strongly linked to depression and anxiety. Temporal associations suggest that social isolation and loneliness likely cause or worsen depression and anxiety. Complementary research suggests that depression and anxiety increase the likelihood of low social connection, which is further addressed in Chapter 4.
- While some research shows no relationship specifically between loneliness and certain health-related behaviors, other studies have found associations of loneliness with lower physical activity, being overweight, higher levels of smoking, and greater alcohol consumption.
- Emerging evidence suggests that social isolation and loneliness negatively affect the quality of life of older adults. However, the existing empirical literature on this relationship is relatively small, and interpretations are limited by variability in the measures and definitions of social isolation and loneliness used.
- Reports of elder abuse, including financial exploitation, physical abuse, psychological (or verbal) abuse, sexual abuse, or outright neglect, are disturbingly common. In the United States there is a lack of infrastructure for reliably measuring this problem.

NEXT STEPS AND RECOMMENDATIONS

Substantial evidence supports the association of social isolation, loneliness, and certain other indicators of social connection (e.g., social support) with an increased incidence of major physical, cognitive, and psychological morbidities; poorer health-related behaviors; and lower perceived well-being or HRQL. Existing evidence suggests that certain aspects of social connection may be especially predictive of certain health outcomes and that the relationship between social connection and health is often bi-directional.

As discussed in Chapter 2, the committee identified the increased funding of basic research as a key to achieving the goal of developing a more robust evidence base on effective prevention, assessment, and intervention for social isolation and loneliness. Specifically, the committee concludes that identifying, prioritizing, and developing ways to translate scientific knowledge of the impacts of social isolation and loneliness on health into effective and efficient clinical and public health interventions (see Chapter 9) first requires a better understanding of how social isolation and loneliness impact health, including the risk factors for social isolation and loneliness (see Chapter 4), the mediators (or mechanisms) by which social isolation and loneliness affect health (see Chapter 5), and the moderators that affect the magnitude of those relationships (see Chapter 5). Furthermore, more needs to be determined about whether and when (e.g., at what stage of the life course, or when the situation is acute or chronic) an intervention will have downstream effects on health outcomes. Therefore, drawing from information in all of these chapters, the committee makes the following recommendation as a strategy to mitigate or eliminate the negative health impacts of social isolation and loneliness:

> **RECOMMENDATION 3-1: Major funders of health research, including the government (e.g., the National Institutes of Health, the Center for Medicare & Medicaid Innovation, and the Patient-Centered Outcomes Research Institute), foundations, and large health plans should fund research to improve the scientific understanding of the links between social connection and health, including the study of risk factors and mechanisms.**

4

Risk and Protective Factors for Social Isolation and Loneliness

Aging, independent of other factors, does not cause social isolation or loneliness. However, people who are 50 years of age and older are more likely to experience many of the risk factors that can cause or exacerbate social isolation or loneliness, such as the death of loved ones, worsening health and chronic illness, new sensory impairment, retirement, or changes in income. The relationships between risk factors and social isolation or loneliness can be bi-directional in that being socially isolated or lonely can affect health, while these same health conditions can make experiencing social isolation or loneliness more likely. This chapter focuses on the risk factors for social isolation and loneliness while also providing some context regarding the health impacts of these two factors, reflecting the frequent bi-directionality of these relationships. (See Chapters 2 and 3 for a fuller discussion of the health impacts of social isolation and loneliness.) When considering the risk factors for social isolation and loneliness, it should be noted that some factors may increase the risk of negative health effects while other factors may lower those risks. Mechanisms and moderators will be discussed in Chapter 5.

This chapter reviews the risk and protective factors for social isolation and loneliness, including predisposing physical health factors (e.g., chronic diseases, functional impairments); psychological, psychiatric, and cognitive factors (e.g., depression, anxiety, dementia); socio-cultural factors (e.g., social supports, disruptive life events); and social environmental factors (e.g., transportation, housing). The chapter then summarizes the risks of social isolation and loneliness among specific subpopulations. As described in earlier chapters, research outcomes pertaining to social connection have included a variety of related terms; the specific terms used in individual studies are noted throughout the chapter for greater clarity. It should be kept in mind that the material presented in this chapter provides a

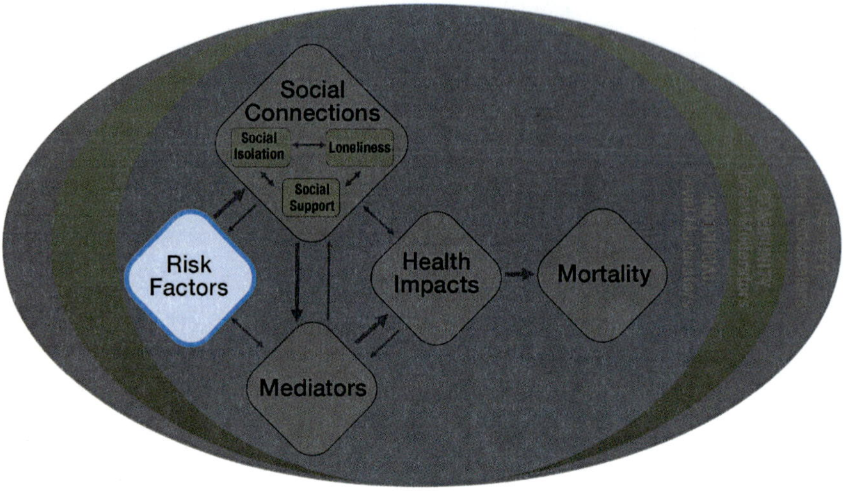

FIGURE 4-1 Committee's guiding framework with focus on risk factors.

summary of the relevant published literature rather than a comprehensive review of these topics. Gaining a broad understanding of risk factors for social isolation and loneliness and also elucidating which factors are most closely linked to them can lead to new initiatives to improve health outcomes at primary, secondary, and tertiary stages of prevention. This chapter represents the portion of the committee's guiding framework related to risk factors (see Figure 4-1). Given the complexity of the terminology used in relation to social isolation and loneliness, a reminder of key definitions is provided in Box 4-1.

PHYSICAL HEALTH FACTORS

Various physical health factors are related to social isolation and loneliness, including many common chronic diseases, impairments, and geriatric syndromes. As mentioned earlier, these relationships are often bi-directional. That is, social isolation or loneliness may increase the chances of developing a chronic health condition (see Chapter 3), while, conversely, a chronic health condition may contribute to social isolation or loneliness by interfering with the quality, quantity, or structure of relationships or by worsening pathophysiological processes. The relationships between combinations of conditions and social isolation or loneliness are less well studied, but having multiple chronic conditions has been associated with a lower participation in social activities (Cantarero-Prieto et al., 2018). Similarly, among older adults discharged after an acute coronary syndrome, a greater number of co-existing chronic conditions has been associated with having a limited social network (Tisminetzsky et al., 2016). This section focuses on the role of physical health as a risk factor for experiencing social isolation or loneliness.

BOX 4-1
Key Definitions

Loneliness: the perception of social isolation or the subjective feeling of being lonely.

Mediators: also known as mechanisms or pathways; the factors that help explain how social isolation or loneliness affects health outcomes.

Moderators: the factors that can influence the magnitude or direction of the effect of social isolation or loneliness on health.

Social connection: an umbrella term that encompasses the structural, functional, and quality aspects of how individuals connect to each other.

Social isolation: the objective lack of (or limited) social contact with others.

Social support: the actual or perceived availability of resources (e.g., informational, tangible, emotional) from others, typically one's social network.

Chronic Disease and Conditions

Roughly 60 percent of all adults and about 80 percent of adults aged 65 and older have at least one chronic disease (e.g., heart disease, diabetes, cancer, stroke), and 77 percent have at least two chronic diseases (CDC, 2019; NCOA, 2019). Research indicates that some chronic diseases and conditions can be risk factors for social isolation and loneliness. There is robust evidence, for example, that cardiovascular disease and stroke can increase the risk of social isolation and loneliness and also of low social support; conversely, there is also research indicating that people who have cerebrovascular or cardiovascular disease may have worse outcomes if they are socially isolated or lonely (Air et al., 2016). The deficits that occur as a result of having a stroke can increase the risk of social isolation, which in turn can affect recovery from the stroke (Alun and Murphy, 2019; Glass and Maddox, 1992; Hinojosa et al., 2011). For example, lasting symptoms of stroke may include visual field deficits and dysphagia, which can impair an individual's ability to interact with others (Cichero and Altman, 2012; Rim et al., 2020).

Other common chronic conditions, such as chronic obstructive pulmonary disease (Castelino et al., 2018) and advanced heart failure (Leeming et al., 2014) as well as many less common and less frequently studied conditions may also increase the risk for social isolation or loneliness. The English Longitudinal Study of Ageing has revealed, for instance, that chronic pain (largely due to musculoskeletal disease) sometimes results in a reduction in physical and social activity, which may lead to social isolation or reduced social participation (Blyth and Noguchi, 2017). A small study of people with wounds infected with methicillin-resistant staph aureus found that fears of infecting someone else or of being rejected made social isolation more likely (Andersson et al., 2011), and older adults living with HIV may face greater social isolation and loneliness as a result of decreased social participation and engagement due to a loss of friends and social networks and to HIV-related stigma (Greene et al., 2018; Greysen et al., 2013; Nachega et al., 2012; Rueda et al., 2014). Others specific conditions that may influence social isolation and loneliness include Parkinson's disease, multiple sclerosis, cancer, and spinal cord injury (Andreadou et al., 2011; Benito-León et al., 2009; Buhse, 2015; Deckx et al., 2014; Newman et al., 2016).

Geriatric Syndromes and Impairments

In addition to specific diseases, geriatric syndromes[1] and impairments may also increase social isolation and loneliness as a result of the associated embarrassment and stigma or because of associated deficits in communication or comprehension, limited functional abilities, or impaired mobility. For example, oral-health-related quality of life is an independent risk factor for loneliness among older adults, possibly due to embarrassment or stigma (Rouxel et al., 2017; Tonetti et al., 2017). These issues may be exacerbated among some racial or ethnic minorities and low-income older populations who lack preventative and corrective dental care (Griffin et al., 2012).

Frailty and Functional Status

Frailty is a medical syndrome that involves a vulnerability to stressors and a greater risk of worse outcomes from new or co-existing conditions. Different frailty assessment tools differ in their questions pertaining to social connection, and some frailty measures lack a social connection question altogether (e.g., the Fried phenotype defined frailty using five criteria: weight loss, exhaustion, low physical activity, slowness, and weakness) (Fried et al., 2001; Galambos, 2017a,b). This variability contributes to an incomplete understanding of the association of frailty with social isolation and loneliness and the extent to which it is bi-directional. Over a 6-year period the English Longitudinal Study of Ageing found that loneliness predicted frailty for men and women, while social isolation predicted frailty only for men (Gale et al., 2018). These findings provide

[1] Geriatric syndromes are "clinical conditions common among older adults that often do not fit into discrete disease categories. Examples include delirium, depression, falls, sensory impairment, incontinence, malnutrition, and osteoporosis. The syndromes tend to be multifactorial and result from an interaction between identifiable patient-specific impairments and situation-specific stressors" (IOM, 2008, p. 43).

evidence for frailty as a health outcome related to low social connections. In a study based on patient interviews conducted 1 week after discharge from a hospital stay, frailty was found to be a risk factor for social isolation (Andreasen et al., 2015). The co-existence of other geriatric syndromes, such as urinary and fecal incontinence, with frailty compounds the specific contribution of frailty to social isolation and loneliness.

Functional status (measured by factors such as gait speed or difficulties in the activities of daily living) is bi-directionally associated with social isolation and loneliness. Loneliness predicts long-term care admission, independent of functional status (Hanratty et al., 2018). Patients' perceived social isolation may moderate the relationship between a chronic illness, such as lower back pain, and the degree of functional impairment that they experience related to that illness (Oliveira et al., 2015). Fear of falling has been associated with the risk of falling, poorer mental health, and social isolation (Kumar et al., 2014). Older adults who restrict their activities or avoid leaving their home due to a fear of falling may increase their risk of becoming socially isolated or lonely (Finch et al., 2014; Parry et al., 2016). A recent study also found an association between frailty and social isolation and a fear of falling in older adults; however, physically frail study participants who were also socially isolated reported having fewer falls than participants who were either physically frail or isolated, but not the two combined (Hayashi et al., 2020).

Incontinence

Urinary incontinence increases the risk of social isolation because individuals tend to avoid activities with limited bathroom access or avoid social contacts altogether (Becher et al., 2013). Among the women surveyed in the National Social Life, Health, and Aging Project (Yip et al., 2013), daily urinary incontinence was associated with often feeling isolated. In one large study urinary incontinence was found also to be associated with greater loneliness, but this effect was largely explained by comorbid depression (Fultz and Herzog, 2001; Ramage-Morin and Gilmour, 2013; Stickley et al., 2017). Fecal incontinence increases the chances of nursing home referral and has effects on social isolation that are similar to those of urinary incontinence (Ditah et al., 2013). Furthermore, the social isolation of caregivers may be affected by the incontinence of their care recipients (Santini et al., 2016).

Sensory Impairment

Hearing loss contributes to both social isolation and loneliness (Davis et al., 2016; Mick et al., 2014; Ramage-Morin, 2016; Strawbridge et al., 2000; Wallhagen et al., 1996). Hearing loss has been associated with being less willing to engage in social interactions, and living in a community where access to hearing health care is limited—such as in some rural communities—can lead to greater isolation than living in an urban community where these services are more accessible (Hay-McCutcheon et al., 2018). Untreated hearing loss has been associated with greater social isolation in the adult population under 70 years of age in particular (Mick and Pichora-Fuller, 2016). Hearing loss as measured by both self-report and an objective measure has been associated with loneliness, particularly among individuals who do not use hearing aids (Mick and Pichora-Fuller, 2016; Pronk et al., 2011). Hearing loss contributes to the broader category of communication difficulty, and such difficulty often has multi-factorial causes. Communication disorders have been linked to social isolation, reduced social participation, and higher rates of loneliness (Palmer et al., 2016).

Visual impairment is associated with loneliness and may be moderated by self-efficacy, which may thus be a target for intervention (Alma et al., 2011). Self-reported visual impairment is associated with social isolation, even after adjustment for demographics, chronic illness, functional limitations, and disability, and it may be a stronger predictor of social isolation than a clinical measure of acuity (Coyle et al., 2017). Furthermore, some data suggest that the spouse of a person with visual impairments is at greater risk for social isolation (Strawbridge et al., 2007).

Dual sensory (vision and hearing) impairment has been associated with loneliness (Guthrie et al., 2018). In one study, the highest rates of loneliness—17 percent—were in the group that experienced dual sensory impairment in addition to cognitive impairment, while the group without any impairments had a 9 percent prevalence of loneliness (Guthrie et al., 2018). Both impairments are associated with worse quality of life, in part due to the mechanism of social isolation (Schneider et al., 2011; Tseng et al., 2018). Even olfactory dysfunction may be associated with loneliness (Sivam et al., 2016).

PSYCHOLOGICAL, PSYCHIATRIC, AND COGNITIVE FACTORS

Psychological symptoms, syndromes, and stressors can all influence whether an individual experiences loneliness or becomes socially isolated. Several of these factors, including anxiety and depression as well as cognitive factors such as dementia, are briefly discussed below. The impacts of social isolation and loneliness on subsequent depression and anxiety and on cognitive decline and incident dementia are summarized in Chapter 3.

Anxiety and Depression

Social isolation and loneliness are more common in older adults with depressive and anxiety disorders than in their non-depressed and non-anxious peers (Evans et al., 2018; Lim et al., 2016). Psychiatric disorders such as major depression, generalized anxiety disorder, and social anxiety disorder have been shown to increase the risk of developing loneliness during middle and late adulthood

(Domènech-Abella et al., 2019; Falk Dahl and Dahl, 2010; Lim et al., 2016; Luo et al., 2012; McHugh Power et al., 2020). Loneliness, in turn, has been linked to increasing social isolation (likely due to the negative social biases and avoidance characteristic of lonely individuals) and to higher rates of depression and anxiety over time (Cacioppo et al., 2010; Domènech-Abella et al., 2019; Luo et al., 2012).

The relationship between depression and loneliness is bi-directional, and these constructs are closely associated. Yet, depression and loneliness are not the same. Depression, particularly major depression, is a clinical syndrome characterized by persistent feelings of sadness or loss of interest and such symptoms as sleep problems, decreased appetite, loss of energy, difficulty concentrating, and suicidal thoughts. Loneliness is not a core diagnostic feature of depression but may be an associated symptom. In some older adults, depression is accompanied by broad deficits in social function and well-being, including high levels of loneliness, low social support, and fewer social connections (Barger et al., 2014; Domènech-Abella et al., 2017). In other older adults depression has been associated with high levels of loneliness that are unrelated to social network size, the level of social support, or individual factors such as personality traits and cognitive function (Domènech-Abella et al., 2017; Evans et al., 2018; Peerenboom et al., 2015). Loneliness may stem from depression-related cognitive biases in which social interactions are appraised more negatively or experienced as less rewarding (Burholt and Scharf, 2014; Lewis et al., 2017). Older adults with generalized anxiety disorder may also be vulnerable to high levels of loneliness even with levels of social contacts that are equivalent to those without anxiety (Evans et al., 2018). Personality characteristics, such as extraversion, neuroticism, and resilience, have been shown to increase the risk of loneliness as well as to moderate this risk in the setting of depression and anxiety (Peerenboom et al., 2015; Teo et al., 2013a; von Soest et al., 2020; Wagner et al., 2016).

Cognitive Function and Dementia

Social withdrawal and other changes in social function are recognized features of dementia in neurodegenerative disorders such as Alzheimer's disease, frontotemporal dementia, Parkinson's disease, and Lewy body dementia (McKhann et al., 2011). These changes can also arise in pre-dementia stages of impairment when neurocognitive deficits are less severe or not yet apparent (d'Oleire Uquillas et al., 2018; Donovan et al., 2016; Ismail et al., 2016).

Primary deficits in the core cognitive domains such as memory, reasoning, or language skills may degrade social function. With increasing cognitive impairment, individuals often disengage from community groups and reduce their social ties as they are experiencing parallel functional losses in other aspects of daily living (Morris, 1993). This global process culminates in severe deficits in comprehension, communication, and interpersonal function in late dementia (Reisberg et al., 1982).

Neurodegenerative disorders may also give rise to specific impairments in such social processes as interpreting information from faces (social perception), recognizing the thoughts and feelings of others (theory of mind), displaying empathy and regulating emotions (emotional processing), and behaving within social norms (Desmarais et al., 2018).

Altered neuropsychiatric function may also impair social functioning in individuals who are affected by neurodegenerative disorders. For example, social withdrawal may be part of a broader apathy syndrome, a neuropsychiatric state that is common across dementia types (Lanctôt et al., 2017). Misperceptions or overestimations of social threat may predispose a person with dementia to agitation and aggression (Rosenberg et al., 2015). Anxiety or depressive symptoms may underlie or contribute to social avoidance or withdrawal (Geda et al., 2013).

A small number of studies have examined the experience of loneliness in persons with dementia. A single population-based study of 589 Swedish old adults with a mean age of 84 years found that loneliness was more prevalent in those with dementia (33 percent) than in those without dementia (22 percent) (Holmén et al., 2000). Dementia caregivers, particularly spouses, are also at risk for greater loneliness and depression both during the course of disease and after the caregiving ends (Adams, 2008; Eloniemi-Sulkava et al., 2002). In semi-structured interviews of 70 persons with early-stage dementia and their caregivers, the study participants with dementia spoke of experiencing relationship loss and of the importance of having meaningful relationships and people to converse with (Moyle et al., 2011). The loss of memory function was acknowledged as a barrier to social relationships, whereas an involvement in arts, crafts, and music was identified as a way of reducing feelings of loneliness (Moyle et al., 2011). Caregivers tended to perceive loneliness from observed emotions and behaviors even if loneliness was not explicitly expressed by the person with dementia (Moyle et al., 2011).

Other research in dementia care has led to the concept of "unmet needs" among persons with dementia who are unable to communicate or fulfill their own basic needs (Black et al., 2013; Cohen-Mansfield, 2001). This work has provided insights into the importance of social relationships to persons with dementia, even in late stages. In a review of studies of persons with dementia living in nursing homes, those interviewed identified meaningful relationships and support for grief and loss as two of their eight main concerns (Shiells et al., 2019). The residents with advanced dementia in particular expressed having a fear of loneliness. Many of these participants wrongly believed that family had not visited them even when they had (Cahill and Diaz-Ponce, 2011). In a separate study, 70 percent of nursing home residents with dementia reported feelings of loneliness (Cohen-Mansfield et al., 2015).

Studies of agitated behaviors in nursing home settings have found that verbal agitation (e.g., constant requests for attention, complaining, screaming) was more common in nursing home residents who were cognitively impaired (Cohen-Mansfield and Libin, 2005) and in those who were lonely (Cohen-Mansfield et al., 2015). An understanding of behavioral symptoms as a form of distress related to unmet needs has led to the development of interventions to reduce loneliness and behavioral symptoms in nursing home residents. In a study of 30 nursing home residents with dementia, both simulated family presence and a music intervention reduced verbal agitation more than usual care (Garland et al., 2007). In a loneliness-focused study of 38 nursing home residents with and without cognitive impairment, individuals who received animal-assisted therapy with either robotic or living dogs, but not those in the control group, reported reduced loneliness ratings (Banks et al., 2008). (See Chapter 8 for more on interventions.)

Loneliness and social isolation are not currently assessed in standard dementia care (Johnston et al., 2011; Sanders et al., 2017), and the established instruments for measuring these constructs have not been validated in persons with dementia. At the same time, there is an emerging interest in understanding how to measure engagement and provide effective opportunities for meaningful activity and engagement in persons with dementia, including those with advanced disease (Cohen-Mansfield et al., 2017).

SOCIAL AND CULTURAL FACTORS

This section explores the societal and cultural factors that can affect how people interact with their environments and whether they experience social isolation or loneliness. Such factors include social support characteristics (including marital status and the quality of relationships with family and friends or pets) and the occurrence of disruptive life events (including bereavement, illness, and retirement).

Social Support Characteristics

Various characteristics of a society, including customs, lifestyles, and values, can affect an individual's everyday interactions—with family members, friends, or complete strangers—and influence how people live their lives and perceive their places in society. This interplay between individuals and their social and cultural milieus has given rise to a wide array of inter-related research areas. The potential impacts of social support networks as well as the influence of different relationships—with spouses and family members, friends and neighbors, or caregivers—are discussed below.

Impact of Social Support Networks

Individuals' social support networks directly affect how they interact with and perceive their environments. The individuals who make up a person's network (e.g., family members, friends, caretakers, spouse, and neighbors) can play important roles in the person's life and lessen his or her chances of experiencing social isolation or loneliness. Having an extensive social network is not required in order to achieve a rewarding social network, but rather the rewards of a social network are greatest when the relationships that do exist are of high quality (Chatters et al., 2018; Cohen-Mansfield et al., 2016; Lauder et al., 2006; Pinquart and Sörensen, 2001; Stokes, 1985). Supportive relationships can decrease self-reported loneliness, while difficult or unfulfilling relationships can increase feelings of loneliness (Cohen-Mansfield et al., 2016; Shiovitz-Ezra and Leitsch, 2010). Lonely older adults (mean participant age = 68.5) reported less frequent sexual activity and reduced feelings of intimacy, although not less frequent sexual thoughts, in a study using items from the UCLA Loneliness Scale; however, the directionality of this association was not determined (Kolodziejczak et al., 2019). Relationships with one's family or spouse have been shown to be beneficial for some facets of health, while relationships with friends, neighbors, community members, and others can help prevent poor mental health and psychological distress (Christakis and Allison, 2006; Fiori et al., 2006; Haslam et al., 2014; Kiecolt-Glaser and Newton, 2001). The totality of these relationships—voluntary and otherwise—can help lead an individual live a life with a sense of meaning, value, and interconnection (Berkman and Glass, 2000).

Family and Marriage

Family can be an important source of social support for older adults, providing social and emotional connection as well as contributing to an individual's financial and physical well-being (Verdery and Margolis, 2017). Individuals who lack family are more apt to be socially isolated and to experience higher rates of loneliness (Verdery and Margolis, 2017).

Marriage can also protect against loneliness and conditions such as poor cognitive function, stress, and dementia; however, the benefits gained from a spousal relationship are proportional to the overall quality of that relationship, including whether a spouse is considered a trusted confidant (Gow et al., 2007; Håkansson et al., 2009; Hawkley and Kocherginsky, 2018; Hawkley et al., 2008; Nicolaisen and Thorsen, 2017; Qualter et al., 2015; Stack, 1998; Victor and Bowling, 2012; Xu et al., 2016). The close, long-term nature of the spousal relationship tends to make an individual's partner the most likely person to provide support if and when assistance is needed (Ha et al., 2019). However, the spousal relationship can be either beneficial or detrimental, as loneliness has been found to be inversely associated with spousal support (Hawkley and Kocherginsky, 2018). In particular, remaining in an unhappy relationship can negatively affect an individual's health and well-being and can be the source of ongoing emotional distress (Evans et al., 2019; Xu et al., 2016). Furthermore, negative spousal behaviors are associated with poorer physical health, and the adverse effects of marital strain are greater at older ages (Bookwala, 2005; Robles and Kiecolt-Glaser, 2003; Umberson et al., 2006).

Relationships with other family members can also affect an individual's likelihood of being lonely, as close family bonds are often the source of social, economic, physical, and other forms of support (Berkman et al., 2000; Redfoot et al., 2013; Verdery and Margolis, 2017). As with other social relationships, the amount of support realized from close familial ties varies depending on the geographical distance between family members, the amount of interpersonal contact (in person or through other means), and each person's willingness to be emotionally and personally invested in maintaining mutually beneficial relationships (Quirke et al., 2019; Verdery and Margolis, 2017). Among older African Americans, family relationships often take precedence over relationships with friends, and social networks tend to be primarily made up of family members (Chatters et al., 2018; Cornwell et al., 2008; Griffin et al., 2006; Taylor et al., 2013). Some families choose to create intergenerational co-residences or live in very close proximity; however, these familial living arrangements are not as prevalent in the United States as in other parts of the world, and their impact on social isolation or loneliness in older adults is mixed (Caputo, 2019; Takagi and Saito, 2019; Teerawichitchainan et al., 2015; Tian, 2016).

Grown children can also provide a measure of support to parents, although their existence or presence is not a panacea for social isolation or loneliness (Cohen-Mansfield et al., 2016; Nicolaisen and Thorsen, 2017). Parent–child relationships are subject to the same limitations described above for social relationships, and therefore these relationships can range in their quality and level of support. Virtual interactions with children and grandchildren are becoming more common, but the success of these interactions is dependent on the computer literacy of the participant (regardless of age), the comfort level with this form of communication, and the availability of and accessibility to computers with reliable Internet access (Cohen-Mansfield et al., 2016). (See Chapter 8 for more on the use of technology.) Increasingly, couples—both unmarried and married—are not having children; in 2018 the number of births in the United States reached its lowest level in 32 years (Hamilton et al., 2019; Verdery and Margolis, 2017). The effect of these demographic dynamics on the rates of social isolation and loneliness among future generations of older adults is unknown.

Single Adults

Single adults—unmarried, widowed, or divorced—may experience social isolation or loneliness differently than adults with partners. While single adults are not destined to be lonely, feelings of loneliness can be more prevalent in this population because of such factors as the lack of a trusted confidant or the lack or loss of a partner (Paúl and Ribeiro, 2009; Theeke, 2009, 2010; Verdery and Margolis, 2017). For others, remaining single is a conscious choice, and many older couples opt to forego marriage and choose cohabitation without marriage (Brown et al., 2012; Copen et al., 2012; de Jong Gierveld, 2004; Verdery and Margolis, 2017). Rates of divorce are also increasing in adults over 50 years of age, with divorce rates highest among individuals who have been married two or more times, among those with less education and a lower income, and among African Americans (Brown and Lin, 2012).

Regardless of the circumstances, single adults are more apt to live alone, which can tend to make them more lonely and isolated than people who cohabitate (Evans et al., 2019; Finlay and Kobayashi, 2018; Perissinotto and Covinsky, 2014). For lesbian, gay, or bisexual individuals, living alone may be a symptom of larger discriminatory practices or societal stigma (Fredriksen-Goldsen et al., 2013; Kim and Fredriksen-Goldsen, 2016). Some older adults who live alone may go for days without seeing or talking with another person (Finlay and Kobayashi, 2018). Living alone should not necessarily be equated with being sequestered from society, however, as many people who live alone still enjoy active social lives and are no more lonely or isolated from friends than those who live with others (Evans et al., 2019). For some, periods of solitude represent opportunities to reenergize, relax, or engage in other pursuits. The disparate reactions to solitude may be explained by differing reasons for being alone; that is, some individuals may choose to be alone, while others may lack opportunities to interact with others.

Friends and Neighbors

Unlike the case with their family members, individuals have choices concerning whom they become friends with, and these non-familial relationships have the potential to affect social isolation or loneliness. Generally, friendships are based on individuals having similar interests, activities, hobbies, experiences, or beliefs and are likely to occur among people in the same peer group (Chatters et al., 2018; Ha et al., 2019). Feelings of loneliness can be minimized by having friends who can be relied on (Henning-Smith et al., 2019). Though some friendships are situational or fleeting, friendships that last into older ages tend to be characterized by relationships between individuals who share similar experiences and backgrounds. These long-term friendships tend to be superior in quality and richness than friendships that have not stood the test of time (Nicolaisen and Thorsen, 2017; Pinquart and Sörensen, 2000). On the extreme end of the friendship continuum are older patients who have been identified as "unbefriended." This term is used to describe individuals who, for example, are incapacitated and unable to make medical decisions for themselves; lack an advanced directive; and lack friends, family, or an authorized surrogate to assist in making medical decisions (Farrell et al., 2017).

Proximity to other individuals can influence whether friendships develop. Neighbors can often provide a measure of support when family members or close friends are not geographically close, but engagement with neighbors tends to be more limited in commitment and scope (Ha et al., 2018; Messeri et al., 1993; Nocon and Pearson, 2000). Communicating with neighbors or others via the telephone can also have an impact on one's sense of social isolation or loneliness. Loneliness was found to be increased in individuals who had fewer daily phone calls; this was most evident for people who received fewer incoming calls (Petersen et al., 2016). Whether one lives in a rural or an urban area can also influence the likelihood and quality of friendships. (See discussions on rural versus urban living later in this chapter.)

Caregivers

With the rapid aging of the population, the number of older adults who need care continues to grow rapidly (NASEM, 2016b). In the 2-year period of 2015–2016, more than 41 million people provided unpaid elder care for adults 65 years of age and older (BLS, 2017). Typical services provided by family and friends range from routine household activities (e.g., housework, food preparation, transportation) to providing direct physical or medical care (e.g., providing exercise, bathing, or toileting assistance or dispensing medication) (BLS, 2017). Most often a spouse, partner, or adult child will fulfill this family caregiver role, but caregiving responsibilities can also be undertaken by other family members (e.g., siblings or elderly parents), friends, neighbors, or volunteers, and they can be provided in private homes, assisted care, or retirement facilities (BLS, 2017; Li and Loke, 2013).

Increasingly, medical care for older adults is taking place in private homes, often for long periods of time. As a result, home care that involves complex and diverse care needs is more often falling on family caregivers with or without assistance from a member of the formal health care workforce (Li and Loke, 2013; Ris et al., 2019). Having care provided in the home can help older adults and their caregivers maintain relationships with family, friends, and others in the community; however, social isolation and loneliness are often byproducts of this arrangement (Evans et al., 2019; Wiles et al., 2012). The quality of the relationship between the patient and an informal family caregiver is an important factor in determining the effectiveness of these arrangements. For example, better relationship quality between patients and their informal family caregivers has been linked to a reduced risk for patient mortality (Hooker et al., 2015). But older adults and their caregivers often must navigate new or different interpersonal roles, responsibilities, or routines and deal with stressful, emotional, and sometimes life-altering changes. These difficult situations can impede communication between older adults and their caregivers or visitors, creating feelings of social isolation or loneliness. This can be especially true if friends' visits taper off over time (Northcott et al., 2016).

In addition to the day-to-day interpersonal challenges faced by family caregivers and older adults, families can also experience negative psychological, financial, and social effects; these effects can be especially acute for female spouses, as they generally bear the largest burden of care (Li and Loke, 2013; Riffin et al., 2019; Zivin and Christakis, 2007). Caregivers commonly suffer from physical issues such as illness, loss of appetite or sleep, or exhaustion as well as mental health issues, trouble maintaining relationships with friends, or difficulty participating in community or social activities (Blum and Sherman, 2010; Dhruva et al., 2012; Haines et al., 2018; Li and Loke, 2013). These difficulties can be compounded by such factors as immigration status, language and cultural barriers, stigma or discrimination issues related to an older adult's sexual orientation, or the specific needs of patients (Kim and Fredriksen-Goldsen, 2016; Kim, H. J., et al., 2016; Moukouta et al., 2017; Shiu et al., 2016). It can be particularly challenging to care for older adults with mobility issues or those who suffer from dementia or other mental illnesses (Riffin et al., 2019).

Human–Animal Interactions

Interacting with an animal or a pet has long been thought to have health-related benefits, but research into the benefits of these human–animal interactions, including their effects on loneliness or social isolation, has had mixed results (Gilbey and Tani, 2015; Krause-Parello and Gulick, 2013; Needell and Mehta-Naik, 2016; Stanley et al., 2014). Needell and Mehta-Naik (2016) examined the impact of pet ownership on the risk and severity of geriatric depression and concluded that "loneliness and social isolation seemed to be ameliorated by pet ownership" (p. 5). Conversely, a review carried out at about the same time that looked at the association between companion animal interactions and loneliness found "no convincing evidence that companion animals can help to alleviate loneliness" (Gilbey and Tani, 2015, p. 195). The studies agree in their observations that research is sparse and insufficient in this area and that many of the available studies are underpowered or inadequately designed.

Other aspects of human–animal relationships may be related to subsequent social isolation or loneliness in older adults. Interactions with animals can promote social interactions and participation; can add structure, routine, meaning, or purpose to an individual's day; can increase exercise and physical activity opportunities; and can provide emotional support (Brooks et al., 2018; Friedmann and Krause-Parello, 2018; Gee and Mueller, 2019; Hui Gan et al., 2019; Mueller et al., 2018). Dogs may serve as a stimulus for social interactions and engagement because daily walks with pets have been found to increase the likelihood of engaging with others and increasing one's sense of community (McNicholas and Collis, 2000; Toohey et al., 2013). A study by Muraco et al. (2018) found that interacting with a companion animal was also associated with increased perceived social support, emotional support, and companionship among older pet owners (older than 65 years of age) in the lesbian, gay, bisexual, and transgender community, especially among individuals who were disabled or who lacked social networks. On the other hand, the emotional difficulties that pet owners may experience when a pet is ill or dies can rival the effects of caring for a sick family member or coping with the trauma of the death of a close relative (Friedmann and Krause-Parello, 2018; Muraco et al., 2018).

Disruptive Life Events

At any age people can experience disruptive life events that alter their interpersonal relations and how they perceive their lives or their feelings of isolation and loneliness. While older adults are not unique in having these life-altering experiences, some disruptive events are more likely to occur, or to occur at a greater frequency, for people over the age of 50. Such disruptive life events include bereavement, illness or poor health, and retirement. Although research on these topics is sparse, it provides insight into how these experiences can disrupt people's lives and how they could lead to social isolation or feelings of loneliness.

Bereavement

The loss of a loved one—be it a child, sibling, spouse, partner, or friend—can result in a critical loss of emotional intimacy and everyday support. Bereavement leads to feelings of sadness and loneliness in grieving relatives and friends, and in some cases these feelings can lead to individuals becoming socially withdrawn, isolated, or depressed and can also affect an older adult's risk for premature mortality (Fried et al., 2015; Holm et al., 2019; Robinaugh et al., 2014; Roelfs et al., 2012). The extent of symptoms associated with grieving can vary depending on the cause of death, when it occurred, the context in which the death occurred, and whether the grieving party believes the deceased individual may have hastened his or her death through habits or lifestyle (Carr, 2009; Fried et al., 2015). Family caregivers may have an especially difficult time after the passing of a loved one under their care because the death may result in the loss of a companion or friend as well as the loss of the personal pride, purpose, or satisfaction they derived from providing care (Holtslander et al., 2017). The loss may be particularly acute when caregivers' responsibilities have compromised their regular social network while they were providing care, thus leaving them with diminished social support or feelings of isolation after the loved one's death (Holtslander et al., 2017).

The death of a spouse typically increases feelings of loneliness in the surviving spouse, and these feelings can act as a gateway to subsequent depressive symptoms (Fried et al., 2015). Many widowed individuals report that loneliness is something they cope with on a daily basis (Fried et al., 2015). Data from more than 500 million persons examining spousal bereavement, which increases the risk of social isolation and loneliness, revealed that, after adjusting for age, widowers had a 23 percent increased risk of death in any given year compared with married people (Roelfs et al., 2012). (See Chapter 2 for additional information on mortality risk.) In another study, late-life bereavement was found to be associated with decreased mortality in widows who had cardiovascular disease and with increased mortality in widowers who did not have cardiovascular disease (Stahl et al., 2016). The authors suggested that the decreased mortality in widows could be due to a decrease in stress or in exposure to suffering or to an increase in self-care after the death of the spouse. Over the long term, however, having been widowed is an enduring risk factor for loneliness in late life, regardless of subsequent marital status (von Soest et al., 2020). Men have a higher likelihood of adjusting poorly to widowhood than women and also have greater feelings of loneliness (Carr et al., 2018). Male veterans may be the exception to this, however; research indicates that some veterans who were exposed to death while serving in the military may experience less loneliness than civilian widowers (Carr et al., 2018). Social support provided by family or friends has been shown to be more helpful for grieving spouses than support from other sources; support from family and friends can help restore function and a sense of cohesion (Chow et al., 2018; Merz and de Jong Gierveld, 2016; Utz et al., 2014). Support is most helpful when it is readily available and when the surviving partner has the opportunity to freely express himself or herself (Merz and de Jong Gierveld, 2016; Utz et al., 2014). Psychological resilience (e.g., emotional stability, extraversion, and conscientiousness) is associated with a more favorable resolution of loneliness in bereaved older adults (Spahni et al., 2015). Addressing the risk factors for loneliness in bereaved individuals may be an important way to reduce the risk of psychiatric morbidity and help shorten the bereavement period and alleviate suffering (Chow et al., 2018; Robinaugh et al., 2014).

Illness and Poor Health

Poor health in older adults has been associated with increased loneliness, and chronically ill individuals are especially vulnerable to becoming socially isolated (Goll et al., 2015; Holley, 2007; Merz and de Jong Gierveld, 2016). Chronic illness is associated with emotional or psychological issues, mobility limitations, a lack of or limitation in transportation or employment options, new or ongoing issues related to coping with disabling conditions, and strained social relationships (Holley, 2007; Warner et al., 2017). In some cases, chronic illness may increase individuals' social support networks and decrease their likelihood of being socially isolated because addressing health issues may increase social interactions in the form of medical or therapy appointments and other health-related activities (Finlay and Kobayashi, 2018).

Functional Impairment or Disability

Individuals with functional impairment or a disability—including physical, mental, intellectual, sensory, or other—face many unique challenges that leave them especially susceptible to being socially isolated or lonely (von Soest et al., 2020).

The degree to which individuals' disability affects how they live their life, and the magnitude to which they are dependent on others for some or all of their needs, have both been found to be correlated with their likelihood of experiencing increased feelings of loneliness or vulnerability (Lykke and Handberg, 2019). Impacts on life satisfaction for those with disabilities or functional impairments have been shown to fluctuate depending on age, gender, residency (rural versus urban), and degree of extraversion (Hudson and Doogan, 2019; Puvill et al., 2019; Repke and Ipsen, 2020; von Soest et al., 2020). The existing social networks of people with functional impairment can impact whether people experience loneliness and to what extent. Unmarried individuals with functional limitations experience higher loneliness than happily married individuals with comparable limitations (Warner et al., 2019). Women with functional limitations have been found to experience greater loneliness if they have strained marital relationships while men may experience increased loneliness if they have overly supportive relationships, and people who lacked contact with friends all experienced greater loneliness (von Soest et al., 2020; Warner et al., 2019).

In general, individuals with greater mobility impairments or functional limitations tend to have fewer friends (Chatters et al., 2018; Ha et al., 2019). Additionally, certain life events (e.g., retirement, illness, death of loved ones or friends) can lead to a marked decrease in an individual's social network; this decrease in friends and in friendships, especially among the oldest older adults, can lead to feelings of loneliness or to becoming isolated (Nicolaisen and Thorsen, 2017). In many cases it is not uncommon for individuals with functional limitations or disabilities to avoid openly expressing feeling of loneliness to others (Wormald et al., 2019).

Employment and Retirement

There is evidence that the relationship between loneliness and occupational function is bi-directional. Loneliness has been shown to be predictive of future work disabilities that occur when mental or physical impairments bring about functional limitations that make it impossible for an individual to perform the duties necessary to maintain paid employment (Morris, 2019). Being lonely can also result in depression, which can then lead to functional limitations and subsequent work disability. Along this pathway, depression can act as a partial mediator between loneliness and work disability.

Retirement can also affect an individual's likelihood of being socially isolated or lonely. The number of post-retirement individuals in the United States is rising quickly, and retired individuals are living longer (Boyle, 2019; Pew Research Center, 2019a). Baby boomers (i.e., those born between 1946 and 1964) make up of 26 percent of the U.S. population, and their exit from the workforce (due to retirement) will dramatically change their lives (Boyle, 2019; Pew Research Center, 2019a). Each day between 2011 and 2030 an estimated

10,000 baby boomers will reach the age of 65, an age when many people are on the cusp of retiring or have already exited the workforce (Pew Research Center, 2019a). Ideally, most of these workers will decide when and under what conditions they will retire, but unplanned exits due to unexpected health problems (either an individual's own health problems or those of a loved one) or employment changes (e.g., downsizing, redundancy, payouts for early retirement) are becoming more frequent (Boyle, 2019; Donaldson et al., 2010; Edge et al., 2017). Whether the decisions to retire is planned or unplanned and whether the retiree believes he or she has a choice in the decision can affect how smoothly the transition between being a paid employee and a retiree progresses (Donaldson et al., 2010; Quine et al., 2007).

Being employed can be protective against loneliness as it provides a convenient social environment for workers (Segel-Karpas et al., 2018). The disruption of these daily social interactions and structured routines upon retirement can lead to subsequent socialization difficulties (Morris, 2019). Workers who are lonely are at an increased risk of having difficulty transitioning to retirement and can experience a worsening of depressive symptoms because they often lack an established social network outside of the workplace (Gum et al., 2017; Segel-Karpas et al., 2018). Some retirees feel a loss of identity without their former job title and responsibilities, and some miss the challenges, demands, or appreciation they received at work (Schaap et al., 2018). For others, retiring can mean more time with family and friends and more enriching social interactions (Schaap et al., 2018). Thus, depending on the individual, retirement can favorably or unfavorably influence social connection and feelings of loneliness.

Factors related to a successful retirement include having good physical and mental health, financial stability, good social integration, the option of retiring by choice, and knowing how to enjoy leisure time (Barbosa et al., 2016; Donaldson et al., 2010; Schaap et al., 2018). In general, most retired people are less lonely than employed workers or people who are simply unemployed, and women typically have an easier time transitioning into retirement than men (Lauder et al., 2006; Perren et al., 2003). Roughly 26 percent of people who retire from their careers end up embarking on second careers, which can be similar to their previous jobs but more likely will involve some type of volunteerism (Boyle, 2019; Cook, 2015). These bridge jobs and volunteer positions help to ease the transition into retired living by allowing people to find new meaning in their post-career lives and can help retirees remain active, fulfilled, engaged, and connected within their communities (Boyle, 2019; Cook, 2015).

Religious and Spiritual Organizations

Many people feel that being part of a religious organization is central to their identity, and such affiliations can also be foundational to a person's social networks. Challenges related to the previously described disruptive life events may lead some older adults to seek supportive social connections through associations with religious organizations (Idler et al., 2003; Levin and Chatters, 1998; Rote et al., 2013). Active involvement in a religious organization can be a source of social support, and this affiliation may help ease an individual's feelings of loneliness or social isolation and, some argue, even make people happier (Gonzales et al., 2015; Rizvi and Hossain, 2017; Rokach, 1996; Strawbridge et al., 2001). The intensity of one's faith may also influence an individual's feeling of loneliness, as individuals who hold stronger religious beliefs may feel less lonely than those who do not hold such strong beliefs (Lauder et al., 2006). Higher levels of social support and social integration have been associated with religious attendance and also with lower levels of loneliness (Rote et al., 2013). Older women are much more likely to be widowed than older men, and religious organizations may help to meet many of their social needs and help them cope with illness (Idler et al., 2017; Strawbridge et al., 2001). Additionally, several studies have found that women are more likely to be active members and experience greater overall benefits from participation in religious organizations, to have stronger social support and social networks, and to generally be less lonely than men (Gray, 2009; Idler et al., 2017; Kirkpatrick et al., 1999; Lauder et al., 2006; Strawbridge et al., 2001). One study did, however, find that men have stronger social networks—defined as the number of close friends and the frequency of interactions with those friends than women (Gallicchio et al., 2007).

SOCIAL ENVIRONMENTAL FACTORS

The interactions between individuals and the environments in which they live, work, and play can profoundly influence their propensities for becoming socially isolated or lonely. This section reviews the relationships of several environmental factors, including transportation and housing situation, with social isolation and loneliness.

Transportation

In 2017 nearly 37 percent of the more than 225 million licensed drivers in the United States were 50 years of age or older (FHWA, 2017). Driving is important for adults who want to maintain independence and mobility; however, declines in physical health or cognitive function or deficits in reaction time or coordination can lead older adults to stop driving (Chihuri et al., 2016; Hwang and Hong, 2018; Johnson, 1999, 2008). Additional reasons for driving cessation include an increased insecurity in driving skills or ability; having had previous car accidents or traffic citations; the high cost of driving; being compelled to comply with requests by family members, friends, or a medical professional; or forfeiting driving privileges in compliance with state driving licensure laws (Johnson, 1999; Ratnapradipa et al., 2018). Driving cessation has been associated with a decrease in social engagement and an increase in social isolation and feelings of loneliness (Barrett and Gumber, 2019; Chihuri et al., 2016; Edwards et al., 2009; Johnson, 1999, 2008). Driving cessation is especially difficult for older adults who live in areas that lack alternative transportation options, such as rural or lower-density neighborhoods (Finlay and Kobayashi, 2018; Herbert and Molinsky, 2019). Without reliable and affordable alternatives to driving, some former drivers may resume their driving despite their initial reasons for stopping (Johnson, 2008).

Impact of Housing or Geographic Location

Different living environments can shape older adults' interactions with their social networks and with their community at large. Whether one's home is a private residence, an apartment, or a room in a retirement community or nursing home, this space—and a person's acceptance of this space—can affect that person's physical, psychological, mental, and financial well-being as well as how attached he or she is to the community (Bekhet et al., 2009; Kemperman et al., 2019). A particular housing situation may represent a risk factor or protective factor for social isolation and loneliness, depending on the specific details and the characteristics of the individual.

Regardless of where or in what type of housing a person lives, the degree of social isolation or loneliness an individual experiences can be affected by whether he or she feels safe in his or her community. Prior direct or indirect exposure to community violence can lead to increased loneliness or a reduction in perceived social support from friends, thus increasing socially isolation (Tung et al., 2019). Even when older adults are motivated to be more socially engaged, living in a high-crime neighborhood can make people reluctant or afraid to leave their residence or engage with others (Portacolone et al., 2018). These concerns can be exacerbated by personal vulnerabilities (such as having chronic health issues or disabilities, limited social ties, or experiencing poverty), derelict or dangerous environmental conditions in the neighborhood, or a lack of opportunity or interest in engaging with other community members (Portacolone, 2018; Portacolone et al., 2018). Furthermore, the rapidly changing demographic trend continues to influence the need for additional, adequate, and appropriate housing for older adults (Herbert and Molinsky, 2019). Though the available research on issues related to housing type or location is sparse and can be somewhat inconsistent, it provides insight into possible links between a person's living arrangement and social isolation or loneliness.

Aging in Place

In 2018 more than 32.9 million households were headed by adults aged 65 and older, and that number is projected to increase by 11.1 million households between 2018 and 2028 (JCHS, 2018; U.S. Census Bureau, 2018). Finding affordable, accessible, and safe housing for older adults will become increasingly challenging (Wick, 2017). Many older adults are choosing to stay in their privately owned houses for personal, practical, and financial reasons, a situation known as *aging in place* (Benefield and Holtzclaw, 2014; Granbom et al., 2014; Herbert and Molinsky, 2019; Pearson et al., 2019; Wick, 2017). Years of shared history and memories become associated with one's home, and leaving can be untenable for some (Granbom et al., 2014). In addition, the desire to remain independent and enmeshed in established social networks close to home can be a compelling reason to stay (Benefield and Holtzclaw, 2014; Herbert and Molinsky, 2019). It should be noted, however, that all housing choices, especially for those with disabilities or special needs, are constrained by financial and other limitations, and staying in one's home is not always a tenable option. Often, accessible housing options are not readily available (Greiman and Ravesloot, 2015).

Aging in place may be both a risk and a protective factor for social isolation and loneliness. While a private home can provide comfort and security, it can also become a hazard if occupants are faced with changes in functional abilities (e.g., trouble walking or navigating stairs) (Herbert and Molinsky, 2019). Aging in place can be isolating if social networks or opportunities for affordable and convenient transportation are not readily available, especially for people who cannot afford sociable leisure activities outside the home (Finlay and Kobayashi, 2018; Herbert and Molinsky, 2019). Changes in physical health can often be accommodated with home modifications (e.g., adding accessible bathrooms or installing ramps) and with increased in-home support services, which provide needed assistance and connection with others, although the expense associated with these accommodations may, in many cases, be cost prohibitive and untenable without outside support (Herbert and Molinsky, 2019; Lane et al., 2019). Assistance from a nurse or supportive caregivers can help aging adults remain in their homes, and the companionship they provide can help alleviate the likelihood of loneliness or isolation for homebound patients (Benefield and Holtzclaw, 2014; Herbert and Molinsky, 2019; Szanton et al., 2019; Taylor et al., 2019). For successful aging in place to occur, a coordinated plan is needed that addresses issues related to health care, housing, financial concerns, social needs, and the use of resources, including technology (Benefield and Holtzclaw, 2014). Older adults who live alone without such support systems in place are more likely to report symptoms related to loneliness and depression (Herbert and Molinsky, 2019).

Co-Housing or Living Groups

A more recent approach to housing may provide some protection against social isolation and loneliness. Resistance to traditional long-term care options and reductions in government resources have led to the development of new and innovative housing options for older adults (Glass and Skinner, 2013; Glass and

Vander Plaats, 2013; Herbert and Molinsky, 2019). Older adults in the United States are increasingly choosing to live in supportive co-housing communities, which can increase these adults' social connections (Glass and Vander Plaats, 2013; Graham et al., 2014; Lubik and Kosatsky, 2019; Wick, 2017). Resident-managed co-housing communities are often intergenerational and feature private units built around a common green space. Inclusion and participation are valued and encouraged as cohabitants share common meals and activities and help with day-to-day operational matters (Glass and Vander Plaats, 2013). Such living arrangements increase the likelihood of socialization opportunities, which can lead to an open exchange of information and ideas, emotional and mutual support, and shared communal coping, and can help alleviate social isolation and loneliness (Glass and Vander Plaats, 2013).

Federally Subsidized Housing and Senior Housing

Subsidized housing and senior housing are options for older adults who may not be able to afford alternative living arrangements. This lower-cost rental option aims to provide general support, assistance for people with disabilities, opportunities for social connections, and security (Taylor et al., 2018b). Compared with community-dwelling non-renters, older adults living in subsidized housing tend to live alone, have lower fixed incomes (averaging about $10,000 per year), have greater functional limitations or disabilities, have more psychiatric conditions, and have more chronic comorbid conditions (Gonyea et al., 2018; Henning-Smith et al., 2019; Parsons et al., 2011; Redfoot and Kochera, 2005; Taylor et al., 2018b). Although subsidized housing communities, senior housing, and retirement communities all offer similar socialization opportunities (e.g., interactions with peers, planned activities, and meeting spaces), studies suggest that loneliness is pervasive among residents living in subsidized and senior housing communities. An estimated 30–70 percent of residents in subsidized housing classify themselves as having high rates of loneliness, compared with only 19–29 percent among older adults living in homes or unsubsidized apartments (Gonyea et al., 2018; Taylor et al., 2018b). The combination of poor health and difficult financial circumstances may be at the root of the loneliness, but other situations that plague some subsidized housing communities (e.g., crime, alcohol and tobacco use, the use of abusive language) may also lead to social withdrawal (Finlay and Kobayashi, 2018; Gonyea et al., 2018; Kemperman et al., 2019). Subsidized housing residents may also experience depression or negative psychological outcomes stemming from the long-term effects of racial discrimination or living lives marked by disadvantage (Gonyea et al., 2018; Park et al., 2018). Other housing options for low-income or homeless individuals (e.g., permanent supportive housing for chronically homeless individuals) are an option for some older adults, but information regarding their impact on social isolation or loneliness is lacking (Henwood et al., 2019).

Retirement Communities

Many older adults transition from private homes to retirement communities, which offer amenities such as social activities, health-related supervision, and 24-hour supervision (Bekhet et al., 2009). The ease and success of an individual's move into such a community has much to do with the person's motivation for moving. For example, such things as the failing health of an individual or the individual's spouse or partner, a need to minimize responsibility, or social isolation and loneliness all can encourage older adults to relocate to a retirement community (Stimson and McCrea, 2004). Alternatively, older adults may move to be with friends, relocate to a specific locale or community, live closer or have more access to medical facilities, feel safer, or live more affordably (Bekhet et al., 2009; Crisp et al., 2013; Stimson and McCrea, 2004). Voluntary moves, when individuals feel they have options and can make their own decisions and maintain autonomy, are more likely to have a positive outcome than non-voluntary moves (Bekhet et al., 2009). Increasingly, retirement communities offer options that allow residents to transition from independent living arrangements to assisted living if needed (Jeste et al., 2019). Yet, these moves are limited to those older adults who have the financial resources to "buy in" to such communities.

Long-Term Care Service Options: Residential Care and Nursing Homes

Locations that offer long-term care services such as adult day care, nursing homes, and residential care provide older adults with a range of health care, personal care, and supportive services. In 2016 long-term care service providers served more than 8.3 million people in the United States, including 1,347,600 in nursing homes and 811,500 in residential care facilities (Harris-Kojetin et al., 2019).

Long-term care providers offer older adults aid with physical functioning and general quality-of-life tasks by providing a wide range of services such as assistance with daily activities, medication management, and health maintenance tasks (Harris-Kojetin et al., 2019; Rijnaard et al., 2016). Many of these organizations aim to provide home-like accommodations by focusing on psychological and social factors (e.g., autonomy and relationships with family, friends, and pets) and the built environment (e.g., comfortable private spaces, helpful technology, personal belongings) (Rijnaard et al., 2016). In some cases, providing person-centered care that includes fulfilling personal preferences related to care and recreation may be helpful in alleviating loneliness in long-term care residents (Andrew and Meeks, 2018). Nevertheless, long-term care can increase social isolation and loneliness for older adults living in such residencies, a portion of whom may be living far from friends and loved ones. Long-term care residents often may not be able to engage in meaningful social interactions and, in some cases, may share a room with people with whom they are not compatible (Trybusińska and Saracen, 2019).

Rural Versus Urban Environments

Compared with adults who live in urban settings, adults who live in rural environments are more apt to face challenges related to the long distances between homes and businesses or medical facilities, limited public transportation options, unreliable or non-existent access to broadband Internet, and access to fewer health care providers (Douthit et al., 2015; Henning-Smith et al., 2019). Research on the relationship of social isolation and loneliness with living in rural versus urban areas has had mixed results. Henning-Smith and colleagues (2019) found that individuals who lived in areas with fewer than 10,000 people reported having more family members they could count on and more friends than urban dwellers, but these same rural residents also said they felt more left out. Individuals who lived in mid-size population areas (up to 49,999 residents) reported less loneliness overall than people who lived in urban environments, but they were more likely to report not having any friends. On the other hand, Mullen and colleagues (2019) failed to find a significant difference in perceived loneliness between rural and urban primary care patients. Finlay and Kobayashi (2018) found that people who lived closer to a city center reported more social interactions than individuals who lived in the suburbs. City dwellers credited those social interactions to daily connections with others in their residential spaces, relationships with building staff or caretakers, and the existence of numerous places for socialization (e.g., parks, stores, movies, libraries, coffee shops) that provided avenues for impromptu social interactions. Generally, study participants in the outer suburbs reported greater loneliness than those closer to the city center, with loneliness decreasing with moves into the inner suburbs and closer to the city center. Many of the inner suburbs lacked communal places in which to gather, and people who lived in the outer suburbs reported that isolation from neighbors and the long distances to opportunities for socialization increased their social isolation and loneliness, although these results were not consistent among study participants.

AT-RISK POPULATIONS

Determining how the lives of older adults aged 50 and over may be affected by social isolation and loneliness is central to the committee's charge; however, the scope of the committee's work also extends to the particular impacts for at-risk (i.e., vulnerable) populations. While it is difficult to specifically define all of the subpopulations or groups of people who would be included as at risk, the committee endeavored to include information pertaining to any special populations for which there is relevant social isolation or loneliness research. Some of these populations include people who were studied on the basis of their racial or ethnic background, sex (i.e., male or female), age, socioeconomic status, health status, or place of residence (e.g., rural, urban). Research pertaining to these populations is included throughout the report. While a fair number of international studies look at the status of at-risk populations in other countries (e.g., Steptoe et al., 2013; Zebhauser et al., 2014), studies focusing on at-risk subpopulations in the United States are sparse. Two populations in the United States that have been researched more extensively than others are immigrants and individuals who identify as part of the gay, lesbian, bisexual, and transgender community. Research pertaining to these two groups is described below.

Immigrants

Evidence suggests that immigrants are more likely to experience social isolation and possibly loneliness than non-immigrants. For example, Latino immigrants have fewer social ties and lower levels of social integration than U.S.-born Latinos (Ramos et al., 2015; Shelton et al., 2011; Steele et al., 2018; Viruell-Fuentes et al., 2013). On the other hand, one study found no difference in loneliness between more and less acculturated Latinos (Gallo et al., 2012). A study of older, highly acculturated Korean immigrants found lower levels of depression in people who had stronger social support networks (Kim et al., 2012).

In general, immigrants experience many stressors that can increase their social isolation, including language and communication barriers; differences in community, family, or intergenerational dynamics; and new relationships that lack depth or history. This social isolation can be especially acute in first-generation older immigrants (Barrington et al., 2012; Curtin et al., 2017; Gerst-Emerson et al., 2014; Miyawaki, 2015). Immigrants also experience physical, cognitive, and mental health consequences associated with increased loneliness, and this can be especially true for women or people who are unmarried or lack a close confidant (Dong and Chen, 2017; Gerst-Emerson et al., 2014). A study in England found that immigrants, including those from Africa, Bangladesh, the Caribbean, China, and Pakistan, had much higher rates of social isolation and loneliness than their nonimmigrant peers, although Indian immigrants were an exception to this finding (Victor et al., 2012). In a Dutch study of immigrants, Moroccan, Surinamese, and Turkish immigrants reported feeling less healthy and more discriminated against than did Dutch natives, and these factors were related to increased loneliness (Visser and El Fakiri, 2016).

Gay, Lesbian, and Bisexual Populations

A small number of studies have found that an individual's sexual orientation can affect his or her feelings of loneliness or social isolation, but the findings are inconsistent. In general, studies have found that gay, lesbian, and bisexual individuals tend to experience more loneliness than their heterosexual peers. For example, in the Swedish National Public Health Survey of more than 79,000 individuals 18–84 years of age, the 1,673 who identified as lesbian, gay, or bisexual reported higher levels of social isolation than did those who identified as heterosexual, and social isolation was associated with increased measures of substance use and psychological distress in these populations (Bränström and Pachankis, 2018). On the other hand, a small study in the Netherlands by Bos et al. (2015) failed to find a similar result in a comparison of primarily middle-aged same-sex and heterosexual couples (median age = 43), and a study by Beam and Collins (2019) did not find that loneliness varied between sexual minority and heterosexual men and women across multiple age ranges.

Several studies have looked at the factors that contribute to loneliness and social isolation among gay, lesbian, and bisexual populations. Jackson et al. (2019) analyzed perceived discrimination and health and well-being in 304 middle-aged and older lesbian, gay, and bisexual individuals (aged 41–85) who participated in surveys in 2010–2011 and 2016–2017. The prospective analysis found that perceptions of discrimination based on sexual orientation increased loneliness. In a study of 912 gay Latino men recruited in bars (primarily aged 20–40 years), experiences of homophobia, racism, financial hardship, and low resiliency all predicted loneliness (Diaz et al., 2001). In a large, nationally representative study of adults in the United States 18 years of age or older, Hatzenbuehler et al. (2011) found that lesbian, gay, and bisexual individuals who were lonely reported higher levels of mood and anxiety disorders than did those who were not lonely. However, the correlation between social isolation and mood disorders differed between those who lived in states with high concentrations of same-sex couples and those who did not. Furthermore, a small study of older lesbian, gay, and bisexual individuals in the Netherlands found that those who had experienced negative social reactions or expected those reactions relative to their sexual preference had the highest levels of loneliness (Kuyper and Fokkema, 2010).

FINDINGS AND CONCLUSIONS

Physical Health Factors

- Physical health risk factors for social isolation and loneliness include many common chronic diseases and conditions, including heart disease, stroke, and cancer.
- The relationships between physical health risk factors and social isolation and loneliness are often bi-directional.
- Functional status (measured by factors such as gait speed or difficulties in the activities of daily living) is bi-directionally associated with social isolation and loneliness.
- Strong evidence links sensory impairment to communication difficulty and, further, to reduced social participation, social isolation, and higher rates of loneliness.
- Hearing loss contributes to both social isolation and loneliness, and remediation of hearing loss has been found to reduce loneliness and improve social functioning.

Psychological, Psychiatric, and Cognitive Factors

- Psychiatric disorders, such as major depression, generalized anxiety disorder, and social anxiety disorder, have been shown to increase the risk of developing loneliness.
- Social isolation and loneliness are more common in older adults with depressive and anxiety disorders than in their non-depressed and non-anxious peers.
- The relationship between depression and loneliness is bi-directional, and these constructs are closely associated. Yet, depression and loneliness are not the same.
- The impairments related to dementia predispose an individual to feelings of loneliness, and caregivers are also at risk for loneliness.

Social, Cultural, and Environmental Factors

- Supportive relationships—especially those with family, friends, and caregivers—can decrease self-reported loneliness, while difficult or unfulfilling relationships can increase feelings of loneliness.
- Losing a spouse is a frequent disruptive event for older adults, particularly for women. Loneliness is a primary symptom of bereavement.
- Research on the benefits of human–animal interactions is mixed.
- Retirement can affect an individual's likelihood of being socially isolated or lonely.
- Social environmental factors such as driving status, housing status, or location can affect the levels of social isolation and loneliness.
- At younger ages men and women experience similar rates of social isolation and loneliness, but women may be at higher risk as they get older.
- Literature focusing on social isolation and loneliness in at-risk subgroups is sparse.
- Gay, lesbian, and bisexual individuals tend to experience more loneliness than their heterosexual peers.
- Immigrants appear more likely to experience social isolation and loneliness than non-immigrants.

5

Mediators and Moderators

The Statement of Task charged the committee to consider "factors that moderate and mediate the links between social isolation/loneliness and health outcomes." By identifying the moderators and mediators of the effects of social isolation and loneliness, one can explore the mechanisms underlying those effects as well as why the effects may differ from one population to another and under which conditions an effect may be stronger or weaker (MacKinnon and Luecken, 2008). Mediators (i.e., mechanisms or pathways) are the factors that help explain how social isolation or loneliness affects health outcomes, while moderators are the factors that can influence the magnitude or direction of the effect of social isolation or loneliness on health. Identifying mediators helps explain the mechanisms, or plausible pathways, by which social isolation and loneliness influence health outcomes, while identifying moderator variables helps to determine whether the health effects of social isolation or loneliness are stronger for some groups than for others.

This chapter represents the portion of the committee's guiding framework related to the mediators and the moderators (largely at the individual level) of the associations between social connections and health outcomes (see Figure 5-1). (See Chapter 1 for more on moderators at the level of the community and society.) Current evidence suggests that there are multiple mediators that each may influence health (see Figure 5-2). This report does not provide an exhaustive review of all known mechanisms. Rather, the following sections summarize the current evidence concerning a few key mechanisms that exert critical roles in explaining the association between social connections and health outcomes. Then the chapter identifies and summarizes the evidence for several variables that have been identified as potential plausible moderators.

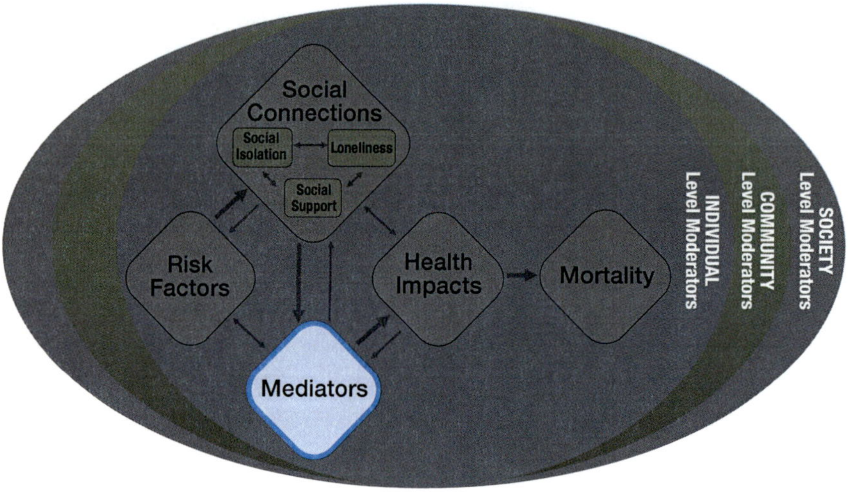

FIGURE 5-1 Committee's guiding framework with focus on mediators and moderators.

As noted in earlier chapters, this chapter uses the term "social connection" as an umbrella term that includes aspects of social isolation, loneliness, and social supports. Social isolation and loneliness are referred to specifically in line with available evidence. Given the complexity of the terminology used in relation to social isolation and loneliness, a reminder of key definitions is provided in Box 5-1.

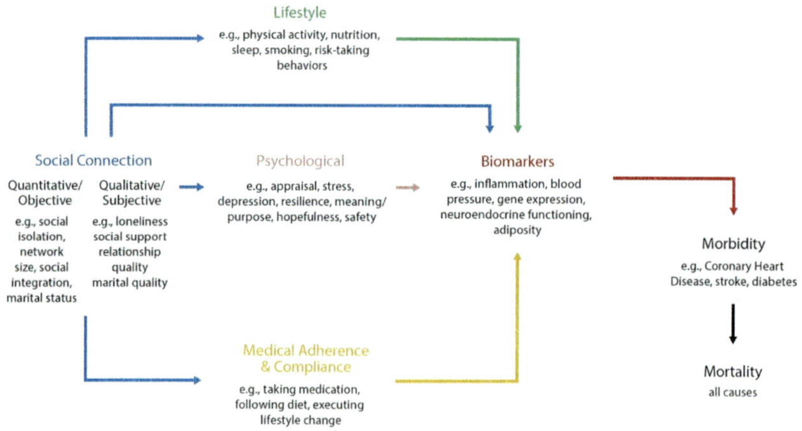

FIGURE 5-2 Possible mechanisms by which social connections influence disease morbidity and mortality.
SOURCE: Holt-Lunstad and Smith, 2016.

BOX 5-1
Key Definitions

Loneliness: the perception of social isolation or the subjective feeling of being lonely.

Mediators: also known as mechanisms or pathways; the factors that help explain how social isolation or loneliness affects health outcomes.

Moderators: the factors that can influence the magnitude or direction of the effect of social isolation or loneliness on health.

Social connection: an umbrella term that encompasses the structural, functional, and quality aspects of how individuals connect to each other.

Social isolation: the objective lack of (or limited) social contact with others.

Social support: the actual or perceived availability of resources (e.g., informational, tangible, emotional) from others, typically one's social network.

MEDIATORS: BEHAVORIAL, PSYCHOLOGICAL, AND BIOLOGICAL MECHANISMS

The mechanisms by which social connection—or the lack thereof—affects the development and course of disease have been elucidated by a robust and growing evidence base. Much of this evidence emerged in the context of examining the protective effects of social relationships and social support; however, this work relates specifically to both social isolation and loneliness. Relevant to social isolation are the experimental studies that randomly assign participants to either a social or an alone condition. In animals, this meant studying some animals housed in isolation versus others housed socially. In humans, many experimental studies examined physiological responses in an individual performing a task (typically stressful) in either the presence of or receiving support from someone (e.g., stranger) and contrasted that with a control condition (e.g., being alone). Later, more nuanced approaches were used to systematically examine aspects of social connection. Examples include testing in the presence of a stranger versus a friend (or other relationship types, such as spouses), having a wide social network versus a small network (even if not present), and observing the effects of perceived availability of social support. Evidence about biological mediators also comes from non-experimental studies. For example, it may not be possible to use random assignments to examine biological responses in everyday life or to study clinical populations. Thus, field studies are often employed in which biomarkers are collected.

Several reviews and meta-analyses link social support to changes in cardiovascular, neuroendocrine, and immune function (Uchino, 2006). Figure 5-2 illustrates different theoretical perspectives of the mechanisms that mediate the relationship between social connection and morbidity and mortality (Berkman et al., 2000; Cohen, 1988; Thoits, 1995; Umberson, 1987). The committee highlights some of these pathways in the following sections.

Health-Related Behaviors (Lifestyle)

As discussed in Chapter 3, heath-related behaviors can mediate the relationship between social isolation or loneliness and health outcomes. Social isolation and loneliness or the characteristics of one's social networks may affect health-related behaviors (e.g., smoking, physical inactivity), which in turn can affect health, either positively or negatively. One study of nearly 8,600 older adults found that "physical inactivity, daily smoking, and poor sleep mediated the association between loneliness and adverse health conditions" (Christiansen et al., 2016, p. 80). As with other factors, health-related behaviors may have a bi-directional relationship with social isolation and loneliness in that health-related behaviors can also exacerbate or reduce social isolation and loneliness. For example, household-based physical activity is associated with reduced social isolation (Robins et al., 2018). In one study with older adults, participation in the SilverSneakers® group exercise program directly decreased social isolation through membership in the program; that is, the greatest impact came from the membership itself in that members were less likely to be socially isolated than nonmembers (Brady et al., 2020). Furthermore, SilverSneakers® members had decreased feelings of loneliness associated with their improved overall health. The practice of tai chi has been associated with reductions in loneliness (Chan et al., 2017; Park and Park, 2010). (See Chapter 9 for more on exercise as an intervention.) Participation in an exercise program for health may lead to reductions in social isolation or loneliness due to the social nature of the program rather than the exercise itself. However, there is some evidence that exercise can help to improve sleep patterns and reduce inflammation (Asian Scientist Newsroom, 2014; Kline, 2014; Park and Park, 2010; Woods et al., 2012).

Sleep

While much of the research on health-enhancing behaviors focuses on smoking, nutrition, and physical activity, a growing body of research points to sleep as vitally important to health. Sleep influences a variety of physical health conditions, including cardiovascular disease, weight gain and obesity, diabetes, and metabolic syndrome, and poor sleep has been associated with an increased mortality risk. Multiple studies have demonstrated a robust association between social support and favorable sleep outcomes, and a lack of social and emotional support significantly predicts insufficient sleep (Kent de Grey et al., 2018; Williams et al., 2016). Social isolation and loneliness have been identified as key factors that alter the quantity and quality of sleep, which in turn influences health and safety at work (Magnavita and Garbarino, 2017). Loneliness has been linked to increased sleep fragmentation and sleep quality, leading to negative effects on metabolic, neural, and hormonal regulations (Cacioppo et al., 2002; Davidson and Rossall, 2015; Hawkley et al., 2010a; Jacobs et al., 2006; Kurina et al., 2011; Valtorta et al., 2016a). Thus, social isolation and loneliness may influence health via poorer sleep, while greater social support may lead to better health via more favorable sleep.

Medical Adherence

One way in which social relationships influence health is through their influence on adherence to medical advice. Adherence, or cooperation with medical treatment recommendations, can have a significant impact on medical outcomes; however, 25–40 percent of individuals are non-compliant, which leads to poorer health outcomes (DiMatteo, 2004; DiMatteo et al., 2000). Support from significant relationships can encourage greater responsiveness to recommendations. A systematic meta-analysis, including 122 empirical studies, examined the effects of structural and functional aspects of social connection on medical adherence (DiMatteo, 2004). The study found that most measures of social connection were significantly related to medical adherence; however, functional measures (e.g., social support) were stronger predictors of adherence than structural measures (e.g., marital status, living alone). When examining social support specifically, practical support more strongly predicted adherence than did emotional support. Thus, being socially isolated and lacking social support significantly reduces medical adherence, which may partially explain poorer health outcomes.

Psychological Pathways

As noted in Figure 5-2 there are several potential psychological pathways by which social connections influence morbidity and mortality. The following sections provide the evidence for stress and depression being examples of these pathways.

Stress

Relationships can help individuals cope with stress through the presence of other people who can provide advice on how to handle a problem (i.e., informational support), provide assistance or resources to handle the actual situation (e.g., tangible support such as a ride, loan, or meal), help the individual feel better (i.e., emotional support), or communicate that one is loved or cared for (i.e., belonging support). The stress-buffering model argues that this social support in turn buffers the pathogenic influence of stress (Cohen and Wills, 1985). A number of studies show that social support attenuates the physiological stress response (Che et al., 2018). Many reviews have looked at the mechanisms by which the stress-buffering effect operates (Brown et al., 2018; Ditzen and Heinrichs, 2014; Hostinar, 2015; Hostinar and Gunnar, 2015; Robles and Kiecolt-Glaser, 2003).

Conversely, not having relationships that one can rely on (i.e., social isolation) in times of need can be expected to result in poorer physiological stress responses. In a systematic review of 11 studies on loneliness, higher levels of loneliness were associated with heightened blood pressure and inflammatory reactivity to stress (Brown et al., 2018). Stress reactivity may be one potential way in which social isolation, loneliness, and social support influences biomarkers of health. It is important to note that the behavioral and psychological mechanisms are not independent and may influence the other. For example, stress can negatively influence health behaviors (e.g., Ng and Jeffery, 2003) while health behaviors (e.g., exercise) can reduce perceptions of stress (e.g., Rejeski et al., 1992).

Anxiety and Depression

Additional research points to other psychological pathways, including anxiety and depression. Several studies have linked social support to lower rates of depression and greater subjective well-being. For example, one study found that that depression increased as in-person social contact decreased and that individuals with lower rates of in-person social contact had "a significantly higher probability of clinically significant depressive symptoms 2 years later" (Teo et al., 2015, p. 2). Furthermore, in older adults both social isolation and loneliness have been shown to independently affect the probability of suffering from depression or anxiety (Domènech-Abella et al., 2019), providing evidence of the bi-directionality of anxiety and depression with social isolation and loneliness. Thus, social isolation, loneliness, and social support may influence health via the impact on these psychological factors, which in turn influence biomarkers of health.

Biological Mechanisms (Biomarkers)

While social connection may influence biological mechanisms via behavioral and psychological pathways, there is also evidence of a direct influence (as noted in Figure 5-2). Indeed, much of the evidence establishing the overall effect of social connection came from studies that adjusted for relevant lifestyle (e.g., smoking, alcohol, physical activity) and psychological (e.g., depression) factors, indicating that social connection influences mortality independently of such factors. Further evidence documents the direct influence that social connection may have on health-relevant physiological pathways.

According to Cole and colleagues (2007), "a large body of epidemiological research has linked characteristics of the social environment to human physical health, but the genomic mechanisms of these effects remain largely unexplored" (p. R189.2). Research is emerging on how social conditions influence gene expression. While most studies of gene expression differences in lonely and socially isolated individuals versus socially connected individuals are not focused on older adults, many studies provide insight as to the role of gene expression in mediating the relationship between social connection and health, and the potential to identify biomarkers as targets for intervention (Cole et al., 2007, 2011, 2015a,b; Murray et al., 2019; Slavich and Cole, 2013). Intersecting with gene expression, activity of the central nervous system may also have a role in mediating the effects of social isolation and loneliness on health (Cacioppo et al., 2014; Canli et al., 2018). The following sections summarize the evidence for several biological pathways, including cardiovascular, neuroendocrine, and immune or inflammatory pathways.

Cardiovascular

Given the strong links that social isolation and loneliness have with risks for cardiovascular disease (see Chapter 3), it is critically important to understand how social relationships influence the underlying molecular processes. Recurring interpersonal experiences and their physiological effects may be an important pathway linking social relationships and coronary heart disease. Loneliness and social stress have been associated with the activation of the hypothalamic–pituitary–adrenocortical (HPA) axis and the sympathetic nervous system, and "repeated and chronic social stress leads to glucocorticoid resistance, enhanced myelopoiesis, upregulated proinflammatory gene expression, and oxidative stress" (Xia and Li, 2018, p. 837), although how loneliness-associated cardiovascular disease may develop as a result of these mechanisms is unclear. Researchers have linked social isolation and loneliness to elevated vascular resistance and heightened blood pressure (Hawkley et al., 2006, 2010b) and to higher rates of metabolic syndrome (Blanquet et al., 2016; Whisman, 2010). Meta-analyses indicate that loneliness is associated with atypical physiological reactivity to acute stress, including exaggerated blood pressure and inflammatory reactivity (Brown et al., 2018). Social isolation is associated with a higher resting heart rate, higher systolic blood pressure, and larger total/high-density lipoprotein cholesterol ratio response to stress (Grant et al., 2009; McCrory et al., 2016).

Strong evidence also links greater degrees of social support to cardiovascular functioning that confers lower risk for disease (Uchino, 2006). This evidence comes from laboratory-based studies that experimentally manipulate social situations, from field studies that monitor cardiovascular function in daily life, and from longitudinal studies that examine the long-term effects of social conditions. Lab-based paradigms examine conceptual links between social isolation, loneliness, or social support and the reactivity hypothesis of disease (Lepore, 1998)—that is, that high levels of cardiovascular reactivity (e.g., blood pressure or heart rate) are related to a higher risk for the development and exacerbation of cardiovascular disease (e.g., Brindle et al., 2018; Chumaeva et al., 2010; Gianaros et al., 2002; Heponiemi et al., 2007; Smith and Jordan, 2015; Uchino et al., 1996). Several studies have also found that particularly for older adults, social support is associated with lower resting blood pressure (Ong and Allaire, 2005; Uchino et al., 1995, 1999). Social support has also been linked to lower ambulatory blood pressure in everyday life (Gump et al., 2001; Linden et al., 1993; Spitzer et al., 1992; Steptoe et al., 2000). Finally, higher cumulative social support has been associated with lower odds of high blood pressure (Hernandez et al., 2014).

Neuroendocrine

The major neuroendocrine systems involved in the stress response are the HPA and the sympathetic adrenomedullary axes. Given that social connections (or the lack thereof) can either blunt or exacerbate stress responses, these may be important pathways to consider. For instance, loneliness is associated with increased HPA activity, specifically an increase in the level of stress-sensitive glucocorticoids (cortisol in humans). Research has linked the HPA axis with trait loneliness (associated with a flattening of the diurnal cortisol curve), daily loneliness (a cortisol awakening response on the following day), and momentary increases in loneliness (momentary cortisol increases in youth who also had high interpersonal stress) (Doane and Adam, 2010). Research in animal models that experimentally manipulate social threat and social isolation has demonstrated that social isolation can have a causal effect on neuroendocrine functioning (Cacioppo et al., 2015a). And loneliness in older adults has been associated with lower cortisol output (Schutter et al., 2017).

Glucocorticoids regulate physiological functions, including immune, metabolic, cardiovascular, and reproductive functioning, as well as neurodegeneration and apoptosis (Cacioppo et al., 2015a; Xia and Li, 2018). This suggests that the association between loneliness and health may be mediated in part by the dysregulation of the neuroendocrine system (Hackett et al., 2012). Conversely, there is a vast literature documenting the buffering effects, or better regulation of the HPA, associated with social bonding and social support. Hostinar and colleagues (2014) provide a review of the psychobiological mechanisms underlying social buffering of the HPA.

Inflammation

Chronic inflammation has been linked to diseases such as heart disease, stroke, some cancers, and autoimmune disorders, so it is possible that there is a common pathway underlying the broad health effects of social connection on multiple disease outcomes. In particular, a meta-analysis of 41 studies (including more than 73,000 participants) established the influence of social connectedness (specifically, social support and social integration) on inflammation (Uchino et al., 2018), suggesting that social connectedness may be implicated in inflammatory-related disease development and exacerbation. Other research has shown that objective markers of social connection may be just as important as individual perceptions in terms of their effects on these health risks. For example, in one study, ratings of an individual's social connections as assessed by friends and family were more predictive of fibrinogen levels (a biomarker of inflammation and cardiovascular risk), than that individual's own ratings (Kim, D. A., et al., 2016). These data suggest that the social connections themselves may have an objective influence on inflammation that is just as important as—if not more important than—the individual's perceptions.

Conversely, a lack of social connections has been linked to worse inflammation. Another review finds

> (1) that exposure to social stressors increases pro-inflammatory activity, (2) that individuals who are more socially isolated (i.e., lonely) show increased pro-inflammatory activity, and (3) that individuals who are more socially isolated show increased pro-inflammatory activity in response to an inflammatory challenge or social stressor. (Eisenberger et al., 2017, p. 242)

In the Midlife in the United States study, a positive significant relationship was seen between loneliness and three systemic inflammation biomarkers—interleukin-6, fibrinogen, and C-reactive protein—after controlling for covariates (Nersesian et al., 2018). This finding is consistent with research that has linked loneliness to stronger inflammatory responses (Cole et al., 2007, 2011; Hackett et al., 2012; Jaremka et al., 2013a; Steptoe et al., 2004).

As mentioned earlier, studies of gene expression may provide insight regarding opportunities for intervention. For example, a small randomized controlled trial showed that a mindfulness-based stress reduction program downregulated the loneliness-related pro-inflammatory gene expression in older adults (aged 55–85) (Creswell et al., 2012).

Summary of the Evidence for Mediators

Social connection has a dose–response effect on physiological risk markers across age groups. Yang and colleagues (2016) used data from four nationally representative longitudinal samples of the U.S. population to assess

> the prospective association of both structural and functional dimensions of social relationships (social integration, social support, and social strain) with objectively measured biomarkers of physical health (C-reactive protein, systolic and diastolic blood pressure, waist circumference, and body mass index) within each life stage, including adolescence plus young, middle, and late adulthood, and compare such associations across life stages. (Yang et al., 2016, p. 578)

They found that "a higher degree of social connection was associated with a lower risk of physiological dysregulation in a dose–response manner in both early and later life" (Yang et al., 2016, p. 578). Conversely, lower social connection (social isolation) was associated with higher risk. This provides strong evidence that social relationships influence health and longevity via these risk markers.

Growing evidence from both animals and humans suggests that the social environment, particularly social adversity,[1] influences the regulation of genes, and it has also been linked to epigenetic changes (Tung and Gilad, 2013). Thus, in addition to the cardiovascular, neuroendocrine, and immune consequences of social relationships, there is now evidence (both correlational and causal) that an individual's social environment plays a critical role in regulating a large number of genes, many of which are also associated with susceptibility to other external stressors and some diseases (Tung and Gilad, 2013).

MODERATING FACTORS INFLUENCING MORTALITY AND HEALTH OUTCOMES

The effects of social connection on mortality risk are well established (see Chapter 2), as is the evidence of plausible biological mechanisms that explain these effects, which has led to a growing interest in factors that may influence the strength or direction of these effects. Examining such moderators helps determine whether some groups may be more affected by social isolation and loneliness than others. The previous section summarized *how* social connection influences health, but the data suggest that biological systems are also influenced by early experiences, developmental factors, and genetics, which can moderate this effect (Ditzen and Heinrichs, 2014; Hennessy et al., 2009; Uchino, 2009a,b). While there may be several other potential moderators, this section specifically considers factors relevant to the committee's Statement of Task, such as age, gender, ethnicity, and socioeconomic status (SES). Furthermore, the evidence concerning relationship quality as a moderator of the association between social connection and health outcomes is described.

Age and Developmental Processes

Naturally, the risk of mortality increases with increasing age. The question arises, however, of whether the effects on mortality of social isolation, loneliness, or social support also increase with age. The meta-analysis by Holt-Lunstad and colleagues (2010) summarized in Chapter 2 synthesized data across

[1] Social adversity includes "acute or chronic exposures which hypothetically would impact on health mainly by directly threatening salient relationships" (Gustafsson et al., 2012, p. 119). Examples include parental loss, mother–infant separation, residential instability, and social isolation (Gustafsson et al., 2012; Tung and Gilad, 2013).

148 prospective studies and found no effect of age, suggesting no difference in the overall effect of various indicators of social connection on mortality risk. However, the majority of these studies used older samples. In a subsequent meta-analysis that focused specifically on the effects of social isolation, loneliness, and living alone on mortality risk, the authors compared the effects among individuals above 65 years old with the effects among younger individuals and found that the mortality risk for those under age 65 was more affected by the social factors than the mortality risk for those over age 65 (Holt-Lunstad et al., 2015). Additional prospective studies have examined the effects of age more directly. For example, a recent study examining social isolation across young, middle-aged, and older adults found a dose–response effect on a variety of health outcomes (Hämmig, 2019). Early life experiences may also influence one's risk trajectory later in life. For example, several studies now demonstrate that adverse childhood experiences have lasting negative consequences (Caspi et al., 2006; Danese et al., 2009; Lacey et al., 2014). Therefore, while the data in this area are not robust, newer evidence seems to suggest that age may moderate the impact of social isolation and loneliness on mortality risk, with greater risk seen among younger ages.

Demographic Factors

Demographic characteristics including gender, SES, and ethnicity all may influence the relationship between social connections and health outcomes.

Gender

Examining the larger literature via available meta-analytic data indicates that the protective effect of social relationships and the risks associated with social isolation broadly and with loneliness and living alone specifically were similar for men and women (Holt-Lunstad et al., 2010, 2015). Despite prior research suggesting that women have larger social networks than men (Antonuci and Akiyama, 1987; Matud, 2004), gender is not a significant moderator of the relationship between social support and mortality. Similarly, when looking just at loneliness across studies of the risk for all-cause mortality, no significant differences were found by gender, though the strength of the association was slightly higher in men than in women (Rico-Uribe et al., 2018). These data suggest that the effect of relationships on mortality from all causes is consistent for both men and women. These results are consistent with work looking at gender differences in the prevalence of loneliness. A meta-analysis by Maes and colleauges (2019) covering nearly 400,000 individuals synthesized the available evidence on gender differences in loneliness across the lifespan and demonstrated nearly a zero overall effect; furthermore, any effect of age was negligible. Thus, levels of loneliness are similar for males and females across the lifespan.

Socioeconomic Status

Given the research suggesting that SES may significantly influence health outcomes, many epidemiological studies statistically control for SES, making it difficult to determine whether the impact of social isolation and loneliness on health and mortality may depend on SES. There is some evidence to suggest that the prevalence of loneliness may differ by SES. For example, one study found that among the (economically) poorest people, older adults were less likely to be lonely than those in the younger groups, while among the richest there was no difference in loneliness by age (Domènech-Abella et al., 2017). Cundiff and Smith (2017) found that the collective effect of recurrent and chronic exposures to a variety of stressful interpersonal experiences (e.g., reduced support, work stress, negative stereotypes) may help explain the increased prevalence of chronic psychosocial vulnerabilities among individuals in lower socioeconomic environments, and further link those psychosocial vulnerabilities to the transient physiological mechanisms (i.e., stress responses) that directly affect coronary heart disease. Nonetheless, the evidence base is not robust, and more large-scale research is needed to further elucidate the potential moderating effects of SES.

Race and Ethnicity

The majority of epidemiological studies do not report effect sizes for social isolation, loneliness, social support, or other aspects of social connection that are broken down by race or ethnicity. Therefore, researchers have not been able to adequately examine this factor meta-analytically. Some evidence suggests that the prevalence of loneliness may differ by ethnicity (Jamieson et al., 2018); however, most of these studies did not examine the moderating effect of ethnicity on health or mortality. Nonetheless, some studies provide some illuminating evidence. For example, one study found that, contrary to expectations, social isolation in older black men did not significantly predict metabolic disorders (Das, 2013). In another study both loneliness and social disconnectedness had a significant negative association with physical and mental health among white older adults; however, among African American older adults social disconnectedness was associated with worse physical health and loneliness and associated with worse mental health (Miyawaki, 2015). One of the strongest studies to date was a 10-year U.S. population-based prospective study that examined ethnic and racial variation in social integration[2] and its effect on mortality among participants of the U.S. National Health Interview Survey (Barger and Uchino, 2017). This study found no significant effect of received social support on mortality among any of the groups (i.e., white, black, Hispanic), but social integration demonstrated a significant effect on survival among all three groups. Consistent with other research, there was

[2] Low social integration scores are a marker of social isolation.

a dose–response effect among whites, but the gradient was flatter among blacks, and a survival advantage was found only at the highest levels of social integration. Among Hispanics the survival advantage was present at all but the lowest levels. Thus, "extreme group contrasts (i.e., contrasting the highest and lowest social integration categories) also obscures different forms of the mortality gradient for black, white and Hispanic participants" (Barger and Uchino, 2017, p. 4).

Relationship Quality

While the absence of others (i.e., social isolation) is detrimental to health, the presence of others may not necessarily be entirely positive or protective. While social relationships can be characterized by a myriad of positive attributes (e.g., intimacy, companionship, nurturance, joy, and compassion), some relationships are characterized by negative attributes (e.g., conflict, insensitivity, jealousy, burden, rejection, neglect, or even abuse) (Rook and Charles, 2017). These attributes may influence the magnitude and direction of the associations between relationships and health. Multiple studies have demonstrated that negativity in social relationship predicts greater risk for mortality (Birditt and Antonucci, 2008; Friedman et al., 1995; Tanne et al., 2004; Tucker et al., 1996). For example, in a study of breast-cancer patients by Kroenke and colleagues (2013), women with small social networks and low levels of social support and small networks had a significantly higher risk of mortality (Kroenke et al., 2013). Additionally, "larger social networks predicted better prognosis after breast cancer, but associations depended on the quality and burden of family relationships" (Kroenke et al., 2013, p. 261). Similarly, poor-quality relationships and relationship strain were found to more than double the risk of depression 10 years later (Teo et al., 2013b). Thus, in medical settings if relationship quality is ignored it may lead to higher risk rather than lower risk.

Indeed, a broad literature documents the protective effects of marriage in terms of reducing risk for mortality (Manzoli et al., 2007; Rendall et al., 2011) and loneliness (Cohen-Mansfield et al., 2016); however, not all marriages are high quality, and there is evidence that marital quality is an important moderator. For example, a meta-analytic review of 126 studies found that marital quality was inversely associated with a variety of health outcomes, including mortality risk (Robles et al., 2014). Similarly, distressed marriages have been associated with poorer immune outcomes (Price et al., 2018) and greater morbidity and mortality risk (Choi and Marks, 2011; Kimmel et al., 2000; King and Reis, 2012; Robles and Kiecolt-Glaser, 2003; Robles et al., 2014). Thus, when assessing for social isolation or loneliness practitioners should not assume a lack of risk based on marital status alone.

Studies done in clinical settings offer evidence that relationship quality can significantly influence treatment adherence. A meta-analysis by DiMatteo (2004) found that adherence to medical regimens was lower in patients from families in conflict and higher in patients from cohesive families. Furthermore, the social conflict that arises as a result of a well-intended efforts to encourage medication adherence (that may be interpreted as nagging or attempts to exert control) has been shown to reduce (rather than increase) medication adherence (Warner et al., 2013). However, another study among people with a chronic illness showed that negative social relations at baseline were associated with decreased risk for mortality (Birditt and Antonucci, 2008), and the authors suggested that this may be due to the buffering effect of social control. Thus, it cannot be assumed that medical adherence will be always be enhanced by increasing family or staff involvement.

There is substantial evidence that the quality of relationships also influences biomarkers of health. For example, studies examining the influences of cardiovascular functioning have found that positivity in social relationships (e.g., support, satisfaction) is associated with protective effects, while negativity (e.g., strain, conflict) and ambivalence in relationships are associated with deleterious cardiovascular functioning (e.g., elevated blood pressure, cardiovascular reactivity) (Birmingham and Holt-Lunstad, 2018; Holt-Lunstad and Uchino, 2019; Robles, 2014). Similarly, poor-quality relationships more than doubled the risk of depression 10 years later (Teo et al., 2013b).

FINDINGS AND CONCLUSIONS

Mediators

- Strong evidence links loneliness, social isolation, and social support to changes in cardiovascular, neuroendocrine, and immune function as well as to the physiological stress response. A lack of social connections has been linked to higher levels of inflammation, which may point to a plausible biological mechanism for the association of social isolation and loneliness with a variety of negative health outcomes.
- Social isolation and loneliness have been linked to decreased quality of sleep, which itself can influence a variety of physical health conditions, including cardiovascular disease, weight gain and obesity, diabetes, metabolic syndrome, and increased risk for mortality.

Moderators

- There is some evidence that demographic factors (e.g., age, gender, ethnicity, SES) moderate the influence of social connection and health. Recent evidence suggests that social isolation and loneliness may carry a higher risk among those under age 65 relative to those over age 65. No reliable gender differences have emerged.
- Both the positive and negative attributes of relationships can significantly influence the magnitude and direction of the association between these relationships and health.

- Higher quality and more numerous relationships is associated with protective health effects and a lower risk of mortality.
- Having poorer quality and fewer relationships is associated with harmful effects on health including higher risk for morbidity and mortality, poorer treatment adherence, and poorer health-relevant biological responses.
- Understanding both the negative and the positive attributes of social relationships is needed to fully understand how these relationships impact health.
- Decreasing social isolation may not reduce risk if attention is not paid to the quality of the relationships; thus, indicators of quality need to be included in assessments.

6

Assessment of Social Isolation and Loneliness in Research

Many measurement tools exist to assess social isolation and loneliness (and other related concepts), but to date most of the established and widely implemented tools have been developed for research purposes. Research using these tools has focused on defining the prevalence, the risk factors, and the health impacts of social isolation and loneliness. More recently, there has been a focus on using these tools to assess the effectiveness of interventions by using measures of social isolation and loneliness as outcomes. (See Chapter 9 for more on interventions.) This chapter will examine the use of different tools related to social isolation and loneliness primarily in the research setting, and it will explore research on the use of information technology to identify individuals at risk for social isolation and loneliness. Chapter 7 will discuss the application of these tools in clinical settings. Given the complexity of the terminology used in relation to social isolation and loneliness, a reminder of key definitions is provided in Box 6-1.

MEASUREMENT OF SOCIAL ISOLATION AND LONELINESS

The concepts of social isolation and loneliness have been defined in different ways (see Chapters 1 and 2), which has led to some variability in how these concepts are measured. When examining social isolation and loneliness in research, a number of tools capture elements of both social isolation and loneliness, which may obscure differences between these two concepts. In addition, in both research and clinical settings social isolation and loneliness may fluctuate over time. This underscores the need for serial testing to better ascertain changes over time,

BOX 6-1
Key Definitions

Loneliness: the perception of social isolation or the subjective feeling of being lonely.

Mediators: also known as mechanisms or pathways; the factors that help explain how social isolation or loneliness affects health outcomes.

Moderators: the factors that can influence the magnitude or direction of the effect of social isolation or loneliness on health.

Social connection: an umbrella term that encompasses the structural, functional, and quality aspects of how individuals connect to each other.

Social isolation: the objective lack of (or limited) social contact with others.

Social support: the actual or perceived availability of resources (e.g., informational, tangible, emotional) from others, typically one's social network.

including the trajectories of these changes and their clinical relevance. However, measures that encompass elements of both social isolation and loneliness or, more broadly, social connection could be advantageous in clinical settings as they may probe both concepts, which would be more efficient, and they could possibly provide a stronger clinical signal. Because of the variability in existing measurement tools for social isolation and loneliness, Valtorta and colleagues (2016b) suggested that these tools can be classified along two dimensions: whether the measure looks at the structural or the functional aspects of social relationships and the degree of subjectivity required by respondents (see Figure 6-1). The researchers examined 54 measurement instruments and found that "tools explicitly designed for measuring loneliness . . . tend to be based on more subjective questions, whereas social network indices primarily use more objective measures" (p. 6).

It is well accepted that the three-item UCLA Loneliness Scale (described later in this chapter) captures loneliness—a subjective self-reported measure. In contrast, the Duke Social Support Index (also described later in this chapter), while classically thought to measure social isolation, does include some subjective questions. Therefore, if a study uses the Duke Social Support Index and says it measures social isolation and not loneliness, the study may incorrectly conclude that it is only social isolation that has an effect or is being

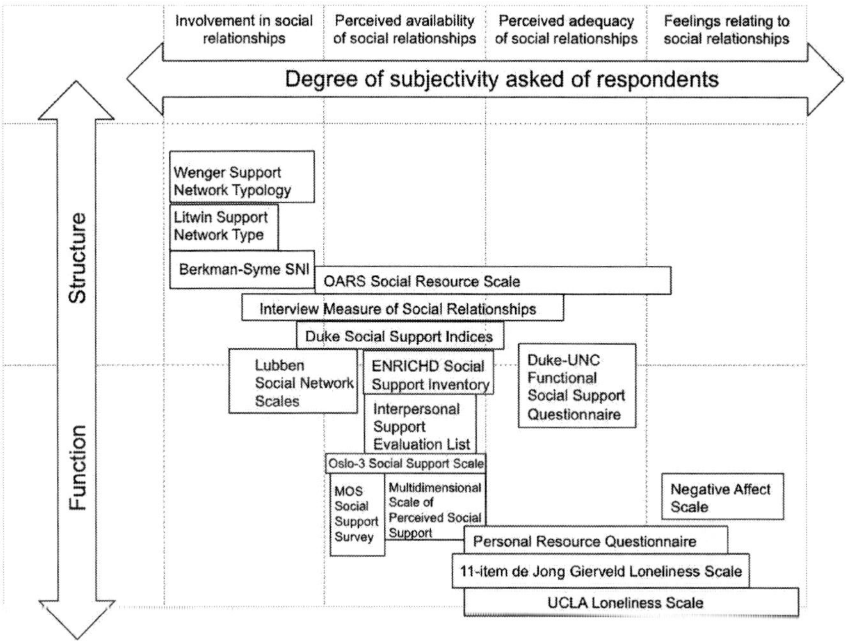

FIGURE 6-1 Multi-item questionnaires compared by structure versus function and for the degree of subjectivity.
NOTE: MOS = Medical Outcomes Study; OARS = Older Americans Research and Service Center; SNI = Social Network Index; UCLA = University of California, Los Angeles.
SOURCE: Valtorta et al., 2016b.

affected. The differences in measurement and how studies report outcomes as being either related to loneliness *or* social isolation may present challenges when comparing studies and even in meta-analyses if the studies are grouped according to how authors define social isolation and loneliness rather than according to the measurement tools used. Some of this variability in measurement likely accounts for the range of prevalence rates and inconsistencies in study conclusions. This creates a landscape in which the effects of social isolation and loneliness on health are demonstrated, but it is not always clear as to which has a greater influence. Because of this, when evaluating the literature it is imperative to examine how social isolation and loneliness are being defined and measured.

The following sections provide a list of and brief explanations for some of the most widely used measurement tools for social isolation and loneliness. The committee emphasizes that this is not a comprehensive list of all available tools and does not represent an endorsement of this committee but rather serves to

BOX 6-2
Berkman–Syme Social Network Index

1. In a typical week, how many times do you talk on the telephone with family, friends, or neighbors?
2. How often do you get together with friends or relatives?
3. How often do you attend church or religious services?
4. How often do you attend meetings of the clubs or organizations you belong to?

NOTE: Marital status is assessed separately and included in scoring.

demonstrate the range of tools being used. Ultimately, one size does not fit all. For any given intervention, the tool picked should be tailored to assess what change in social isolation or loneliness is expected to be affected, over what time period, and whether the effect is sustained. Unless there is compelling evidence to suggest a new measurement tool, researchers and program evaluators should try to use existing and validated tools (see Recommendation 7-1 in Chapter 7). However, questions remain as to how existing tools can be used in clinical settings (for more on this, see Chapter 7).

Berkman–Syme Social Network Index

The Berkman–Syme Social Network Index (see Box 6-2) focuses on the general adult population and measures social integration versus isolation by looking at marital status, frequency of contact with other people, participation in religious activities, and participation in other club or organization activities (Berkman and Syme, 1979). This measure was recommended for inclusion in electronic health records (EHRs) as a measure of social isolation by a prior Institute of Medicine committee (IOM, 2014). (See Chapter 7 for more on EHRs.)

The Revised UCLA Loneliness Scale

The Revised UCLA (R-UCLA) Loneliness Scale is a 20-item, self-administered questionnaire that has become a standard measurement of subjective loneliness (Russell, 1996). The three-item UCLA Loneliness Scale was developed for use in telephone surveys in which questions are posed to the person being assessed (Hughes et al., 2004; see Box 6-3). The three-item scale is being used widely in both research and clinical settings in the United States as a brief assessment of loneliness.

BOX 6-3
Three-Item UCLA Loneliness Scale

Lead-in and questions are read to respondent.

The next questions are about how you feel about different aspects of your life. For each one, tell me how often you feel that way.

1. First, how often do you feel that you lack companionship: Hardly ever (1), some of the time (2), or often (3)?
2. How often do you feel left out: Hardly ever (1), some of the time (2), or often (3)?
3. How often do you feel isolated from others: Hardly ever (1), some of the time (2), or often (3)?

Scoring:
Sum the total of all items. Higher scores indicate greater degrees of loneliness.

SOURCE: Hughes et al., 2004.

Steptoe Social Isolation Index

In a study by Steptoe and colleagues (2013), the authors created an index of social isolation. The index involves a five-point scale, with one point being assigned for each of the following factors:

- Unmarried/not cohabiting
- Less than monthly contact (including face-to-face, by telephone, or in writing/email) with children
- Less than monthly contact (including face-to-face, by telephone, or in writing/email) with other family
- Less than monthly contact (including face-to-face, by telephone, or in writing/email) with friends
- No participation in social clubs, resident groups, religious groups, or committees

People with a score of 2 or more were defined as being socially isolated.

Duke Social Support Index

The Duke Social Support Index is a 35-item measure of various dimensions of social support, including social network (e.g., proximity of family), social interaction (e.g., frequency of interactions), subjective support (e.g., perceptions of relationships), and instrumental support (e.g., availability of help) (Koenig et al., 1993). However, the interview required for this measure is lengthy. As a result, two abbreviated versions of the tool have been developed: an 11-item scale that includes subscales for social interaction and subjective support and a 23-item scale that adds a subscale for instrumental support (Koenig et al., 1993).

Lubben Social Network Scale

The Lubben Social Network Scale is an adaptation of the Berkman–Syme Social Network Index developed to focus specifically on older adults (Lubben, 1988). At that time, Lubben found that marital status and participation in religious activities vary less in the older adult population. Therefore, this 10-item measure focuses more heavily on the quality and frequency of an individual's relationships with family and friends. Lubben and colleagues have published revised versions of the Lubben Social Network Scale including an abbreviated six-item version (Lubben and Gironda, 2003; Lubben et al., 2006).

de Jong Gierveld Loneliness Scale

The de Jong Gierveld Loneliness Scale is an 11-item questionnaire designed to assess both overall loneliness and two specific types of loneliness (de Jong Gierveld and Kamphuis, 1985; see Table 6-1). This scale includes two subscales: a three-item emotional loneliness subscale (aimed at loneliness due to the lack of a close, intimate relationship) and a three-item social loneliness subscale (aimed at loneliness due to the lack of a broader social network) (de Jong Gierveld and Van Tilburg, 2006). As with the R-UCLA Loneliness Scale, the length of this instrument can be challenging to use in large surveys. As a result, a shortened 6-item scale comprising two of the 3-item subscales within the original 11-item questionnaire has been used (de Jong Gierveld and Van Tilburg, 2006; Weiss, 1974; see Table 6-1).

Cornwell Perceived Isolation Scale

Cornwell and Waite (2009) measured perceived isolation by creating a nine-item scale that combines indicators of perceived lack of social support and of loneliness. The first six items came from asking individuals the following questions: "How often can you open up to your family if you need to talk about your worries?" and "How often can you rely on them for help if you have a problem?" (Cornwell and Waite, 2009). These same questions were then asked again in relation to their friends and then in relation to their spouse or partner. The last three items come from the three-item UCLA Loneliness Scale (described above).

TABLE 6-1 Items of the 11-Item (original) and 6-Item (short) de Jong Gierveld Loneliness Scales

Statement	Original Emotional Subscale	Original Social Subscale	Short Emotional Subscale	Short Social Subscale
1. There is always someone I can talk to about my day-to-day problems[a]		X		
2. I miss having a really close friend	X			
3. I experience a general sense of emptiness	X		X	
4. There are plenty of people I can rely on when I have problems[a]		X		X
5. I miss the pleasure of the company of others	X			
6. I find my circle of friends and acquaintances too limited	X			
7. There are many people I can trust completely[a]		X		X
8. There are enough people I feel close to[a]		X		X
9. I miss having people around	X		X	
10. I often feel rejected	X		X	
11. I can call on my friends whenever I need them[a]		X		

[a] Item should be reversed before scoring.
SOURCE: de Jong Gierveld and Van Tilburg, 2006.

For this scale, the authors standardized each item and averaged scores, with a higher score indicating greater perceived isolation.

Campaign to End Loneliness Measurement Tool

The Campaign to End Loneliness (see more on the campaign in Chapters 8 and 9) developed a three-item tool to measure loneliness (see Box 6-4). The guidance for using the tool notes that "the main purpose of this tool is to measure the change that happens as a result of an intervention to address loneliness" (Campaign to End Loneliness, 2019a, p. 12). The tool was developed "in partnership with over 50 older people, service providers, commissioners and housing associations" (Campaign to End Loneliness, 2019a, p. 13).

BOX 6-4
Campaign to End Loneliness Measurement Tool

People are asked to respond to the following questions:

1. I am content with my friendships and relationships.
2. I have enough people I feel comfortable asking for help at any time.
3. My relationships are satisfying as I would want them to be.

Scoring:
The score is a total of responses to the above statements, based on scored responses of strongly disagree (4) / disagree (3) / neutral (2) / agree (1) / strongly agree (0). The higher the score, the greater the degree of loneliness.

SOURCE: Campaign to End Loneliness, 2019a.

MEASURING IMPACT FOR SOCIAL ISOLATION AND LONELINESS

The committee's review of the literature on social isolation and loneliness revealed a number of measurement and interpretation challenges pertaining to prevalence rates and outcomes that need to be addressed. These challenges are summarized in the following sections.

Measuring the Prevalence of Social Isolation and Loneliness

The committee emphasizes the importance of using validated tools in the assessment of social isolation and loneliness (rather than using only parts of existing tools or creating new, unvalidated tools). Validation means that the tool has been shown to accurately reflect the level of social isolation or loneliness (and is not biased). When studying the prevalence of loneliness or isolation, it is most important to choose a measurement tool that matches the research question. For example, if one is looking to establish the prevalence of loneliness in a given population, it is necessary to pick a measurement tool that is validated to measure loneliness rather than other aspects of social connection. (Chapter 7 further discusses the importance of using validated tools in clinical settings.)

Given the confusion surrounding the definitions of social isolation and loneliness, using a validated tool for the specific construct being evaluated is of the utmost importance. Employing an unvalidated tool or, as mentioned previously, a tool that was designed to assess social isolation for a study that is actually examining loneliness, may yield inaccurate results. To address this issue,

Chapter 7 (and Recommendation 7-1 in particular) further discusses the use of validated tools in clinical settings.

Measuring Social Isolation and Loneliness as Outcomes of an Intervention

When seeking to understand whether a particular intervention has an effect on social isolation or loneliness, it is important to choose a measurement tool that can be used both before and after the implementation of an intervention in order to detect and quantify any difference in the score. Although numerous measurement tools are available, in those cases when a researcher seeks to compare the impacts of different interventions, it is important to use the same measurement tool for the different interventions being compared.

In observational or longitudinal studies, it is critical to use a common, standardized assessment at all time-points during the study duration. The length of follow-up and frequency of measurement are particularly important for a few reasons. For example, because social isolation and loneliness may be episodic for some, it is important to have several time periods of measurement in order to determine if observed differences are true reflections of changes in outcomes or if they represent measurement variability or natural fluctuations over time. There is no set standard for the number of time-points or numbers of assessments per unit of time used to determine social isolation and loneliness. As a general principle, having more than two data points (the beginning and the end of the study) can help to reliably measure trajectories of social isolation and loneliness. Because of the large health effects of social isolation and loneliness (see Chapters 2 and 3), studies with longer follow-up periods that can demonstrate sustained effects during an intervention (and even months after an intervention) will be more useful. (See Chapter 9 for more on interventions.)

Overall Measure Quality

As is discussed in more detail in Chapter 7, concerns exist regarding the quality and relevance of current tools, and particularly as to whether the tools developed decades ago can fully capture the expectations and values of older adults today. This is likely to be especially relevant for measures of social isolation as modes of interaction have changed significantly in recent years and decades. For example, questions about living alone or participation in religious activities may not fully reflect preferences in today's society. Also, alternative modes of communication to the "telephone" (e.g., social media, instant messaging, video conferencing) may not be fully captured in these measures. On the other hand, measures of loneliness may not be influenced by social changes because responses are subjective to the current context. While current tools may have limitations, the committee asserts that the use of existing validated tools is important to advance the role of the health care system in addressing social isolation and loneliness (see Chapter 7).

Furthermore, researchers need to strive toward a goal of measure development and evaluation in this space to ensure that the available tools for social isolation and loneliness can fully capture the experience of today's older adults.

IDENTIFICATION OF INDIVIDUALS AND POPULATIONS AT RISK

In addition to the measures described above, information technology offers the possibility of detecting or predicting patterns of social isolation and loneliness in older adults. This can be done without using specific tools or measurement scales. For instance, data mining can be used to assess or predict patterns of social isolation and loneliness (Austin et al., 2016); to this end various sources of data have been explored, including passive monitoring sensors, wearables, and programs to track social media. However, the development of algorithms to accurately predict social isolation or loneliness has proved challenging because of the lack of a specific outcome measure that is available at a large scale in EHRs or other sources of data (e.g., hospital readmission or death). One benefit may be that for both research and clinical settings this could reduce the burden on individuals, providers, and researchers in terms of the time needed to answer certain questionnaires.

Prediction

Multiple approaches exist for identifying individuals at risk for social isolation or loneliness, including self-referral, community referral, formal assessments, and predictive analytics. In health care, predictive analytics have been widely used to enable better decision making and to support preventive care (Wang et al., 2018). For example, one hospital system used predictive analytics on data from medical sensors to predict patients' movements and monitor their actions throughout their hospital stay, allowing the health system to provide services more efficiently, optimize operations, and reduce medical risk (Wang et al., 2018). The section on predictive analytics in Chapter 7 describes opportunities for health care systems to develop predictive strategies based on the vast datasets within health information systems.

Identifying Social Isolation and Loneliness at the Individual Level

In clinical research, machine learning[1] technologies have been used to analyze social media data to predict depression (Eichstaedt et al., 2018), suicidality (Braithwaite et al., 2016), and posttraumatic stress disorder (Coppersmith et al., 2014). Natural language processing (NLP)[2] technologies and machine learning

---

[1] Machine learning, a subset of artificial intelligence, refers to the "algorithms, tools, and techniques that give computers the ability to learn from experience and data" (CTA, 2018, p. 21).

[2] Natural language processing is "technology that produces conversational text or speech understandable by humans" (CTA, 2018, p. 21).

are also being used to examine EHR data to identify individuals at risk for a variety of behavioral issues, including suicidality (Walsh et al., 2018). Given the lack of standardization for assessing social isolation and loneliness in clinical documentation, researchers have used NLP techniques to identify mentions of social isolation in clinical notes. In one study, investigators used validated scales and expert opinion to develop a lexicon representing concepts related to social isolation (Zhu et al., 2019). Among the terms in the algorithm were "lack companionship," "isolated," and "feel left out." The algorithm was tested in a dataset of clinical notes from 1,057 prostate cancer patients, and the performance was evaluated using chart review as a gold standard. The algorithm correctly identified 36 cases of social isolation, and an additional 4 cases were determined to be false positives. Reviewers found one false negative in a sampling of the algorithm's negative cases. In another study, NLP was used to analyze transcripts of psychotherapy sessions to identify symptom and diagnostic information using not only language but also interactional variables such as turn-taking in the conversation between provider and patient (Gaut et al., 2017).

Some health care organizations use fields in the EHR to document "living alone" as a proxy for social isolation. Given the many life circumstances implied by living alone (e.g., being independent), these data alone are of little use in identifying patients at risk for negative outcomes related to social isolation and loneliness (LaWall et al., 2019). (See Chapter 7 for more on the use of information technology in clinical settings.)

Population-Level Identification and Targeting

In general, technologies that analyze large public and private datasets are being used both in and out of clinical settings to identify target groups of individuals according to behavioral characteristics, which has raised various ethical and social concerns (Eubanks, 2018; Zuboff, 2019). For example, in industry, video games and other Web-based mobile interventions are designed for targeted appeal and subsequent loyalty. However, there is a dearth of research on how individuals experiencing social isolation and loneliness are targeted by such industry interventions. That is, the outcome of the product design could encourage increased use of their products, leading to increased social isolation or loneliness.

Key ethical issues related to the use of large datasets to predict social isolation and loneliness include the violation of privacy and the creation of new, harmful stereotypes, though various other ethical concerns may also arise, depending on the way in which identification is conducted and used for targeting.

Implications and Ethical Concerns

While the use of data to identify, predict, and potentially mitigate social isolation and loneliness is considered promising by many, some concerns exist about the ways in which data might be used and the ways in which assessment may be ethically problematic. This section will consider various ethical issues concerning the measurement and monitoring of social isolation and loneliness. The ethical considerations described here pertain not only to research studies examining social isolation and loneliness but also to clinical practice and the implementation of interventions or strategies by health care organizations. This list is not comprehensive, and serious thought should be given to other potential ethical concerns that may arise due to the nature of a specific assessment tool or monitoring program.

Informed Consent

Informed consent is a requisite for all clinical care, beginning with the assessment of the problem and continuing through any provided treatment or intervention (whether social or medical in nature). Adequate informed consent entails ensuring that a patient understands the facts of the medical issue at hand, the implications of choosing to treat or forgo treatment, and the potential risks and benefits of the assessment or treatment. Informed consent enables older adults to weigh the pros and cons of an intervention. Informed consent is ongoing and provides an opportunity for older adults to have a dialogue with their practitioners about the course of their treatment (Price et al., 2012; Reid et al., 2018). Individuals are considered capable of providing consent only if they have adequate reasoning faculties and are in possession of all the relevant facts. It is possible that older adults with cognitive limitations such as dementia or memory loss may not be able to give informed consent, and in this case individuals with proxy status or legally authorized representatives (such as family members or spouses) may be asked to provide consent. In situations when a person is not fully able to make a decision but still not quite at the surrogate decision-making stage, a joint decision-making model can be invoked in which trusted family members or legally authorized representatives or both assist the older adult with the decision-making process, taking into consideration the person's past and present wishes (Galambos et al., 2018; Nuffield Council on Bioethics, 2009). It is important to note, however, that for assessments in health care settings (e.g., questions about smoking and other health care risks), while patients have the option to not answer questions, clinicians would rarely provide informed consent for each question asked.

Autonomy

In addition to issues of informed consent, a variety of bioethical principles relevant to the use of data for the assessment of social isolation or loneliness also need to be considered. Broadly speaking, the concept of autonomy stipulates that individuals have the right to make their own decisions about what entails "living a good life." In medicine specifically, patients are understood to have the right to make decisions regarding what medical care or procedures they accept and the circumstances surrounding that care. Importantly, autonomous decision making is free of outside coercion. In order for a patient to make an autonomous decision, he or she must understand the potential risks and benefits of a given procedure and the likelihood of the procedure's success. Notably, it is possible for individuals to lose the ability to make autonomous decisions if they are suffering from mental or cognitive deficits and are unable to fully grasp the implications of a medical procedure or treatment.

Regarding social isolation and loneliness, as social relationships typically fall outside of the realm of medical care, some individuals may object to the health care system assessing—or "judging"—their relative levels of social isolation or loneliness. For example, respecting an older adult's autonomy may mean respecting a person's choice to live alone or to be alone. In these situations, periodic assessment and monitoring of older adults' social isolation and loneliness may be the approach that is required to respect their living preferences. (See more in Chapter 7.)

Privacy

With the increasing digitalization of information and health records, concerns about medical privacy have become more widespread. Respecting individual privacy entails ensuring that health information is captured and stored in a protected way and that protected health information is not shared without an individual's specific approval. The Privacy Rule, part of the U.S. federal law known as the Health Insurance Portability and Accountability Act (HIPAA), gives individuals rights over their own protected health information and sets rules and limits on who can access and share or receive that information when it is documented in electronic format. Health care staff are required to comply with such regulations when sharing any information in the health record, including any assessment information on social isolation and loneliness. It is also important that older adults be given the opportunity to designate how and with whom their health information should be shared. Once an understanding is reached about information sharing, the necessary permissions and releases should be documented. A periodic review of these sharing preferences should occur and any changes be noted formally.

Individuals experiencing isolation or loneliness may feel embarrassed or uncomfortable acknowledging their isolation to others, and it is possible that individuals might experience stigma after being labeled as "lonely" by a health care provider. Because of this potential harm from stigma, it is extremely important that information about isolation captured in the health record be treated as protected health information. An older adult should be provided the opportunity to determine how and with whom assessment information on social isolation and loneliness is shared. Initial and periodic clarification as to whom older adults select to have access to this information will help ensure that information is shared within the parameters set by the older adult.

Additionally, the way in which patients' data are used in research also falls under HIPAA and other related human-subjects research protections.

Beneficence and Non-Maleficence

The principles of beneficence and non-maleficence are related, though they are not the same. Beneficence requires that medical procedures be provided with the intent of doing good for the patient and serving in the patient's best interest, and it demands that health care providers continuously maintain their own skills and knowledge in order to provide the best treatment for their patients. Non-maleficence refers to making sure that medical procedures and treatments do not harm patients nor others in society (Beauchamp and Childress, 2013). Both are core moral principles that are incorporated into health professions' codes of conduct. When applied in the area of social isolation and loneliness, these principles require knowledge of the adverse risks and benefits associated with the intervention under consideration and with alternative courses of action as well as the risks and benefits of not intervening at all (Bantry-White, 2018; Beauchamp and Childress, 2013; Reid et al., 2018).

Additionally, concerns about the exploitation of individuals suffering from isolation or loneliness must be taken into account when considering possible assessment tools or interventions. It is possible, for instance, that individuals who are isolated are more susceptible to exploitation or abuse (physical, emotional, or financial). It is also possible that certain technologies might exploit lonely or isolated elders, such as robo-calls, phishing emails, or other financial scams. And it is possible that technologies used to identify individuals at risk of isolation or loneliness could be exploited for commercial marketing and monetary gain.

Populations at Risk

Certain populations, such as low-income, minority, and lesbian, gay, bisexual, and transgender elders, may be disproportionately affected by the social determinants of health. It is critical to have assessment tools for social isolation and loneliness that do not further exacerbate inequalities between minority or at-risk groups and the general population. One way to ensure ethical assessment is to implement assessments across entire practice populations, rather than targeting specific subgroups. Focusing on groups of a particular social status may have negative implications for trust in the health care system and could very well be unethical in certain circumstances. In addition, assessing populations more broadly allows for a focus on primary prevention.

As mentioned in the above section on privacy, assessment might involve stigmatizing the conditions of social isolation and loneliness, which is an undesirable outcome for various reasons: individuals may avoid seeking help for social isolation or loneliness if they are embarrassed or ashamed, leading to negative health consequences, and the implementation of assessment for social isolation or loneliness might itself bring about the creation of new, harmful stereotypes. For example, public health campaigns have been successful in reducing the prevalence of smoking in the American population. However, much of this success has to do with shaming individuals who smoke cigarettes. Shaming individuals for health issues that may be out of their control (like social isolation and loneliness) could be extremely harmful.

FINDINGS AND CONCLUSIONS

- The concepts of social isolation and loneliness have been defined in different ways, which has led to variability in how these concepts are measured.
- Picking assessment tools that match the research question or intervention is critical.
- The length of time for follow-up in an intervention is an important part of determining the clinical utility of an outcome.
- The use of standardized and validated measurement tools will help build a more robust evidence base in which results are comparable to other studies.
- Measures developed decades ago may not appropriately account for newer modes of interaction and communication (e.g., social media, instant messaging, video conferencing).
- More effort is needed to update existing measures as well as to develop better instruments for assessing social isolation and loneliness that can fully capture the experience of today's older adults.
- Technological advances such as machine learning, EHRs, and predictive analytics show promise as potential ways to identify social isolation and loneliness.
- A variety of ethical concerns are associated with measuring and assessing an individual's levels of social isolation and loneliness. As further work is done to identify individuals at risk of isolation or loneliness and to identify promising treatments for these conditions, serious consideration should be given to ethical issues that might arise from the use of a specific assessment tool or intervention technique.

7

Role of the Health Care System

As discussed in Chapters 2 and 3, the health consequences of social isolation and loneliness are significant across the age spectrum and worsen as people age. Specifically, as discussed in Chapter 2, data from 148 studies with more than 300,000 participants showed that being socially connected was associated with 50 percent increased odds of survival (Holt-Lunstad et al., 2010). Additionally, as discussed in Chapter 3, a meta-analysis of 23 studies using 16 longitudinal datasets found that poor social relationships (e.g., social isolation, loneliness) increased the risk of developing coronary heart disease and stroke, independently of traditional cardiovascular disease risk factors (Valtorta et al., 2016a). Given the significant evidence for the negative impacts of social isolation and loneliness on the health of older adults, this chapter explores the role of the health care delivery system in identifying and addressing social isolation and loneliness.

Recognition of the role of the health care system in addressing social isolation and loneliness is not new. In 1985 Jones et al. drew attention to the role of physicians in addressing loneliness, noting:

> General practitioners have unique opportunities to reduce the suffering caused by loneliness. The lonely elderly consult their doctors more often (because of their higher degree of physical disability), and so general practitioners are the professional group most likely to come into contact with the lonely person. By listening to lonely patients and gaining their confidence, the doctor can refer them to appropriate bodies such as the social services, voluntary organizations, neighbourhood schemes and local churches. (Jones et al., 1985, p. 139)

BOX 7-1
Key Definitions

Loneliness: the perception of social isolation or the subjective feeling of being lonely.

Mediators: also known as mechanisms or pathways; the factors that help explain how social isolation or loneliness affects health outcomes.

Moderators: the factors that can influence the magnitude or direction of the effect of social isolation or loneliness on health.

Social connection: an umbrella term that encompasses the structural, functional, and quality aspects of how individuals connect to each other.

Social isolation: the objective lack of (or limited) social contact with others.

Social support: the actual or perceived availability of resources (e.g., informational, tangible, emotional) from others, typically one's social network.

In 2018, Helen Stokes-Lampard, the chair of the Royal College of General Practitioners in the United Kingdom, expressed the following to this committee:

> I know as a clinician and as a physician that I cannot solve the problems of my patients' lives with respect to their social challenges, but if I identify them, if I recognize that those problems are impacting adversely on health, then it is my responsibility to call that out, to signpost people to help.

Given the complexity of the terminology used in relation to social isolation and loneliness, a reminder of key definitions is provided in Box 7-1.

HEALTH CARE ACCESS AND UTILIZATION

Older adults are particularly high-volume and high-frequency users of the health care system, especially as compared with younger groups. The 2008 Institute of Medicine (IOM) report *Retooling for an Aging America: Building the Health Care Workforce* found that adults over age 65 use a disproportionate number of health care services, stating

> Although older adults make up only about 12 percent of the U.S. population, they account for approximately 26 percent of all physician office visits, 47 percent of all hospital outpatient visits with nurse practitioners, 35 percent of all

> hospital stays, 34 percent of all prescriptions, 38 percent of all emergency medical service responses, and 90 percent of all nursing-home use. (IOM, 2008, pp. 3–4)

Research on the impact of social isolation and loneliness on health care utilization and access is limited, and it has had mixed results. While the available research indicates that social isolation and loneliness among adults lead to a heightened focus on utilization, few studies have examined access issues for older adults who are isolated or lonely. Extensive research has been conducted in countries outside the United States, including Australia, Ireland, New Zealand, and the United Kingdom. These studies can be used as a foundation to inform what we know about how social isolation and loneliness affect access and utilization. However, the U.S. health care delivery system is very different from those of other countries, so it is necessary to conduct research within the United States in order to elucidate issues of particular concern to the U.S. health care system. As noted previously in this report, the existing evidence base shows that a variety of indicators are used to evaluate social isolation and loneliness, including the strength of an individual's relationships and social networks, a person's living arrangements, and a person's psychosocial functioning. Similarly, health care utilization is often determined differently in different studies, with readmission rates, length of hospital stay, number of hospitalizations, the use of outpatient services, and primary care visits being examined in various studies. Furthermore, some types of increases in utilization are desirable (e.g., preventive care) while other types of increases in utilization (e.g., hospital readmissions) are not desirable.

Evidence of Increased Utilization

Social relationships are one of many factors that affect health care utilization. Social isolation and loneliness have been found to be associated with an increased rate of hospital readmissions, perhaps as a result of the individual having a smaller social support network to contact when health care issues emerge (Hawker and Romero-Ortuno, 2016; Valtorta et al., 2018b). A similar finding was noted in a study of older American veterans enrolled in a psychogeriatric program (Mistry et al., 2001). However, other evidence suggests a higher number of previous hospitalizations among those with larger family networks (Ha et al., 2019). Social isolation and loneliness have also been associated with increased hospitalizations among older adults and older veterans (Gerst-Emerson and Jayawardhana, 2015; Greysen et al., 2013; Jakobsson et al., 2011), and social isolation has been linked to an increase in Medicare spending, primarily on costs associated with inpatient care and skilled nursing facility care (Flowers et al., 2017; Shaw et al., 2017). However, these spending patterns changed when adjusted for socioeconomic and health status. Despite the increased use of health care, these individuals experiencing social isolation and loneliness are more vulnerable to adverse outcomes and are a greater risk of death (Shaw et al., 2017).

Older adults who have been identified as being at risk for social isolation and loneliness experience longer length of stays when hospitalized (Hawker and Romero-Ortuno, 2016; Mitchinson et al., 2008; Valtorta et al., 2018b), which may be due to having smaller social networks and less social support to provide post-hospitalization care (Mitchinson et al., 2008; Valtorta et al., 2018b). Chronic loneliness is also positively associated with increased physician visits, with the physician–patient relationship providing both social support and medical treatment (Gerst-Emerson and Jayawardhana, 2015). In behavioral health settings, adults (not limited to older adults) living with family make greater use of rehabilitative and social care services, including day care, rehabilitation, socialization, and work-related activities; by contrast, those living alone have a higher number of home visits (Donisi et al., 2013). In one study of veterans enrolled in a psychogeriatric program, the veterans with higher social connections reported increased access to services (Mistry et al., 2001). Living with others and having a stronger social system may serve as a motivator to participate in health care services.

Evidence of No Impact on Utilization

Some studies have found that having fewer social supports has limited to no impact on health care utilization by older adults. In one study, older patients with weaker social relationships did not place greater demands on ambulatory care (as defined by physician visits and community- or home-based services) (Valtorta et al., 2018b). In addition, social isolation (as measured by living alone) was not a predictor of potentially preventable readmissions to hospitals (LaWall et al., 2019). Flowers and colleagues (2017, p. 5) found "no difference in outpatient use or spending for socially isolated Medicare beneficiaries." Living alone may actually provide some protective health factors, and having such a living arrangement may be an indicator of a person's level of independence or personal preferences.

Evidence of Decreased Utilization

There is limited evidence indicating a decrease in health care utilization by those older adults who are socially isolated and lonely. In particular, there is some evidence for a lower use of preventive health services (an undesirable decrease in usage), including mammograms, dental visits, immunizations, colonoscopy, general practitioner visits, and an exercise program for joint pain (Vozikaki et al., 2017). Loneliness has been linked to lower Medicare spending when adjusted for health status (Shaw et al., 2017). However, these examples of decreased usage could be a reflection of fewer supports and resources being available to enable such individuals to access outpatient and preventative services.

Concerning prevention, a connection exists between an individual's level of physical activity and his or her use of health care. Engagement in a physical activity program was found to be associated with fewer emergency room visits and hospital visits (Jacobs et al., 2013). In that study, participants who became more active were more likely to be male with higher self-reported health and functional independence and reduced rates of loneliness. Engagement in physical activity programs, while beneficial, may be more challenging for older adults who have chronic health conditions and more functional impairments and who are at risk for loneliness. (See Chapter 9 for more on physical activity programs as an intervention for social isolation and loneliness.)

Primary Care and Utilization

As discussed above, social isolation and loneliness affect the quantity and type of health care services used by older adults. Among community-dwelling older adults in the United States aged 60 and older, one study found that chronic loneliness (defined as being lonely at two points of time over 4 years) was a predictor of an increased number of both physician visits and hospital visits; the correlation was independent of sociodemographic variables, subjective and objective health measures, depressive symptoms, insurance status, and financial situation (Gerst-Emerson and Jayawardhana, 2015). Reporting feelings of chronic loneliness and having higher rates of health care utilization were associated with a variety of factors, including depressive symptoms, being married, having difficulty with activities of daily living (e.g., bathing, toileting, dressing), having a higher number of chronic conditions, and having at least a high school or GED-level of education (Gerst-Emerson and Jayawardhana, 2015).

These examples suggest that individuals living with social isolation or loneliness are more likely to use outpatient, emergency department, and inpatient services. However, there is no evidence that these individuals will isolate themselves from the benefits of primary care, and, in fact, loneliness is associated with increased visits to the physician's office (Gerst-Emerson and Jayawardhana, 2015). Comprehensive and advanced primary care settings serving older adults are well suited to the task of caring for individuals living with social isolation and loneliness and could ultimately help link these individuals to effective interventions.

For example, a collaborative of practice-based networks in Colorado and Virginia assessed the prevalence of loneliness and associated characteristics and behaviors through a survey of registered adult patients presenting for routine primary care (Mullen et al., 2019). The prevalence of loneliness for individuals 65 years and older screened during the study period was 11 percent. As had been found in other studies, loneliness was associated with an increase in health care utilization across outpatient, emergency department, and inpatient settings and also with poorer health status. The study found no evidence that loneliness was associated with individuals isolating themselves from primary care. The authors concluded that "the primary care setting has the potential to identify solutions and implement interventions" (Mullen et al., 2019, p. 113).

Long-Term Care Settings and Utilization

The literature on utilization related to social isolation and loneliness among older adults in long-term care (LTC) settings is scant. One study of data from the National Study of Caregiving and the National Health and Aging Trends Study demonstrated that a sense of community engagement was a significant predictor of likelihood of older adults remaining in the community (Moon et al., 2018). Flowers and colleagues (2017, p. 5) found that "socially isolated individuals were 29 percent more likely to use [skilled nursing facility (SNF)] care and their monthly SNF costs were $75 higher on average." The authors suggested one explanation, being that these individuals may lack adequate support following a hospital stay, and therefore require higher use of SNFs for rehabilitation. Shaw and colleagues (2017) similarly found that social isolated individuals used more SNF care. They noted that "future study of social isolation in managed care and nursing home populations is warranted" (p. 13).

Data from other countries also suggest that social connection affects utilization in LTC settings. Godin and colleagues (2019) examined "the association between social vulnerability and the odds of [LTC] placement within 30 days of discharge following admission to an acute care facility" (p. 1) among patients with acute respiratory illness admitted to hospitals in Canada. The authors created a social vulnerability index, which included attention to social support, living situation, and social engagement, among other factors. They found that

> at younger ages (e.g., 70 years), social vulnerability was associated with lower odds of LTC placement for those who were the frailest, while at older ages (e.g., 90 years), social vulnerability was associated with increased odds of LTC placement in those adults who were non-frail or only mildly frail but did not impact odds of LTC placement among the frailest participants. (Godwin et al., 2019, p. 9)

Another Canadian study of residents of assisted living facilities showed that those with poor social relationships had a significantly increased risk for placement in a nursing home (Maxwell et al., 2013). Data from the English Longitudinal Study of Ageing showed that loneliness predicts LTC admission, independent of functional status (Hanratty et al., 2018).

Factors Associated with Access

A limited number of studies have examined access to health care and its relationship with social isolation and loneliness. A lack of transportation resources limits one's ability to get to medical appointments, for instance, and living in remote areas limits an individual's social networks and other resources, including rural health services (Hadley Strout et al., 2016; King and Dabelko-Schoeny, 2009). Moreover, for lesbian, gay, and bisexual older adults, living in rural communities has been found to reduce social networks (King and Dabelko-Schoeny, 2009). As people experience functional declines and adverse health events, access to resources is further compromised by increased isolation (King and Dabelko-Schoeny, 2009).

Having better and more robust social networks makes it more likely that individuals will make greater use of health and social services, as demonstrated in the Village model, a consumer-driven housing model for aging in place in which the coordination of needed health and social services is provided by the residents and delivered within these communities (Graham et al., 2014). Greater access to services, including to health care, was associated with the use of companion resources (e.g., friendly visiting, check-in calls), volunteer involvement, and attending social activities. However, the benefits were lessened for those who had worse self-reported health. As noted earlier, Ha and colleagues (2019) found that those with larger family networks are likely to have had a higher number of previous hospitalizations. In these cases, family served as the primary source of support during times of medical need and provided more people to call on to access care.

Summary of the Evidence on Access and Utilization

The results of studies of the impact of social isolation and loneliness on health care access and utilization are mixed, with the evidence suggesting an association between loneliness and an increased use of inpatient care, more doctor's visits, increased re-hospitalizations, and longer length of stays. Persons with larger social networks tend to rely more on outpatient services (as opposed to inpatient stays) than those with smaller networks. Physical functioning and health status are linked with both social isolation and loneliness. Older adults who are higher functioning and have higher perceived health status have more options to be socially connected. The oldest of the older adults appear to have fewer options for social connection, thus placing them at greater risk. Furthermore, most of the research examines utilization at the systems level, not at the level of the individual, and therefore individual characteristics (such as the impact of comorbidities like depression) are not the focus of the analysis. Issues of access such as transportation, geographical location, and socioeconomic status all contribute to an individual's risk for social isolation and loneliness.

SOCIAL DETERMINANTS OF HEALTH AND THE HEALTH CARE SYSTEM

Targeting the major social and behavioral risk factors for health offers a way to improve population health and even reduce health disparities. Healthy People,[1] a program of the U.S. Department of Health and Human Services,

[1] For more information, see HealthyPeople.gov.

"provides science-based, 10-year national objectives for improving the health of all Americans" (HHS, 2019a). The program establishes benchmarks and monitors progress in order to:

- Encourage collaborations across communities and sectors,
- Empower individuals toward making informed health decisions, and
- Measure the impact of prevention activities (HHS, 2019a).

Addressing the social determinants of health is a priority in the *Healthy People 2020* agenda (HHS, 2019b). Social cohesion is noted as a key issue within the determinant area of social and community context and social support.

On a macro level, public health and managed care organizations affect large populations of older adults through policy and programs (e.g., the fully integrated Medicare and Medicaid special needs plans). These health plans are structured to take a holistic and comprehensive approach to addressing the social determinants of health. For example, one of the social risk factors observed most frequently by those in the Care Wisconsin program was limited social supports (Fouad et al., 2017). Gottlieb et al. (2016) assessed the efforts of 25 geographically dispersed Medicaid managed care organizations (MMCOs) that designed programs to address the social needs of beneficiaries. The authors suggest that one way to address the non-medical factors related to health is to design programs that are integrated into clinical settings. However, the authors found that MMCOs are "not yet systematically engaged in comprehensive [social determinants of health] strategies to improve health or change health care utilization patterns" (Gottlieb et al., 2016, p. 374).

On an individual level, older adults in the United States will ideally experience first-contact care that is comprehensive, continuous, and coordinated through the primary care experience. Comprehensive and advanced primary care delivers significantly more high-value care and better health care access and experience than typical primary care without significantly altering the overall volume of outpatient, emergency department, or inpatient visits (Levine et al., 2019). Newer models of primary care have built on this success. A 3-year primary care medical home intervention, which included a shared savings initiative that created incentives for specific structural transformation, resulted in statistically significant improvements in performance on selected quality measures in all-cause and ambulatory care–sensitive emergency department visits as well as a reduced use of specialty care and higher rates of ambulatory primary care visits (Friedberg et al., 2015). Comprehensive primary care delivered to Medicare beneficiaries aged 65 years or older has been shown to be associated with fewer emergency department and hospital admissions as well as lower Medicare expenditures per beneficiary per month (Bazemore et al., 2015; O'Malley et al., 2019). Assessing the social determinants of health (including social isolation and loneliness) is key to comprehensive primary care.

Primary Care and Assessment of Social Determinants of Health

Many health care delivery systems are exploring the feasibility and impact of practice-based strategies to identify and address such social determinants of health as social isolation and loneliness. The 2019 National Academies consensus study report *Integrating Social Care into the Delivery of Health Care* noted that "patients visiting health care organizations are increasingly being asked to answer social risk screening questions in the context of their care and care planning" (NASEM, 2019, p. 38). However, the study also notes that collecting data on social determinants of health in the health care setting "may be affected by unconscious or implicit biases held by program leaders and practitioners" (NASEM, 2019, p. 38).

When Tong and colleagues (2018) evaluated the experience of clinicians conducting assessments for social needs (e.g., transportation, food access, housing, social connections), they found three themes that were associated with positive outcomes:

1. knowing the patient better,
2. understanding the patient's social circumstances, and
3. addressing self-management through such steps as exercise and dietary counseling, addressing financial barriers to medications, and helping with transportation.

However, the process of screening was labor intensive, and the yield varied by how well the clinician knew the patient over time and the willingness of patients to discuss their social needs. The individuals in a practice who may need such assistance most may be the least likely to come in for assessment. Furthermore, if needs are found, connecting patients to resources in the community is difficult.

Tong and colleagues (2018) took a targeted approach to the clinician screening of a subset of registered patients who resided in a geographic region likely to predispose those living there to having social needs. In this study, 57 percent of the targeted cohort visited the practice during the study period and agreed to screening. Of these, more than 70 percent reported at least one social need, yet only 3 percent of those individuals accepted assistance with meeting that need. The authors suggest that the limited number of individuals who were willing to receive help may represent a manageable first step for primary care clinicians who may be otherwise overwhelmed by the volume and prevalence of social needs within the population of patients served by their practice. However, because the approach only addresses those who are willing to participate in an intervention, additional consideration is needed concerning how to address those who are in most need of intervention but who may not initially be willing to participate.

Adding assessments of the social determinants of health to busy health care practices may be considered a burden. In the United Kingdom, Walters et al. (2017) studied the feasibility of embedding a health and social risk appraisal tool into the electronic health records (EHRs) of five English National Health Service primary care practices. The Well-Being Interventions for Social and Health study assessed 454 community-dwelling people aged 65 and older. The fact that the "already burdened" practices were interested in implementing the tool and willing to implement it universally was a positive finding. However, Walters and colleagues (2017) expressed concern that the subset of patients who completed the case-finding tool may not be representative of the needs of the entire population served. They concluded that a practice-based case-finding approach may limit access to services for the high-risk populations who need them, such as the poor, severely ill, and homebound. Furthermore, in a study of strategies for collecting data on the social determinants of health for the EHR, "clinicians did not want to collect [social determinants of health] data themselves, preferring to transfer that responsibility to another team member" (Gold et al., 2017, p. 6). Concerns were also raised about the impact on workflow.

Researchers are considering how informatics might be used to make social determinants of health data collected in the EHR accessible, the use of implementation science to address program development and deployment, and natural language processing to identify information related to the social determinants of health, such as an individual patient experiencing social isolation, in clinical notes (Bazemore et al., 2018; Hripcsak et al., 2015; Zhu et al., 2019). (See later in this chapter for more on the EHR.)

The following sections highlight the general opportunities and challenges related to the clinical assessment of social isolation and loneliness.

CLINICAL ASSESSMENT OF SOCIAL ISOLATION AND LONELINESS

The evidence strongly indicates that social isolation and loneliness affect health. Because of this, the health care sector has a role to play in identifying individuals at risk for, or already experiencing, social isolation and loneliness in order to mitigate the health consequences. However, clarity is needed about whether the best approach is a formal screening process or identification of these issues within the patient population. The differences between screening and identification and why the committee chose to highlight these differences are discussed below.

General Principles of Screening

The National Institutes of Health suggests that screening tests can help detect conditions or illnesses early in an illness course or before symptoms are apparent (NIH, 2017). The purpose of such screening is thus to decrease the risks of certain illnesses, their complications, and their related mortality. Other definitions of screening are:

> Screening is the process of identifying healthy people who may have an increased chance of a disease or condition. The screening provider then offers information, further tests, and treatment. This is to reduce associated risks or complications. (Public Health England, 2019)

> Screening refers to the use of simple tests across a healthy population in order to identify individuals who have disease, but do not yet have symptoms. (WHO, 2019a)

However, all tests have associated risks and benefits, and the determination of when a screening test is warranted is a source of much debate. The U.S. Preventive Services Task Force reviews the evidence and makes recommendations about whether a particular screening test has sufficient support to be widely adopted into clinical practice.[2] The task force focuses on primary prevention (i.e., when there are no symptoms or signs of the illness or behavior). To date, the majority of screening recommendations by the task force have focused on disease-specific or medication-specific concerns. There are few, if any, categories of screening that relate to the social determinants of health in general or certainly for social isolation and loneliness specifically. Thus, there are currently no recommendations for screening for social isolation and loneliness at a national level.

Ultimately, the basic concept underlying screening is that the early detection of risk factors or of early disease will result in better clinical or public health outcomes. See Box 7-2 for criteria commonly used to determine if screening is warranted.

Screening Versus Assessment for Social Isolation and Loneliness

Loneliness and social isolation have high prevalence rates in adults over age 60 (see Chapter 1) and have been linked to significant health consequences and increased mortality risk (see Chapters 2 and 3), which indicates that it might be valuable to have a national standard or recommendation for screening for social isolation or loneliness. Ultimately, however, the value of such a standard or recommendation will depend on several factors, not just the prevalence and health consequences of social isolation and loneliness, but also whether there is a potential treatment or way to mitigate risks in such situations as well as the potential risks of screening and its possible unintended consequences (Garg et al., 2016). Several elements of the Wilson and Jungner criteria (see Box 7-2) support screening for social isolation or loneliness. However, at present there is a lack

[2] For more information, see https://www.uspreventiveservicestaskforce.org/Page/Name/about-the-uspstf (accessed December 16, 2019).

BOX 7-2
Wilson and Jungner Classic Screening Criteria

- The condition sought should be an important health problem.
- There should be an accepted treatment for patients with recognized disease.
- Facilities for diagnosis and treatment should be available.
- There should be a recognizable latent or early symptomatic stage.
- There should be a suitable test or examination.
- The test should be acceptable to the population.
- The natural history of the condition, including the development from latent to declared disease, should be adequately understood.
- There should be an agreed-upon policy on whom to treat as patients.
- The cost of case finding (including diagnosis and treatment of patients diagnosed) should be economically balanced in relation to possible expenditure on medical care as a whole.
- Case finding should be a continuing process and not a "once and for all" project.

SOURCE: Wilson and Jungner, 1968.

of the sorts of policies and data needed to guide clinicians in making decisions about specific treatments or interventions (see Chapter 9). Furthermore, a review of the existing literature finds no high-quality studies demonstrating that social isolation and loneliness can be prevented through primary prevention, although there are some promising secondary and tertiary prevention areas of research (see Chapter 9). Because of the paucity of literature on successful interventions for specific populations, it is difficult to conclude that formal screening protocols for social isolation and loneliness could reduce prevalence rates or negative health consequences. Yet, because of the high prevalence rates and broad-reaching health effects, the committee concludes that the health care system is well poised to develop methods and processes for identifying social isolation and loneliness in health care settings, even if the methods do not rely on a formal screening protocol. As such, the committee concludes that it is more appropriate to talk about the *identification* of loneliness and isolation as risk factors for health consequences rather than about how to *screen* for social isolation and loneliness.

Specific Concerns for Clinical Assessments

Similar to the concerns about clinician burden that were raised earlier in this chapter, some people have voiced concerns that charging health care providers with identifying social isolation and loneliness or their risk factors among patients may create a burden by asking providers to identify social problems that cannot be readily fixed. However, a recent study examining clinician burnout demonstrated that when clinicians felt they had the needed support to address problems such as social isolation, burnout rates were actually lower (De Marchis et al., 2019a).

As the health care delivery system mobilizes to incorporate assessments and, as the research develops, to integrate interventions for the social determinants of health, some researchers are cautioning that not all patients may view primary care interventions of this type as positive. Kharicha and colleagues (2017) found that individuals identified as lonely often did not perceive primary care and community interventions as desirable or helpful and that they perceived a stigma in being labeled as lonely. In particular, many participants did not see loneliness as an illness and therefore did not see a role for primary care physicians, whom they perceived as not being able to help with non-physical problems. "For many, loneliness was a complex and private matter that they wished to manage without external support" (Kharicha et al., 2017, p. 1733). However, another study found that a strong majority of adults reported screening for (or, in the committee's preferred language, identification of) risk to be appropriate; as such, a fear of stigmatization should not necessarily be considered as a barrier to implementation (De Marchis, 2019b).

Assessment Tools

Chapter 6 describes many of the tools used in research settings to measure social isolation or loneliness. Unfortunately, few if any implementation studies examine how to use these tools in clinical settings or define which are the most favorable tools to use in specific settings or populations. The committee suggests that a logical approach would be to consider how and why the tool is being used. For example, in health care encounters if clinicians are seeking to determine how to improve health care outcomes or how to reduce the risk of negative health care outcomes, it may be necessary to identify both social isolation and loneliness. In order to compare certain groups (e.g., by age or high-risk attribute), defining the target population (i.e., those who are isolated versus those who are lonely) will help determine what demographic factors underlie the context for their social isolation or loneliness. Another aspect of choosing the best tool is having a framework or theory of change. For example, is the intervention intended to decrease loneliness, to decrease social isolation, or both? Answering this question will help determine whether to use questions related to social isolation, loneliness, or other composite measures.

Implementing Assessment Tools

Despite the limited data on implementation, when health care providers are adapting or selecting research tools for clinical settings they can consider various general factors that are important to the successful implementation of an identification tool. These include the amount of training required to administer the tool; whether a tool can be administered by clinicians and, potentially, ancillary staff and other clinical team members; the time required to administer the tool; and the tool's availability and validation in other languages. Using this framework and working with the available evidence, the committee concluded that the existing tools likely to have the greatest success in clinical settings are the Berkman–Syme Social Network Index (for measuring social isolation) and the three-item UCLA Loneliness Scale (for measuring loneliness). (See Chapter 6 for descriptions of these measures.) No composite measurement tools have been designed specifically to measure the overarching rubric of social connection (although some may approximate this). The three-item UCLA Loneliness Scale alone does not get into the details of the quantification of isolation; similarly, the Berkman–Syme does not delve into the subjectivity of loneliness.

As noted in Chapter 6, concerns exist regarding the relevance of current tools, and particularly as to whether the measures developed years or decades ago can fully capture the expectations and values of older adults today. This is likely to be especially relevant for measures of social isolation as modes of interaction and social preferences have changed significantly in recent years and decades. Some have suggested using "living alone" as a proxy measure for social isolation and loneliness. However, as living alone may be a distinct or even positive experience, particularly for those who choose to live alone, and as it does not necessarily capture the distress of loneliness, this question by itself may not be sufficient to fully capture the health risks or the entire context of those experiencing social isolation or loneliness. Similarly, the Berkman–Syme measure, for example, has a single question that focuses specifically on religiosity and participation in religious group activities, which may create a bias against those who do not participate in religious groups but do participate in other social activities with equal benefit. Furthermore, the Berkman–Syme measure also only asks about "telephone use," which may not account for other modes of communication in today's society such as texting and video calling. Another drawback of many of these tools is their limited testing and availability in other languages.

Predictive Analytics

Advances in health technologies, including the digitization of medical records, has resulted in vast amounts of data from both "formal" sources, such as clinical tests and imaging, and "informal" sources, such as wearable consumer devices and health-tracking applications in smartphones. This explosion of population-level data, coupled with an emphasis on evidence-based medicine, has led to increasing investment in predictive analytics in health care. These technologies include machine learning and statistical risk scoring and have been widely used to enable better decision making and support preventive care (Wang et al., 2018). (See Chapter 6 for more on the use of these technologies to identify social isolation and loneliness.)

Data for predictive analytics can be gathered from a variety of sources, including various types of information captured in the EHR, such as visit patterns, medications, and patient portal messages; retail activity such as prescriptions filled or over-the-counter medications purchased; social media and internet usage, including search history data;[3] and physical activity monitors such as wearable sensors and other consumer health devices. Other sources of data that may be of use for predictive analytics are information captured in files maintained in social service agencies and, in the future, outcomes data from the widespread implementation of assessment tools for social isolation and loneliness and for potentially precipitating life events (Weissman et al., 2020).

Additional Implementation Needs for Clinical Assessment

In addition to selecting the right tools for the valid clinical assessment of social isolation and loneliness, it is also necessary to determine:

- who should receive the assessment (i.e., everyone or just those most at risk),
- who should conduct the assessment,
- the ideal frequency of assessment for different subpopulations, and
- the appropriate interventions, referrals, and follow-up care.

When social isolation or loneliness are identified, it may be appropriate to assess for other potential co-existing conditions (e.g., depression, safety concerns, cognitive impairment) and to engage in advanced care planning, particularly if the individual has no friends. That is, advanced care planning may be needed in situations in which the individual is not capable of making his or her own medical decisions but has no surrogates to make those choices. In addition, follow-up will be needed to determine the severity and the individual's response to any potential interventions or resources provided. This may be done at the next clinical encounter. No literature currently delves into the appropriate frequency of measurement, but following more established models (e.g., depression screening) may be a reasonable comparison. Also, the initiation of an intervention may depend heavily on the individual's willingness to participate in such an intervention (as is true for many issues of health care and adherence to treatment). Finally, it is critical for health care systems to maintain these assessments in easily identifiable locations

[3] A recent study of the Google search histories of those admitted into the emergency department found in the week leading up to admission, more than 50 percent of those patients searched for information about their symptoms or nearby hospitals (Asch et al., 2019).

in the EHR. (See the next section for more on documentation of social isolation and loneliness in the EHR.)

TECHNOLOGY AS INFRASTRUCTURE FOR COORDINATION AND INTERVENTION

The IOM Committee on the Recommended Social and Behavioral Domains and Measures for Electronic Health Records was commissioned "to identify domains and measures that capture the social determinants of health to inform the development of recommendations for Stage 3 meaningful use of electronic health records" (IOM, 2014, p. 5). EHRs facilitate the systematic implementation of evidence-based interventions in clinical practice. Large-scale EHR products include modules for tracking the social determinants of health. Features can be customized within the modules, which also include functions for facilitating follow-up and linking to community agencies.

The IOM committee issued its reports in two phases: first, an identification of domains and criteria for inclusion and, second, specific measures in each domain along with issues and opportunities related to the implementation of the measures. The criteria for domain selection included

1. strength of the evidence associating the domain with health;
2. usefulness of the domain for decision making, monitoring, and research;
3. availability of standardized measures;
4. feasibility of using the measures in a clinical setting;
5. sensitivity of personal information; and
6. accessibility of data from other sources.

The domains selected include (1) sociodemographic, (2) psychological, (3) behavioral, (4) social relationships, and (5) neighborhoods and communities. The domain "social connections and social isolation" was described as an item not routinely collected in clinical settings but nonetheless a crucial domain for inclusion, with the evidence supporting its inclusion equivalent to the evidence supporting the inclusion of race, education, physical activity, tobacco use, and neighborhood characteristics.

The measures recommended in the Phase 2 report (IOM, 2014) are included in Table 7-1. Importantly, the committee concluded that the Berkman–Syme Social Network Index could be adopted into EHRs (IOM, 2014). The inclusion of this information in the EHR may vary according to clinical setting (e.g., primary care, inpatient, emergency department), and decisions about its use in EHRs will need to take into account the purpose of the information, how it is used, how to track it over time, and how to ensure it is easily viewable and extractable. Some EHRs have modules for the social determinants of health that enable structured documentation and presentation of the data. Additional options for

TABLE 7-1 Recommended Domains and Measures from the Institute of Medicine Committee on the Recommended Social and Behavioral Domains and Measures for Electronic Health Records

Domain/Measure	Measure	Frequency
Alcohol use	3 questions	Screen and follow-up
Race and ethnicity	2 questions	At entry
Residential address	1 question (geocoded)	Verify every visit
Tobacco use	2 questions	Screen and follow-up
Census tract-median income	1 question (geocoded)	Update on address change
Depression	2 questions	Screen and follow-up
Education	2 questions	At entry
Financial resource strain	1 question	Screen and follow-up
Intimate partner violence	4 questions	Screen and follow-up
Physical activity	2 questions	Screen and follow-up
Social connections and social isolation	4 questions	Screen and follow-up
Stress	1 question	Screen and follow-up

NOTE: Domains/measures are listed in alphabetical order; domains/measures in the shaded area are currently frequently collected in clinical settings; domains/measures not in the shaded area are additional items not routinely collected in clinical settings.
SOURCE: Adapted from IOM, 2014.

locations to capture these data in the EHR include the history review, the review of systems, or "flowsheets" or "questionnaires" that are already seamlessly incorporated into intake workflows. In order to highlight the clinical significance of loneliness and social isolation in the EHR, a best practice includes adding loneliness or social isolation to problem lists with their corresponding *International Classification of Diseases, Tenth Revision* (ICD-10) codes.

The IOM committee's report outlined several potential implementation issues related to the general capture, storage, and use of data that are self-reported or externally sourced (e.g., from community agencies or national surveys). The concerns discussed in the report included privacy, data quality, and the burden imposed on clinicians by incorporating additional data collection into the clinical workflow. The report had a pragmatic emphasis on choices that enable action in clinical settings, but it stopped short of making recommendations related to the communication and coordination infrastructure (e.g., between medical and community-based service providers) that would be needed to implement interventions to address issues related to social determinants for individual patients or groups.

This infrastructure issue was subsequently taken up by the Robert Wood Johnson Foundation's (RWJF's) report *Using Social Determinants of Health Data to Improve Health Care and Health: A Learning Report* (DeMilto and Nakashian, 2016). This report identified four key barriers to the widespread use of social determinants of health data for improving health:

1. lack of knowledge and consensus on measures,
2. resource and power differences between social services and health care organizations,
3. lack of effective multi-sector collaboration, and
4. rigid technology systems.

The RWJF report argues for sharing data across sectors and suggests that EHRs may not be the right tool for this purpose. Research has shown that effective coordination among community agencies, including health care organizations, requires not only an information architecture, but also a process for maintaining a social connection among the agencies (DeMilto and Nakashian, 2016).

While information systems and other digital tools provide a platform to facilitate the assessment and documentation of social isolation and loneliness and, ultimately, to inform action at an organizational level, there are many well-documented challenges related to the use of information technology infrastructure. A number of these challengers were identified by the National Academies consensus study report *Integrating Social Care into the Delivery of Health Care*, including varying degrees of access to digital infrastructure, a lack of data standards and interoperability, and privacy and security considerations (NASEM, 2019).

The key challenge in implementing effective interventions is linking the information to actions such as outreach, intervention, and follow-up (see Figure 7-1). This requires the following:

1. Incorporating assessment data into clinical workflow.
2. Establishing evidence-based clinical decision-support protocols for action that are based on assessment findings.
3. At the local level, establishing an infrastructure for connections with community resources.
4. Using the infrastructure for communication with other clinical providers to support patients transitioning among clinical settings, including secure electronic messaging that protects patient privacy when available.
5. Communicating with patients via patient portals and personal health records when available.

Between 2016 and 2018 Kaiser Permanente Northwest (KPNW) used a combination of EHR capabilities and patient navigators to screen more than 11,000 patients for the social determinants of health. The aim of this KPNW initiative was to better understand the connections needed to address patients' non-clinical needs and to understand the impact on health outcomes of meeting those needs

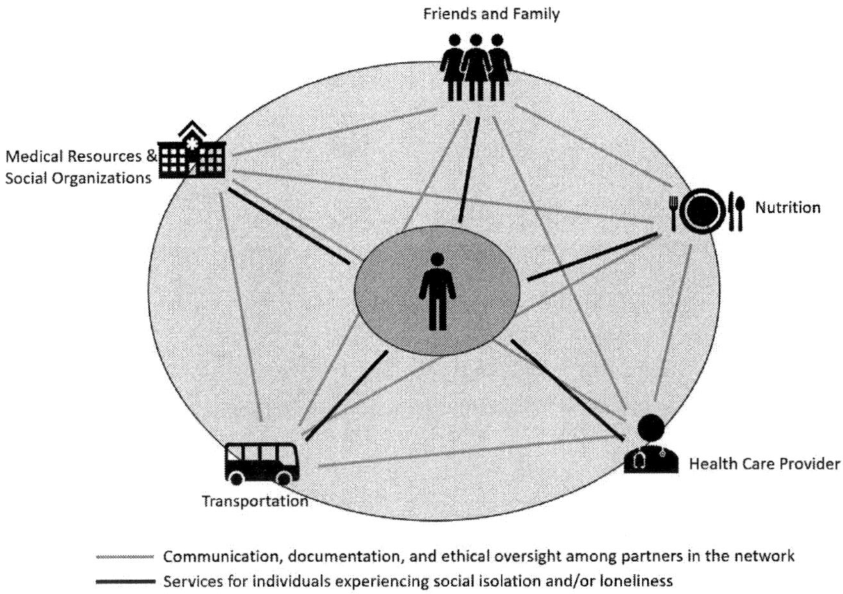

FIGURE 7-1 Sustained intervention for social isolation and loneliness depends on a social and technological infrastructure for coordinated action.

(Friedman and Banegas, 2018). In a parallel process, OCHIN, Inc., a nonprofit health care innovation center in Oregon, reported on the process that was used and the lessons that were learned through the implementation of a social determinants of health screening tool across a network of more than 400 federally qualified health centers in the KPNW region, taking advantage of the KPNW tool's social isolation domain and questions (Gold et al., 2017). Researchers identified several considerations for using the tool, including striking a balance between standardized data collection and the need to adapt to local context, identifying patients who do not want assistance, determining a method for updating lists of local resources and referrals, and accommodating different staffing structures.

FINDINGS AND CONCLUSIONS

- Evidence strongly indicates that social isolation and loneliness have an adverse impact on health. Therefore, the health care sector should play a role in identifying individuals at risk for, or already experiencing, social isolation and loneliness in order to mitigate their health consequences.
- Evidence suggests an association between loneliness and increased use of inpatient care, more health care provider visits, increased re-hospitalizations, and longer length of stays.

- Access to services is influenced by factors such as transportation, geographical location, and socioeconomic status, all of which may be associated with social isolation and loneliness.
- The health care system is well poised to develop and evaluate methods and processes to identify social isolation and loneliness in health care settings.
- It is more appropriate to consider and plan for the *identification* of loneliness and social isolation as risk factors for health consequences than to consider how to *screen* for social isolation and loneliness.
- The current identification tools most likely to be successfully implemented in clinical settings are the Berkman–Syme (for measuring social isolation) and the three-item UCLA Loneliness Scale (for measuring loneliness).
- More effort is needed to update existing measures as well as to develop better instruments for assessing social isolation and loneliness in clinical settings that can fully capture the experience of today's older adults.
- A key aspect of selecting a tool for use in clinical settings is standardization within a specific organization so that everyone within the organization uses the same tool or set of tools rather than resorting to different tools, everyone uses validated tools, and everyone refrains from using only parts of existing tools or creating a new, unvalidated tool.
- Advances in health technologies, increases in data collection, and an emphasis on the use of evidence-based medicine have led to the application of predictive analytics to various health concerns. Predictive analytics may also be of value for identifying individuals at risk for social isolation and loneliness.

NEXT STEPS AND RECOMMENDATIONS

Chapters 2 and 3 show the strength of the evidence for the mortality and morbidity impacts of social isolation and loneliness on older adults. As such, the committee concludes that the health care system has an important role to play in the identification in clinical settings of social isolation and loneliness in older adults. In fact, a single interaction with the health care system may represent the only touchpoint for the most isolated and lonely older adults. For example, a home health worker may provide the only face-to-face interaction for an older adult who is housebound, has no family, and does not belong to a religious institution or social group.

However, no single clinical indicator (or measure) serves as a marker for the presence or risk of social isolation or loneliness. Because of the scarcity of literature on effective interventions (see Chapter 9), it is premature to conclude that formal screening for social isolation and loneliness could reduce prevalence rates or negative health consequences. Yet, because of the high prevalence rates (see Chapter 1) and extensive health effects (see Chapters 2 and 3) of social isolation and loneliness, the committee concludes that the health care system is well poised to begin the process of developing methods to identify social isolation and loneliness in health care settings, even if providers are not using a traditional screening approach. By first identifying those at highest risk, and potentially whether their social isolation or loneliness is acute or chronic, clinicians and health care researchers may be able to use these findings to target appropriate clinical and public health interventions to individual patients as well as to target high-need regions and populations served by a practice or health care system. Furthermore, this will support a stepwise approach to care that includes the identification of individuals at risk, the provision of education, and, ultimately, intervention. Finally, for many older adults who are socially isolated or lonely, health care providers may be able to identify underlying causes for the social isolation and loneliness that may be addressed through established evidence-based practices. For example, as discussed in Chapter 4, hearing loss is associated with social isolation and loneliness. In this case, a practitioner would be able to make appropriate referrals to a hearing health specialist. While some question the value of identifying individuals at risk for social isolation and loneliness when in many cases specific, effective interventions have not been developed, the committee recognizes that many health care providers and professionals are already implementing programs for social isolation and loneliness, and so program developers need to understand best practices for identifying at-risk individuals to engage in these programs. Finally, within this context, the committee emphasizes that the preservation of an individual's own decisions regarding his or her life is essential as a guiding principle for all interventions, including assessment. Therefore, the committee identifies the following goal and recommendations:

GOAL: Translate research into health care practices in order to reduce the negative health impacts of social isolation and loneliness.

RECOMMENDATION 7-1: Health care providers and practices should periodically perform an assessment using one or more validated tools to identify older adults experiencing social isolation and loneliness and to initiate potential preventive interventions after having identified individuals at elevated risk due to life events (e.g., loss of someone significant, geographic move, relevant health conditions).

- **In the case of older adults who are currently socially isolated or lonely (or at an elevated risk for social isolation or loneliness), health care providers should discuss the adverse health outcomes associated with social isolation and loneliness with these older adults and their legally**

appointed representatives. Providers should make appropriate efforts to connect isolated or lonely older adults with needed social care.

- **For older adults who are currently socially isolated or lonely, health care providers should attempt to determine the underlying causes and use evidence-based practices tailored to address those causes (e.g., hearing loss, mobility limitations).**

As discussed in Chapter 6, there are a variety of established tools to measure social isolation and loneliness, each with different strengths and weaknesses. Despite the limits of the evidence base concerning how to best implement these tools in clinical settings, the committee concluded that an important aspect of selecting a tool for use in clinical settings is standardization. This means that within a specific health care system or organization, all clinicians would use the same tool or set of tools rather than resorting to different tools; they should also use only validated tools and refrain from using only parts of existing tools or creating new, unvalidated tools. While the committee recognizes that some variation in choice of appropriate tools may be necessary for assessing certain specific populations or health conditions, it emphasizes that the chosen measurement tool needs to match the research question. (That is, if assessing for loneliness, for instance, the tool needs to be validated specifically for the measurement of loneliness, as opposed to other indicators of social connection.) Furthermore, the committee notes that the thresholds for identifying socially isolated or lonely older adults and their risk of health impacts will vary with the tool used and the health profile of the person being assessed. While there are limitations to current tools, the committee asserts that the use of existing validated tools is necessary in order to address social isolation and loneliness more fully in clinical settings. However, the committee recognizes that more effort is needed to update existing tools and develop better tools that can fully capture the experience of social isolation and loneliness among today's older adults.

The committee also notes that more research related to assessment is needed to evaluate the ethical implications and unintended consequences of assessments as well as to determine specific implementation parameters, including

- who should receive the assessment,
- who should conduct the assessment,
- the ideal frequency of assessment for different subpopulations, and
- the appropriate interventions, referrals, and follow-up care.

A variety of mechanisms for performing these assessments may need to be explored, including the Medicare annual wellness visit; hospital discharge planning; pre-admission, quarterly, or other assessments for long-term care settings;

or other opportunities in which assessment for social isolation and loneliness may be incorporated.

Linking those who are implementing new interventions in clinical settings with formally trained researchers early on can help ensure robust research design. Therefore, in order to improve the evidence around the use of specific tools in clinical settings, the committee makes the following recommendation:

RECOMMENDATION 7-2: Health care systems should create opportunities for clinicians to partner with researchers to evaluate the application of currently available evidence-based tools for assessing social isolation and loneliness in clinical settings, including testing and applications for specific populations.

Finally, the committee concludes that assessment data should be included in clear locations in the EHR. Therefore, the committee makes the following recommendation:

RECOMMENDATION 7-3: The committee endorses the recommendation of previous National Academies reports that social isolation should be included in the electronic health record or medical record.

As noted in both this chapter and Chapter 6, the committee recognizes limitations of current measures of social isolation (e.g., Berkman–Syme) in capturing current modes of interaction. However, as stated previously the committee asserts that the use of existing validated tools is necessary in order to move forward. The measures used and captured in the EHR need to be updated as better measures are developed. The committee further notes that research will be needed to determine how to best integrate information from patients' assessments into their health record in order to make determinations about future care and the identification of risk (see Recommendation 9-4 in Chapter 9 for the need for more research on interventions in clinical settings).

8

Education and Training

Relatively little attention has been paid by public health officials and other medical professionals to the importance of loneliness.

—Gerst-Emerson and Jayawardhana (2015)

Members of the health care workforce (including professionals and direct care workers) are vital in the effort to prevent, identify, reduce, and eliminate the negative health impacts of social isolation and loneliness in older adults. This chapter addresses the education and training of this workforce. In addition to the imperative to increase the knowledge and skills of those employed by the health care delivery system, this chapter considers the opportunity to increase awareness and knowledge about social isolation and loneliness among patients, families, caregivers, volunteers, and the community at large. Given the complexity of the terminology used in relation to social isolation and loneliness, a reminder of key definitions is provided in Box 8-1.

FRAMEWORK FOR THE ROLE OF EDUCATION IN CATALYZING CHANGE

The committee developed a framework to explain the role of education in addressing issues of social isolation and loneliness (see Figure 8-1). The framework emphasizes catalyzing change in clinical care delivery with the goals of preventing, ameliorating, and eliminating social isolation and loneliness in older adults and addressing the health effects of chronic social isolation and loneliness. Clinical care provides an important—and underused—opportunity to address

BOX 8-1
Key Definitions

Loneliness: the perception of social isolation or the subjective feeling of being lonely.

Mediators: also known as mechanisms or pathways; the factors that help explain how social isolation or loneliness affects health outcomes.

Moderators: the factors that can influence the magnitude or direction of the effect of social isolation or loneliness on health.

Social connection: an umbrella term that encompasses the structural, functional, and quality aspects of how individuals connect to each other.

Social isolation: the objective lack of (or limited) social contact with others.

Social support: the actual or perceived availability of resources (e.g., informational, tangible, emotional) from others, typically one's social network.

social isolation and loneliness in older adults. All types of health professions and careers need to be involved, and the necessary changes can be catalyzed through various types of education, including direct care worker education, lifelong learning by health professionals and direct care workers, and public educational campaigns. All learners need to understand how the educational and training context for social isolation and loneliness either creates higher risk or provides avenues for mitigating these problems. This context includes

- The impact of national standards and policy priorities;
- Current education and training approaches;
- How health system design can change practice behaviors and facilitate treatment strategies (e.g., through partnerships with academic environments and communities); and
- How payor policies facilitate or impede addressing social isolation and loneliness.

NATIONAL STANDARDS AND POLICY PRIORITIES

At the highest level, national standards and policy priorities can influence and shape the education of the formal health care workforce. As each profession sets its own standards for education and practice, the topics of social isolation and

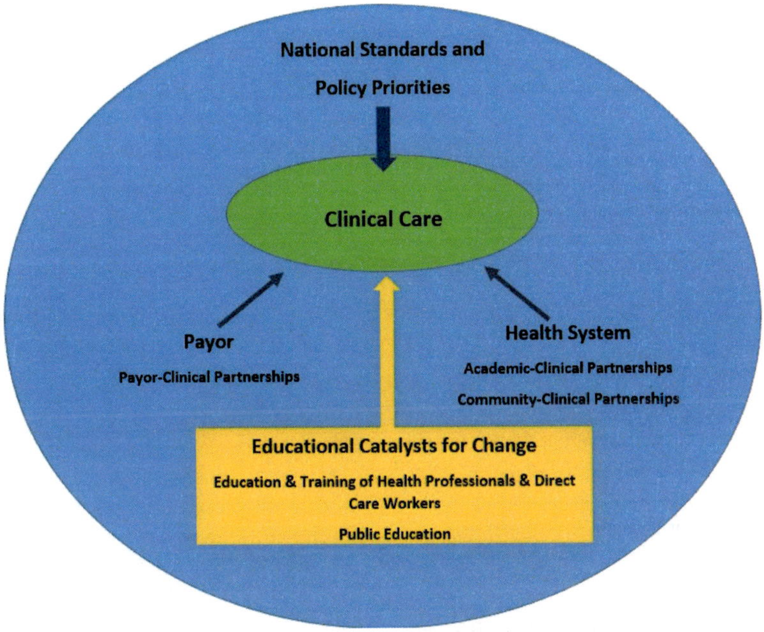

FIGURE 8-1 Framework for educational catalysts for change.

loneliness can be incorporated into the standards and competencies expected of students. The compelling evidence base for the health effects of social isolation and loneliness provide faculty and educational leaders with a strong rationale for including this content in educational programs. The following sections highlight several opportunities for influencing the education and training of the formal health care workforce.

Interprofessional Groups

Many interprofessional groups related to the care of older adults need to be partners in improving education and training related to social isolation and loneliness among older adults. Such groups include (but are not limited to) the American Geriatrics Society, the Society for Post-Acute and Long-Term Care Medicine, LeadingAge, the Eldercare Workforce Alliance, and other service provider organizations. The following sections provide examples of a few key partners specifically engaged in professional education.

The Interprofessional Education Collaborative (IPEC), formed in 2009 by a group of health professions education associations to develop a set of competencies for interprofessional education (IPEC, 2016), could address social isolation and loneliness through its focus on team-based approaches. The four initial competencies and sub-competencies developed by IPEC were updated in 2016 to reflect interprofessional collaboration as the primary organizing construct and to focus more clearly on population health. The updated competencies emphasize collaboration with others outside of the formal health care system. This updated format is particularly germane to addressing social isolation and loneliness in older adults because much of the support needed may come from other sectors, including sources within neighborhoods and communities. Because the interventions needed to address social isolation and loneliness draw on so many different professions and disciplines, including a variety of frontline workers such as direct care workers and community health workers, volunteers, and family caregivers (sometimes called informal caregivers), it would be particularly helpful when promulgating recommendations to note their relevance to the IPEC competencies.

Beyond Flexner[1] is an interprofessional group that promotes the inclusion of social determinants of health into all health professions curricula (Kaufman, 2016). Mullen (2017) argued that social, economic, and geographic conditions are fundamental in determining the presence or absence of health inequities and therefore that all health professions schools should educate students about the importance of the social mission. The name, Beyond Flexner, is intended to signify the inclusion of the social mission and learning experiences related to social determinants of health that go above and beyond the biologically and clinically based educational model the founders of this movement assert is currently in use. This social mission could incorporate issues related to social isolation and loneliness and expand health professions education around these issues.

Englander and colleagues (2013) proposed a framework composed of eight domains that they recommended for use within medical education. The domains, developed to be sufficiently broad to be applicable to any health profession, have been adopted by one nurse practitioner residency program (Flintner and Bamrick, 2017) and are being discussed for use in nursing education more broadly (AACN, 2019). The eight domains are:

1. patient care;
2. knowledge for practice;
3. practice-based learning and improvement;
4. interpersonal and communication skills;
5. professionalism;
6. systems-based practice;
7. interprofessional collaboration; and
8. personal and professional development (Englander et al., 2013, pp. 1091–1092).

[1] In 1910, Abraham Flexner issued a report (now known as the Flexner report) that criticized the quality of medical education at that time and resulted in a reorganization of the medical education system (Flexner, 1910).

The prevention and treatment of the health impacts of social isolation and loneliness in older adults fits within several of these domains. For example, incorporating evidence-based recommendations to prevent or ameliorate social isolation and loneliness in older adults fits within the domains of patient care, interpersonal and communication skills, system-based practice, and interprofessional collaboration.

The Academy for Gerontology in Higher Education (AGHE) is a membership organization of colleges and universities that offer education, training, and research in the field of aging. Interdisciplinary in nature, the goals of AGHE include educating society about aging, preparing service delivery people who work with older adults, and providing leadership on policies and issues related to higher education (AGHE, 2019). AGHE develops, promotes, and publishes gerontology competencies for undergraduate and graduate education. These recommended competencies include foundational competencies, interactional competencies, and contextual competencies (AGHE, 2014). For example, the foundational competencies are in the areas of the biological aspects of aging, the psychological aspects of aging, and the social aspects of aging. Content about social isolation and loneliness could be included within these three aspects of aging and would serve to prepare the workforce with tools to recognize social isolation and loneliness, to understand its impact on older adults, and to ameliorate it. One interactional competency is interdisciplinary and community collaboration. Community collaborative competency work could focus on solutions to address social isolation and loneliness from an interdisciplinary perspective. Finally, the contextual competencies include well-being, health, and mental health as one contextual competency and social health as another. Social isolation and loneliness could be integrated within these competencies. AGHE could provide the leadership to promote social isolation and loneliness in its recommended competency content, and infusion across curriculum standards and within the structure of the AGHE competencies would be possible.

National Goals for Health and Well-Being

The Healthy People national goals provide yet another opportunity for encouraging the inclusion of content related to social isolation and loneliness in health professions education as well as in programs aimed at practicing clinicians and other professionals who care for older adults. Since 1990 Healthy People goals have been developed for each decade, and social cohesion is one of the topics addressed in the section on social determinants of health for *Healthy People 2020* (HHS, 2019b). Foundational principles and overarching goals have already been proposed for *Healthy People 2030*, and the specific goals and objectives are under development at this time (HHS, 2019c). Healthy People goals provide important directions for health professions education. Although the goals and objectives are not educational standards, they influence curricula because they represent national priorities. The overarching goals for *Healthy People 2030* are based on a vision of "a society in which all people can achieve their full potential for health and well-being across the lifespan" (HHS, 2019c). Addressing social isolation and loneliness fits clearly within this broad vision.

An Individual Health Professions Response

Making the prevention and treatment of social isolation and loneliness in older adults a priority of individual health professions is another important strategy. One example has occurred within the social work profession, with the American Academy of Social Work and Social Welfare having adopted the elimination of social isolation as one of its grand challenges (Lubben et al., 2015, 2018). The Grand Challenge initiative[2] provides a framework for disseminating evidence-based strategies to solve important social problems and to bring a range of stakeholders together in designing multifaceted solutions. The benefits of grand challenges, such as this one developed by the social work profession, are that they provide a focus, bring leaders to the table, provide a framework for collaboration and interdisciplinary engagement, capture public interest, attract resources, and promote diplomacy (Uehara et al., 2013). The success of this initiative will depend on participation across professional groups, organizations, and communities (Uehara et al., 2013). Indeed, social isolation and loneliness in older adults is a complex issue that will benefit from cross-sector collaborative initiatives such as this.

CURRENT EDUCATION AND TRAINING OF THE HEALTH CARE WORKFORCE

In 2016 an ad hoc committee of the National Academies of Sciences, Engineering, and Medicine (the National Academies) developed a framework for educating health professionals to address the social determinants of health (NASEM, 2016a; see Figure 8-2). The committee concluded that there should be "a holistic, consistent, and coherent framework" of education and training that promotes a systems-based approach aligned across health, education, and other sectors in partnership with communities (NASEM, 2016a, p. 4). This call for a unified approach (based on the three pillars of transformative learning, dynamic partnerships, and lifelong learning) is especially important for a health care workforce concerned with social isolation and loneliness in older, vulnerable populations. Many health professions stress the incorporation of the social determinants of health in general into curricula for students and trainees. However, the nontraditional components of education recommended by the 2016 committee (e.g., experiential learning, collaborative learning, an integrated curriculum, continuing professional development) are not universally deployed.

[2] For more information, see https://grandchallengesforsocialwork.org/about (accessed December 16, 2019).

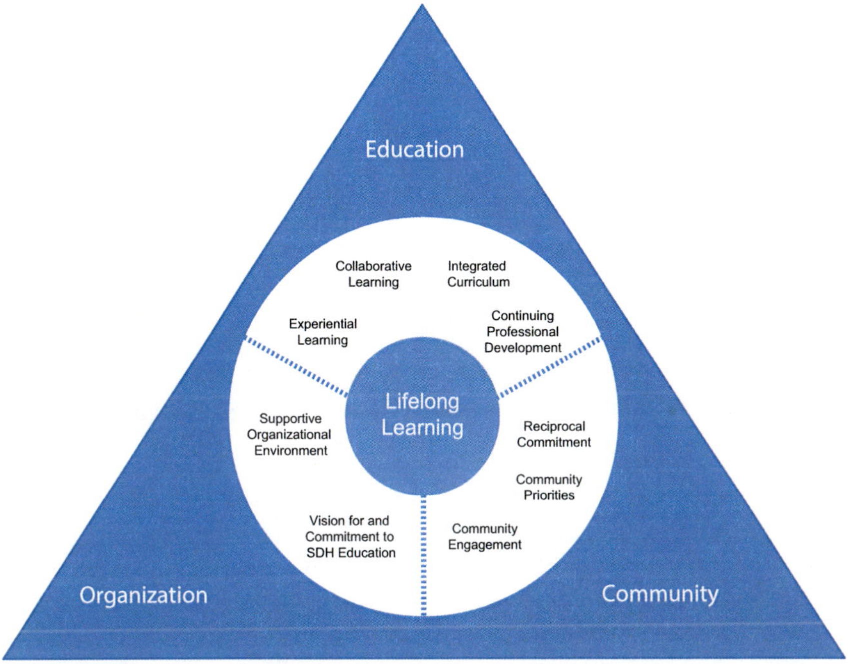

FIGURE 8-2 Framework for lifelong learning for health professionals in understanding and addressing the social determinants of health.
NOTE: SDH = social determinants of health.
SOURCE: NASEM, 2016a.

The 2019 National Academies consensus study report *Integrating Social Care into the Delivery of Health Care* discusses the role of education in developing a workforce that can understand and address social factors and recommends the incorporation of competency-based curricula on social care into health professions and continuing education programs (NASEM, 2019). The following sections expand on that report's recommendation and highlight specific examples and opportunities for the education and training of the health care workforce on issues related to the social isolation and loneliness of older adults.

Health Professions Education

Many individual professions have paid attention to the education and training of their own professionals about the social determinants of health in general. However, except for a few notable examples, little is known about the level of education and training provided on the particular effects of social isolation and loneliness. Aside from formal education programs, the role of certification may be explored as a way to foster the infusion of these topics into the education and training of health care professionals. The committee recognizes that adding more requirements may add to burden and burnout among health care professionals. However, given the significant impact of social isolation and loneliness on health, the committee asserts that all of these potential options need to be explored as ways to impart critical knowledge. Several examples of these efforts are described below.

Educational Efforts by Individual Professions

The Accreditation Council for Graduate Medical Education sets standards for accrediting U.S. graduate medical education programs and the institutions that sponsor them. The common program requirements for residency govern the professional development of physicians. Program directors are required to "design and conduct the [residency] program in a fashion consistent with the needs of the community" (ACGME, 2018, p. 9). Each program "must understand the social determinants of health of the populations they serve and incorporate them in the design and implementation of the program curriculum" (ACGME, 2018, p. 9). Similarly, "residents must demonstrate an awareness of and responsiveness to the larger context and system of health care, including the social determinants of health, as well as the ability to call effectively on other resources to provide optimal health care" (ACGME, 2018, p. 21). The common program requirements do not specifically address social isolation and loneliness.

The American Association of Colleges of Nursing publishes the *Essentials* documents that delineate expected core outcomes of nursing education at the baccalaureate, master's, and doctor of nursing practice levels (AACN, 2006, 2008, 2011). While the *Essentials* documents are broad, they clearly indicate the expectation that nurses care effectively for all age groups, including older adults. For example, *Baccalaureate Essentials* (AACN, 2008) states that nurses care for people of all age groups, with special attention to "older adults and the very young" (p. 32). The document also indicates that care should be holistic and account for patient and family preferences and community concerns and that professionalism in nursing involves integrating physical, emotional, and social concerns. Finally, this document indicates that nurses provide a link between hospitals and community environments and supports the importance of nurses' roles in assessing social and psychological needs as well as physical health needs and making referrals to community services as needed. *Master's and Clinical Doctoral Essentials* similarly focuses on comprehensive care based on a full biopsychosocial model that includes the social determinants of health (AACN, 2006, 2008). Similarly, the National League for Nursing has identified competencies for graduates of nursing education programs that address the full age continuum and a holistic approach to caregiving (AACN, 2011).

The Council on Social Work Education's Educational Policy and Accreditation Standards (EPAS) sets forth guidelines for professional competence. These standards are used to accredit baccalaureate and master's level social work programs (CSWE, 2015). The EPAS consists of nine competencies that are guided by a person-in-environment framework, a global perspective, and respect for human diversity (CSWE, 2015). These competencies outline the importance of working with diverse populations within the context of relationship building, interprofessional teamwork, and inter-organizational collaboration. Engagement, assessment, and intervention occur within the intersection of multiple factors, including age, class, culture, disability and ability, ethnicity, gender, gender identity and expression, immigration status, marital status, political ideology, race, religion and spirituality, sex, sexual orientation, and tribal sovereign status. The focus on these factors reinforces the importance of understanding and recognizing the influence of the social determinants of health on the lifelong development of individuals (CSWE, 2015). The EPAS outlines the role that social workers have in assessing and intervening within a practice context that includes working with individuals, families, groups, organizations, and communities toward mutually agreed-upon goals (CSWE, 2015). These competencies reinforce the expectation that social workers are trained to attend to the social and psychological needs of older adults and their families within the context of health and social service settings. Social workers are trained to serve as a bridge to the broader community and are well positioned to make connections between health providers and the larger social service community (CSWE, 2015).

Additionally, the social work profession, under the auspices of the Council on Social Work Education through its Gero Ed Center, developed a Geriatric Social Work Competency Scale with Lifelong Leadership Skills (CSWE, 2019). This scale lists skills recognized by gerontological social workers as important to social workers in their work with and on behalf of older adults and their families. Designed to be used at the baccalaureate, master's, and post-masters levels of curriculum, it is used for pre–post evaluations of education and field training. Students are rated in four areas of competence:

1. Values, ethics, and theoretical perspectives
2. Assessment
3. Intervention
4. Aging services, programs, and policies (CSWE, 2019)

The assessment of social support and human connections is one of the factors that is included in the assessment competency section. Adding content on social isolation and loneliness to the intervention competence could strengthen social work practitioners' response to at risk older adults.

National Geriatrics Training Program

National training programs in geriatrics, such as the Geriatrics Workforce Enhancement Program (GWEP) funded by the Health Resources and Services

Administration, provide another potential opportunity for improving education and training on social isolation and loneliness in older adults. GWEP provides grants "that improve health care for older adults and maximize patient and family engagement to health professions schools, health care facilities, and programs leading to certification as a certified nursing assistant."[3] Key goals of the program are to "educate and train the primary care and geriatrics workforce to care for older adults in integrated geriatrics and primary care models," and "to partner with community based organizations to address gaps in healthcare for older adults, promote age-friendly health systems and dementia-friendly communities, and address the social determinants of health."[4] Social isolation and loneliness could be explicitly incorporated into some of these programs, particularly as a key social determinant of health.

Role of Certifications

Certification exams use standards of practice as the basis for exam questions and could include questions about social isolation and loneliness. Specialty gerontologic certification exams are available in, for example, medicine, nursing, physical therapy, psychology, and pharmacy. Certification examinations and credentials are also available for more specific areas, such as diabetes educators (NCBDE, 2019), although none exist for addressing social isolation and loneliness. The development of a certification exam related to preventing and treating social isolation and loneliness, either as a stand-alone exam or by including items related to this topic on a currently existing gerontologic exam, is a potential opportunity for emphasizing the importance of this area.

Direct Care Worker Education and Training

Direct care workers are the paid front line of long-term care in the United States, providing critical, daily support to millions of older people and people with disabilities. As a result, direct care workers, of which there were 4.3 million in 2017 (PHI, 2018a), are well positioned to support older people nationwide in addressing social isolation and loneliness. As interventions directed at social isolation and loneliness in older adults gain traction, direct care workers will need to be properly trained, educated, and supported.

Governing and shaping the direct care workforce are a variety of broad and inconsistent state and federal training requirements in addition to an under-resourced training and public education landscape. The current training for the direct care workforce rarely explicitly addresses social isolation and loneliness in older adults.

[3] See https://bhw.hrsa.gov/grants/geriatrics (accessed December 16, 2019).

[4] See https://www.americangeriatrics.org/programs/gwep-coordinating-center (accessed December 17, 2019).

Core Competencies

Ideally, a set of core competencies—manifested as knowledge, skills, and abilities—form the foundation of training for direct care workers, delineating the capabilities that workers should acquire and demonstrate in order to effectively provide care. An array of public and private actors in the long-term care field have created core competency skill sets for direct care workers, which vary widely in terms of content areas (and other aspects). While none of these competency sets explicitly address social isolation and loneliness, many of them include related areas that could allow for more focused attention on these two topics. For example, the Centers for Medicare & Medicaid Services direct service workforce core competencies include a competency area of "community inclusion and networking" (CMS, 2014, p. 7). The following two skill statements are included under that competency area:

1. The direct service worker "encourages and assists individuals in connecting with others and developing social and valued social and/or work roles based on his or her choices," and
2. The direct service worker "supports the individual to connect with friends and to live and be included in the community of his or her choice." (p. 7)

The National Alliance for Direct Support Professionals' direct support professionals competencies includes a section on "community living skills and supports" and notes that "the competent [direct care worker] supports the participant in the development of friendships and other relationships" (NADSP, 2016, p. 5).

Training Requirements and Credentialing

Direct care workers are subject to an array of federal and state training requirements, which vary widely in terms of their duration and content (among other dimensions) across different direct care occupations, states, and service delivery models.[5] While these requirements need significant improvement, they provide opportunities to expand the skills of direct care workers on social isolation, loneliness, and older adults. For example, federal guidelines for home health aides require that the aides must be trained in the "physical, emotional, and developmental needs of and ways to work with the populations served by the Home Health Agency, including the need for respect for the patient, his or her privacy

[5] Federal regulations today require that home health aides and nursing assistants receive at least 75 hours of training, including at least 16 hours of supervised practical or clinical training. They must also complete 12 hours of continuing education every 12 months. Only 17 states and the District of Columbia surpass this 75-hour requirement, and only 6 states and the District of Columbia meet the 120-hour standard encouraged by the Institute of Medicine (IOM, 2008). Personal care aides have no federal training requirement, and state-level requirements vary considerably, typically with little to no uniformity across programs or requirements on duration, content, and methods (PHI, 2019a,b).

and his or her property."[6] Similarly, the federal guidelines for nursing assistants require that workers be trained in the "mental health and social service needs" of older adults.[7] Guidelines for both direct care occupations could specify social isolation and loneliness as priority topics.

Personal care aides—the largest-growing segment of the direct care workforce—lack any federal training requirement and have few state-level requirements (PHI, 2019c). A number of states require the use of state-sponsored curricula or training outlines that set forth detailed training content for specific segments of the direct care workforce. Compared with broad regulatory requirements, these curricula and outlines are more prescriptive in terms of their content, instruction methods, and competency assessment, and they could be updated to address social isolation and loneliness in older adults. A few notable examples:

- New York's curricular outline for personal care aides covers the emotional well-being of consumers (i.e., "safety and security including emotional security") (NYSDOH, 2002, p. 61).
- Virginia's curricular outline covers the basic physical and emotional needs of consumers, including "love and belonging" (VDMAS, 2003).
- Arizona's Principles of Caregiving curriculum addresses social isolation and loneliness in multiple areas, including in a section on the "emotional impact of aging" (Arizona Direct Care Initiative, 2011).
- Washington State's state-sponsored curriculum encourages home care aides to help consumers stay socially connected. The curriculum also emphasizes the aide's role in the emotional well-being of consumers (WSDSHS, 2009).
- Maine's personal support specialist curriculum refers trainees to a companion textbook for content on social isolation (MDHS, 2003).

Other Members of the Health Care Workforce

Aside from health care professionals and direct care workers, many other members of the health care workforce may be especially important to addressing social isolation and loneliness because they are natural connectors of the health care system with the local communities. Community health workers (CHWs) are

> lay members of the community who work either for pay or as volunteers in association with the local health care system in both urban and rural environments. CHWs usually share ethnicity, language, socioeconomic status, and life experiences with the community members they serve. (NIH, 2014)

CHWs have been shown to be particularly effective in creating linkages between communities and the health care system and in providing health education

[6] 42 CFR § 484.36—Condition of Participation: Home Health Aide Services. 82 FR 4504.

[7] 42 CFR § 483.152—Requirements for Approval of a Nurse Aide Training and Competency Evaluation Program. 56 FR 48919, 75 FR 21179.

and informal counseling, particularly for underserved communities (HRSA, 2007). While CHWs typically come from the communities in which they serve and often serve as advocates for the individuals in these communities, patient navigators (or patient advocates) tend to be based within the health care system. Patient navigators help patients acquire necessary information and services that may affect their health care (NCI, 2011). For example, patient navigators may assist patients with setting up appointments, reaching out to insurers, and connecting to needed social supports. Case managers (or care managers) focus particularly on coordinating health and social care for individuals with complex needs either in health care systems or with social service agencies (NASEM, 2019). These health care workers and others can serve an important role in connecting the health care system with community-based services.

PUBLIC HEALTH CAMPAIGNS

Public education campaigns can be a powerful method for raising awareness of and support for key issues, among other objectives. For example, public education campaigns have addressed various health topics, including tobacco use; nutrition, physical activity, and obesity; heart disease and stroke; diabetes; and Alzheimer's disease, among others (NIH, 2019). Such campaigns are used to "help health care professionals, practitioners, and the general public make informed decisions about their health and the health of their patients" (NIH, 2019).

Public education campaigns are often undertaken by specific health care professions and occupations. For example, nonprofit organizations in the direct care sector have used public education campaigns to:

- focus attention on the growing workforce shortage in home care at the national and state levels,
- support specific policy goals,
- reach workers with information about their rights and benefits, and
- explore future solutions for the full elder care workforce (EWA, 2019; PHI, 2018b, 2019d).

The following sections highlight examples of the use of campaigns to spread awareness of issues related to aging in general as well as social isolation and loneliness in particular.

Public Education and Framing Strategies for Aging

Public education campaigns have been increasingly used in the aging and long-term care sector to raise awareness about the realities of aging, the variety of challenges and opportunities facing older people, and the demand for a strong elder care workforce. In recent years, these campaigns have sought, among other goals, to change perceptions of aging through personal stories of older people, to connect the millennial generation to aging-related concerns, and to inspire policy makers to address the worsening shortage in home care workers (Snelling, 2019).

More broadly, an extensive body of research and applied practice exists to guide communications planning, strategy, and evaluation across social issues, identifying effective techniques for defining and establishing clear goals, objectives, audiences, and evaluation measures. When designed properly, public education campaigns can shape public policy by raising awareness, increasing the numbers of champions and supporters, building constituents, strengthening public will, and sparking policy change. These campaigns can also influence such characteristics as awareness, salience, attitudes and beliefs, self-efficacy, social norms, and behavioral intention and change (Communications Network, 2008).

Furthermore, social scientists and strategic communications experts have recently created and tested a variety of approaches to promoting strong, positive messaging regarding health and older adults and to reducing harmful ideas that perpetuate problematic representations of older adults. This emerging trend builds on a body of research and practice focused on "collective action framing" in social movements worldwide—intentional, large-scale efforts to transform how the public at large understands societal problems, solutions, and related actions (Benford and Snow, 2000). Two current examples related to health and aging are an effort to provide guidance on how to discuss the social determinants of health, led by the Robert Wood Johnson Foundation (RWJF), and the Reframing Aging Project, which seeks to improve messaging about aging and to reduce ageism, led by the FrameWorks Institute, a nonprofit organization focused on advancing ways to communicate about science (FrameWorks Institute, 2019; RWJF, 2010). The two efforts both created research-tested approaches and practical tools for the public and private sectors to frame concerns about health (the RWJF project) and aging (FrameWorks), guiding the creation of effective, strength-based narratives on the topics. Of note, the Reframing Aging Project was steered by a group of leading organizations in the aging services field: AARP, the American Federation for Aging Research, the American Geriatrics Society, the American Society on Aging, the Gerontological Society of America, Grantmakers in Aging, the National Council on Aging, and the National Hispanic Council on Aging (FrameWorks Institute, 2019).

Despite the potential and the proliferation of these types of approaches, researchers and communications strategists have not produced any easily available, research-tested frames, messages, or communications campaigns and tools that are specific to social isolation and loneliness in older adults—a fact that limits strategic, collective action on this pressing concern.

Education by Campaigns and Coalitions Specifically for Social Isolation and Loneliness

As the complexities of mitigating social isolation and loneliness are increasingly acknowledged, some stakeholders support large-scale campaigns and coalitions to disseminate information and best practices. The increased visibility from such media campaigns has the potential to change public attitudes and social norms, which in turn could indirectly influence behavior change (Holt-Lunstad et al., 2017).

Campaign to End Loneliness (UK)

The Campaign to End Loneliness, a large-scale media campaign, was founded in the United Kingdom in 2011 with the goal of sharing research, evidence, and knowledge in order to connect individuals and communities across the country (Campaign to End Loneliness, 2019b). The campaign is hosted by Independent Age, a charitable organization focused on the well-being of older people, and it is supported by the National Lottery Community Fund, the Calouste Gulbenkian Foundation, the Tudor Trust, and donations from the general public. The campaign has created a series of toolkits, research briefs, and events to raise awareness among public health and health care practitioners about the deleterious health effects of social isolation and loneliness. The campaign has also created the Learning Network (Campaign to End Loneliness, 2019c), which links like-minded organizations, distributes the latest research on social isolation and loneliness, and shares examples of best practices for addressing loneliness, but does not necessarily perform evidence-based assessments of these practices on their own. The campaign has been relatively successful in distributing information and bringing loneliness to the front of public discourse. An evaluation of the campaign's outreach efforts found that 84 percent of National Health Service health and well-being boards targeted by the campaign had implemented written strategies for addressing loneliness (Cupitt, 2013).

AARP Foundation Connect2Affect

The AARP Foundation has partnered with the Gerontological Society of America, Give an Hour, n4a, and UnitedHealthcare to launch a campaign, Connect2Affect, to address social isolation and loneliness (AARP Foundation, 2019). The major goal of the campaign is to create a network of resources that meets the needs of anyone who is socially isolated or lonely and that helps build the social connections that older adults need to thrive. The campaign has helped to increase awareness of the impact of social isolation and loneliness on older adults, to provide information on service and training resources, and to create networks. The National Good Neighbor Day[8] is an example of a community impact activity associated with this campaign.

[8] For more on the National Good Neighbor Day, see https://connect2affect.org/goodneighborday (accessed December 18, 2019).

CHANGING PRACTICE BEHAVIORS

While education is one method for catalyzing change, dissemination and implementation science has shown that an individual's (or group's) knowledge of what to do is never enough to institutionalize and sustain change. (See Chapter 10 for more on dissemination and implementation.) Educating users about evidence-based practices (EBPs) is a necessary but not sufficient step to change practice, and didactic education alone does little to change practice behavior (Forsetland et al., 2009; Giguère et al., 2012). Users of the EBPs need to know the scientific bases for EBP recommendations and to have the knowledge and skills to carry out such practices, and health system design and payor policies need to support the implementation of these recommendations.

Lifelong learning opportunities are vital for the ongoing development of health care workers who interact with older adults. Given that the evidence base is continuing to develop in the area of social isolation and loneliness, those working with older adults, families, and communities will need ways to learn about future research developments in this area. Multiple modalities are available for lifelong learning, including just-in-time learning, Web-based modules and webinars, other forms of online learning, conference presentations, and journal articles (IOM, 2009).

Certain roles and responsibilities already present in health systems can be modified to address social isolation and loneliness in older adults. Discharge planning, case management, and transitional care planning are examples of the sorts of roles and functions that can be used to directly address the assessment of and interventions for social isolation and loneliness. Discharge planning and case management are most often provided by social workers and registered nurses. Transitional care planning may be provided by advanced practice nurses and master's-prepared social workers (Altfeld et al., 2013; Alverez et al., 2016; Eaton, 2018; Naylor et al., 2018). For instance, Naylor et al. (2018) developed a transitional care model designed to prevent rehospitalizations and health complications in older adults with chronic illnesses. An advance practice nurse provides a thorough assessment prior to the discharge and leads the discharge and home follow-up process. Given the extensive nature of the pre-discharge assessment, screening for social isolation and loneliness could be integrated into the assessment process. If social isolation and loneliness are detected in the screening, intervention and follow-up could occur in the community as part of the community visits.

In the Bridge model (Altfeld et al., 2013; Alvarez et al., 2016) a social worker with a master's degree connects with the patient and family prior to discharge. Inpatient and outpatient providers are also connected with the patient and family to reinforce the continuity of care. This model encourages attention to the social determinants of health, and as social needs are identified, the social work care coordinator addresses them in both health care and community-based settings. Using this model, social isolation and loneliness could be identified before discharge and addressed throughout the care transition process and as the patient integrates back into the community. For example, current team-based models for identifying frail patients in hospitals (through the use of multi-dimensional assessments) could serve as models for the identification of social isolation and loneliness in the inpatient setting (Ansryan et al., 2018; Borenstein et al., 2013, 2016). Strassner et al. (2019) describe a study planned in Germany that will prepare general practitioners to provide holistic disease management services for frail older adults. These services will include assessments of loneliness, suggesting that the inclusion of this aspect of managing chronic conditions is gaining interest. Team-based approaches to helping older adults manage care over a period of time provide multiple perspectives for incorporating social isolation and loneliness into care plans. (See Chapter 7 for more on the role of the health care system.)

As noted in the 2019 National Academies consensus study report *Integrating Social Care into the Delivery of Health Care*, "Understanding the role each member of an interprofessional team plays . . . is important for ensuring effective collaboration among team members and for maximizing their ability to address patients' social needs" (NASEM, 2019, p. 77). This approach can be adopted when designing education and training models to address social isolation and loneliness. Collaboration and coordination among all members of a health professional team is a critical component in education and training initiatives.

Health Systems: Academic–Clinical Partnerships

Academic–clinical partnerships can catalyze evidence-based practice (Noel et al., 2019). Education and research on the causes and outcomes of social isolation and loneliness in older adults, screening tools, assessment strategies, and effective interventions need to be connected with clinical practice in ways that accelerate improvements in practice, change systems of care when needed, influence payment systems, increase health, and highlight successful teamwork among health professionals, direct care workers, and community members. The 2016 report *Advancing Healthcare Transformation: A New Era for Academic Nursing* highlights the importance of intentional and systematic academic–practice partnerships in catalyzing improvements in nursing care (AACN, 2016). Alberti et al. (2018) noted that action planning with communities is more likely to generate lasting results in health equity than are less intentional partnerships. The use of relevant clinical guidelines, such as those promulgated by the Hartford Institute for Geriatric Nursing's *Depression in Older Adults* (Harvath and McKenzie, 2012), and the development of specific guidelines targeted to the treatment of social isolation and loneliness in older adults can help improve practice. Boston College's Institute on Aging is another example of an academic–practice partnership, with its emphasis on interdisciplinary education, research, and community partnerships. One product of this Institute is BC Talks Aging,[9] which is a series of modules with

[9] For more information on BC Talks Aging, see https://www.bc.edu/centers/ioa/videos.html (accessed December 17, 2019).

free access, developed by established scholars on topics related to aging, and one of these modules specifically addresses social isolation and loneliness. The aim of BC Talks Aging is to provide learning opportunities on aging issues for social workers, nurses, and other health practitioners in the field (BCIA, 2019).

Partnerships between clinical organizations and community organizations are essential to ensuring that a full range of services and care are available for older adults at risk for social isolation and loneliness. The 2019 National Academies consensus study report *Integrating Social Care into the Delivery of Health Care* notes the importance of developing cross-sector coalitions and describes the success of multi-sector coalitions in improving health delivery. One successful partnership described in the report was between Johns Hopkins University and the Homewood Community Partners Initiative, which led to the establishment of health enterprise zones, aligning and increasing activity coordination with health departments, health providers, and community organizations. The impact of this partnership was a reduction in inpatient hospital visits resulting in a net cost savings of $93.39 million (NASEM, 2019).

Health Systems: Payor–Clinical Partnerships

Critical to the adoption of clinical interventions is understanding payor policies and inviting payors to the table when changes may be needed. The 2018 Alliance of Community Health Plans (ACHP) report *Accelerating the Adoption of Evidence-Based Care: Payer Provider Partnerships* found that collaboration among high-performing health plans to influence provider behavior can accelerate the dissemination and adoption of EBPs. Although the research by ACHP did not specifically address social isolation and loneliness, the report highlighted examples of consensus building, customized education, tools, and access to extensive training as a means to disseminate and promote accelerated delivery of evidence-based care best practices across diverse types of payor–provider partnerships (ACHP, 2018).

The 2019 National Academies consensus study report *Integrating Social Care into the Delivery of Health Care* concludes that if social care is to be properly addressed in health care, health care financing structures need to recognize the importance of the unique contributions of team members and to ensure adequate reimbursement of clinical partnerships (NASEM, 2019).

FINDINGS AND CONCLUSIONS

- Educating health care professionals, direct care workers, and the general public on the health impacts of social isolation and loneliness is essential.
- National standards and policy priorities influence the education of the formal health care workforce. Social isolation and loneliness can be incorporated into these standards and priorities in order to raise awareness and educate current and future health professionals about these topics.

- Formal and informal education, lifelong learning, and educational campaigns can catalyze change by facilitating learners' knowledge of the risk factors for social isolation and loneliness and how to prevent and ameliorate these problems.
- Despite limited research on the effectiveness of selected interventions for social isolation and loneliness, health professionals need to learn core content in areas such as the prevalence of social isolation and loneliness, morbidity and mortality related to social isolation and loneliness, risk factors, assessment strategies, referral options and processes for making and following up on referrals, ways to support and encourage older adults and their significant others, partnering with community agencies, and program development and evaluation. This content crosses disciplinary lines and could be included in team-based instruction.
- No certification credential currently exists for health professionals who address social isolation and loneliness in older adults. A unique certification process or questions added to existing gerontologic certification exams could motivate more health professionals to address these topics in depth.
- Direct care workers are the paid front line of long-term care in the United States and are well positioned to support older people in addressing social isolation and loneliness. Providing education and training to these workers about social isolation and loneliness is essential to their ongoing work.
- Although personal care aides are a growing segment of the direct care workforce, there is a lack of federal and state training requirements for this sector. Instructive curricula and outlines for personal care aides should be created or updated in order to recognize social isolation and loneliness in older adults.
- Researchers and communications strategists in the United States have not produced easily available, research-tested frames, messages, or communications campaigns and tools specific to social isolation and loneliness in older adults, which limits strategic, collective action on this issue.
- Addressing social isolation and loneliness is a community-wide concern and requires that health professionals, direct care workers, and members of the community work together to achieve solutions.

NEXT STEPS AND RECOMMENDATIONS

Broadly based workforce development needs to account for the entire range of the health care workforce within formal degree and postgraduate programs for health professionals and in training programs for direct care workers and community members. Education and training of the health care workforce about addressing social isolation and loneliness will require a broad approach similar to the one used to educate the workforce about addressing the social determinants of health. It will be necessary to educate and train all members of the health care workforce, including professionals, direct care workers, community health workers, volunteers, family caregivers, and members of the larger community, such as police officers and mail carriers, who provide a broad array of services to or regularly interact with older adults.

Improving Overall Awareness

The 2019 National Academies consensus study report *Integrating Social Care into the Delivery of Health Care* noted that "activities seeking to increase social and health care integration frequently begin with elevating and sustaining awareness about the influence of social risk and protective factors on health outcomes" (NASEM, 2019, p. 36). Based on the significant evidence base concerning the health and medical impacts of social isolation and loneliness (see Chapters 2 and 3), the committee concluded that, as with other public health issues of the same magnitude, a critical step toward preventing, mitigating, or eliminating those impacts will be to improve awareness among the general public and, specifically for this report, among the health care workforce itself. The committee therefore offers the following goal and related recommendations.

GOAL: Improve awareness of the health and medical impact of social isolation and loneliness across the health care workforce and among members of the public.

RECOMMENDATION 8-1: The U.S. Department of Health and Human Services should advocate for including measures of social isolation and loneliness in major large-scale health strategies (e.g., Healthy People) and surveys (e.g., National Health Interview Survey).

RECOMMENDATION 8-2: Health and aging organizations, relevant government agencies, and consumer-facing organizations should create public awareness and education campaigns that highlight the health impacts of social isolation and loneliness in older adults.

- **Health care systems, associations representing all types of health care workers (e.g., American Medical Association, American Nurses Association, American Psychological Association, National Association of Social Workers, American Geriatrics Society, American Association for Geriatric Psychiatry, associations representing direct care workers); health-related organizations (e.g., American Heart Association); consumer-facing, health-related organizations (e.g., AARP); aging professional associations (e.g., American Society on Aging, Gerontological Society of America); aging services organizations (e.g., area agencies**

on aging, state departments on aging); and organizations working with at-risk older adults (e.g., National Hispanic Council on Aging) should actively communicate information about the health impacts of social isolation and loneliness through print and digital media.

- **Organizations representing health plans and providers should include consumer-friendly information about the health impacts of social isolation and loneliness in their repository of patient resources (e.g., where the organization provides information about the self-management of various chronic diseases).**

A large-scale, public–private sector investment could build awareness and support among the various clinicians, direct care employers and workers, and community members about the need to address social isolation and loneliness in older adults, creating a groundswell to develop comprehensive training and educational programs. These types of campaigns could have several audiences and purposes. For example, given that direct care workers often have the most interaction with the most vulnerable populations of older adults, the direct care sector could create public education campaigns that build awareness and support among direct care employers and workers about the health impacts of social isolation and loneliness. In addition, groups such as the Frameworks Institute could create a research-based framing strategy—similar to the Reframing Aging initiative—that assists in developing effective, strength-based frames and messages on social isolation and loneliness in older adults, including more vulnerable populations.

Strengthening Education and Training

While research-based evidence is not yet available to support curricular content on specific interventions for social isolation and loneliness in older adults (see Chapter 9), enough is known about the health impacts to warrant broad curricular recommendations for all health professions and careers. Health professions students need to learn about the prevalence of social isolation and loneliness in older adults, about its health outcomes and risk factors, and also about how to assess for these problems. The move toward more comprehensive geriatric assessments by interprofessional teams (e.g., Borenstein et al., 2016) provides an ideal opportunity for evaluating social isolation and loneliness. One example of an evidence-based assessment guide that can be helpful is Fulmer SPICES, which was developed as part of the Nurses Improving Care for Health System Elders project (Fulmer, 2007). This guide provides assessment criteria for hospitalized older adults for six key problems: "sleep problems, problems with eating and feeding, incontinence, confusion, evidence of falls, and skin breakdown" (p. 40). While social isolation and loneliness are not included, each of these key problems can lead to or result from social isolation and loneliness and can indicate the need to look more deeply into causative factors and outcomes. The Fulmer SPICES tool can be used in conjunction with an evidence-based assessment tool that assesses social isolation and loneliness to gauge the influence of social isolation and loneliness on patient health.

Health professionals also need to learn how to work directly with older adults and their significant others to support and encourage ways to prevent or reduce social isolation and loneliness. They need to know how to make and follow up on referrals to community services that may be helpful or that may specifically be intended to address social isolation and loneliness. This includes learning to work with direct care workers (e.g., home health aides, personal care workers), community health workers, family caregivers, and lay community members as part of a team-based approach to helping older adults. They also need to learn how to work with community partners to develop, implement, and evaluate programs for preventing and ameliorating social isolation and loneliness in older adults. Competency in each of these areas will become increasingly important for health professionals as systems of care are developed for preventing and intervening with social isolation and loneliness in older adults. Therefore, the committee offers the following goal and recommendations:

GOAL: Strengthen ongoing education and training related to social isolation and loneliness in older adults for the health care workforce.

RECOMMENDATION 8-3: Health professions schools and colleges as well as direct care worker training programs should include education and training related to social isolation and loneliness in their curricula, optimally as interprofessional team-based learning experiences.

- **Health education and training programs should include information on clinical approaches to assessing and intervening when an older adult is at risk for social isolation and loneliness.**
- **As evidence on effective interventions develops, health education and training programs should provide education on integrating care related to social isolation and loneliness into clinical practice and as part of discharge planning, care coordination, and transitional care planning with community organizations.**

RECOMMENDATION 8-4: Health professional associations should incorporate information about the health and medical impacts of social isolation and loneliness on older adults in their advocacy, practice, and education initiatives.

- **Health professional associations should include social isolation and loneliness in conference programming, webinars, toolkits, clinical guidelines, and advocacy priorities.**

RECOMMENDATION 8-5: Health professional associations, membership organizations, academic institutions, health insurers, researchers, developers of education and training programs, and other actors in the public and private sectors should support, develop, and test different educational and training approaches related to the health and medical impacts of social isolation and loneliness in older adults across different segments of the health care workforce (including health care professionals and direct care workers) in order to determine the most effective ways to enhance competencies. In addition to initial clinical education, these approaches should apply to professional education, continuing education modules, online learning, and other forms of lifelong learning.

Concerning the above recommendations the committee notes that, as discussed in Chapter 10, depending on the complexity of the knowledge to be disseminated or the evidence-based practices to be implemented, a variety of teaching strategies can be considered, including train-the-trainer programs, high-fidelity simulation, and ongoing point-of-care coaching (Brownson et al., 2018a; Titler and Anderson, 2019). Additionally, resource materials could be made available to faculty for inclusion in health professions courses. This information should be included in formal education programs, continuing education, and just-in-time learning. Other educational opportunities include the dissemination of information and resource availability through presentations at scientific meetings and webinars, publications in peer-reviewed journals, toolkits, and other forms of media. Toolkits should contain enough detail for use in practice, including modules, slides, reading materials, interactive exercises, case studies, and other tools that can support a variety of health professional education programs. Real-time and archived webinars and podcasts with faculty development materials to support the inclusion of content and learning activities could be helpful. Aside from developing educational opportunities specific to social isolation and loneliness, the committee recognizes that there are existing educational opportunities that could incorporate issues of social isolation and loneliness, such as those focused on the social determinants of health and those that address the inclusion of social care needs into clinical practice. Finally, as the evidence for interventions evolves, these educational and training opportunities need to expand to include new and updated evidence-based practices for preventing, assessing, and treating the negative health and medical impacts of social isolation and loneliness.

9

Interventions

Varied approaches have been used to mitigate the negative health impacts of social isolation and loneliness. This chapter first describes a number of large-scale efforts to review the effectiveness of interventions for social isolation or loneliness, with a focus on several approaches that are specific to health care settings. Next, the role of technology is considered, both as an intervention tool and a factor that exacerbates or contributes to social isolation and loneliness. Then, ethical issues pertaining to interventions are discussed and potential sources of funding for interventions are explored. The committee notes that educational approaches and awareness campaigns may be considered a type of intervention; however, these topics are covered in Chapter 8. Finally, the committee suggests ways to reframe interventions using a public health approach. Given the complexity of the terminology used in relation to social isolation and loneliness, a reminder of key definitions is provided in Box 9-1.

LARGE-SCALE REVIEWS OF INTERVENTIONS

Several studies and projects have examined interventions intended to ameliorate social isolation or loneliness specifically, or their associated health impacts; these interventions have generally not been limited to health care providers or settings (see Table 9-1). An extensive review of all interventions for social isolation and loneliness outside of the health care setting (e.g., efforts to create intergenerational communities) is beyond the scope of this report. However, the committee discusses these large-scale reviews here

BOX 9-1
Key Definitions

Loneliness: the perception of social isolation or the subjective feeling of being lonely.

Mediators: also known as mechanisms or pathways; the factors that help explain how social isolation or loneliness affects health outcomes.

Moderators: the factors that can influence the magnitude or direction of the effect of social isolation or loneliness on health.

Social connection: an umbrella term that encompasses the structural, functional, and quality aspects of how individuals connect to each other.

Social isolation: the objective lack of (or limited) social contact with others.

Social support: the actual or perceived availability of resources (e.g., informational, tangible, emotional) from others, typically one's social network.

for two reasons: first, most of these large-scale reviews do not separate interventions by setting and therefore the committee wanted to capture as much evidence on the effectiveness of interventions as possible; second, health care professionals and others will likely need to be aware of efforts in the community for possible referral.

Most of these large-scale reviews note the poor quality of the evidence concerning the effectiveness of such interventions. In particular, the authors of these reviews note several weaknesses in the study designs, including a lack of long-term follow-up, a limited range of ages included among "older adults," variability in the definitions of social isolation and loneliness, variability in the measurement tools and outcome measures used, and small sample sizes. Several studies reported that successful interventions tended to have certain key features, including the active participation of older adults, having an educational focus, and using a group-based approach.

In addition to reviews in the published literature, there have been other efforts to assess interventions for social isolation and loneliness among older adults (again, not limited to health care settings). The committee summarizes several of these efforts other than the studies listed in Table 9-1 in the following sections.

TABLE 9-1 Published Reviews of Interventions for Social Isolation and Loneliness

Author	Focus	Number of Studies	Key Findings	Recommendations
Findlay (2003)	Social isolation in older adults	17	• Most effective interventions involve high-quality training of intervention facilitators, active participation of older adults in planning, implementation, and evaluation, and use of existing community resources	• Evaluation should be built into intervention • Funding needed to evaluate sustainability and long-term benefits
Cattan et al. (2005)	Social isolation and loneliness in older adults	30	• Educational and social activity group interventions that target specific groups were most effective • Most effective interventions involve active participation of older adults • Unclear if home visits, befriending, or one-on-one interventions are effective • Substantial differences in target groups, measurement tools, and outcome measures	• Need for better study design • Need to draw on qualitative, observational, and multilevel evaluations to determine the transferability of evidence
Dickens et al. (2011)	Social isolation in older adults	32	• Interventions with a theoretical basis and active participation of the older adult appeared more likely to be effective • Group-based activities appeared to be more effective than one-on-one interventions • Substantial differences in definitions • Many studies had poor reporting and quality	• Encourage more randomized trials • Adhere to reporting guidelines • Include rigorous process evaluations
Masi et al. (2011)	Loneliness in all ages	50	• Interventions that address maladaptive thinking were most effective • Group-based interventions were no more effective than individual-based interventions • Most intervention studies are aimed at adults over age 60	• Future studies need to acknowledge that social isolation and loneliness are not the same concept • Control groups needed, but this might pose ethical problems • Consider ethics of randomized study designs • More attention needed for the role of technology

continued

TABLE 9-1 Continued

Author	Focus	Number of Studies	Key Findings	Recommendations
Centre for Policy on Ageing (2014)	Loneliness in all ages	72	• Key elements of success: group interventions with educational focus or specific support function, targeting a specific group, engagement of the participant, use of existing services, having a theoretical basis, and using technology	—
Cohen-Mansfield and Perach (2015)	Loneliness in older adults	34	• Variable results on effectiveness of one-on-one interventions as compared to groups • Methodological flaws are common: different groupings of age, small sample sizes, qualitative analyses • Use of technology is effective • Educational programs focused on social networks maintenance and enhancement appear to be effective	• Establish efficacy of specific approaches before starting more complex comparative studies • Research needed on cognitively impaired older adults —
Gardiner et al. (2018)	Social isolation and loneliness in older adults	38	• Group interventions are not necessarily more effective than one-on-one approaches • Elements of successful interventions: adaptability to local context, including input from the target population, and approaches that engage the individual	• Need better understanding for the mechanisms by which interventions affect social isolation and loneliness • Urgent need for research on cost-effectiveness of different approaches

AARP Foundation Catalog Project

The AARP Foundation commissioned Jessica Retrum of Metropolitan State University to do research toward the ultimate goal of creating "an interactive tool designed to serve as a resource catalog for evidence-based or promising practices to address loneliness and social isolation in older adults."[1] In her analysis, Retrum examined both published and unpublished interventions. Unpublished interventions were collected by outreach to groups that had previously contacted the AARP Foundation. Tables 9-2 through 9-5 describe the interventions evaluated in this review, categorized by target population, intervention level, intervention type, and the rigor of the evaluation in order to give a sense of the breadth of these interventions.

Retrum found that the most effective interventions included

- Specific targeting of socially isolated individuals;
- A multi-systemic approach;
- Active participation of the older adults; and
- Having a sound theoretical basis.[2]

Furthermore, Retrum noted[3] the following persistent challenges to the evaluation of interventions for social isolation and loneliness:

- A limited number of studies quantifying the impact of interventions;
- A shortage of randomized controlled trials (RCTs) and quasi-experimental studies;
- Variability in the concepts being measured;
- A targeting of either the general community or individuals who are "easy to find"; and
- Difficulty in recruiting those who are extremely isolated or lonely.

The committee noted that many of these studies, both published and unpublished, did not indicate that they had used a validated tool (as described in Chapter 6). Rather, many of these interventions assessed impact through qualitative interviews, surveys, and internally designed measurement tools.

[1] Presentation by Jessica Retrum to the committee on February 27, 2019.

[2] Retrum, J. 2017. PowerPoint presentation—*A review of interventions: Addressing social isolation in older adults.* In Public Access Files for the Committee on the Health and Medical Dimensions of Social Isolation and Loneliness in Older Adults (received December 21, 2018).

[3] Retrum, J. 2017. PowerPoint presentation—*A review of interventions: Addressing social isolation in older adults.* In Public Access Files for the Committee on the Health and Medical Dimensions of Social Isolation and Loneliness in Older Adults (received December 21, 2018).

TABLE 9-2 Target Population

Catalog	Totals	General Older Population	Health-Related Issue/Condition	Vulnerable Group	Residents in a Setting
Literature Review Interventions	92	37	7	31	17
Unpublished Interventions	48	13	10	22	3

SOURCES: Retrum, 2017; American Public Health Association (APHA) data (used with permission from APHA). In Public Access Files for the Committee on the Health and Medical Dimensions of Social Isolation and Loneliness in Older Adults (received December 21, 2018).

TABLE 9-3 Intervention Level

Catalog	Totals	One-on-One	Group	Community
Literature Review Interventions	92	27	41	24
Unpublished Interventions	48	31	13	3

SOURCES: Retrum, 2017; American Public Health Association (APHA) data (used with permission from APHA). In Public Access Files for the Committee on the Health and Medical Dimensions of Social Isolation and Loneliness in Older Adults (received December 21, 2018).

TABLE 9-4 Intervention Type

Catalog	Totals	Intentionally Addresses	General Social Activity/Engagement	Environment Change/New Resource (e.g., transportation, neighborhood safety)
Literature Review Interventions	92	41	55	39
Unpublished Interventions	48	27	21	12

SOURCES: Retrum, 2017; American Public Health Association (APHA) data (used with permission from APHA). In Public Access Files for the Committee on the Health and Medical Dimensions of Social Isolation and Loneliness in Older Adults (received December 21, 2018).

TABLE 9-5 Rigor of Evaluation

Catalog	Totals	1	2	3	4	5
Literature Review Interventions	92	0	18	22	31	21
Unpublished Interventions	48	10	4	30	4	0

NOTE: On a scale of 1 to 5, 1 = lowest, 5 = highest.
SOURCES: Retrum, 2017; American Public Health Association (APHA) data (used with permission from APHA). In Public Access Files for the Committee on the Health and Medical Dimensions of Social Isolation and Loneliness in Older Adults (received December 21, 2018).

Agency for Healthcare Research and Quality Rapid Review

In 2019 the Agency for Healthcare Research and Quality (AHRQ) conducted a review to "rapidly evaluate the effect of interventions targeting social isolation/loneliness in community-dwelling older adults (60 years and older) on outcomes of social isolation/loneliness, health, and health care utilization" (Veazie et al., 2019, p. ii). The researchers focused on 16 individual studies, but only half of these studies were deemed to be of good or fair quality. Ultimately, the researchers found limited evidence that the interventions significantly affected health outcomes. Two studies related to health services access interventions were found to be of poor quality. The researchers noted several challenges overall with the evidence base, including differences in constructs and measures, the overall poor quality of the studies (based on their quality assessments of study design), short follow-up periods, a lack of measurement of health care utilization or potential harms, and a failure to control for confounders. The researchers also noted that most studies were conducted outside of the United States. The report includes several recommendations for improving the quality of the evidence base, including

- "Collaborate with health systems, payers, and patient advocacy groups to agree upon standardized definitions and measures for social isolation and loneliness. As mentioned previously, social isolation is currently measured with myriad constructs and measures, which complicates the ability to draw conclusions between social isolation and health outcomes" (Veazie et al., 2019, p. 14).
- "Recruit and report results for a diverse population . . . to determine important population differences" (Veazie et al., 2019, p. 15).

Campaign to End Loneliness

The United Kingdom's Campaign to End Loneliness (see more in Chapter 8) noted that "in recent years there have been a number of attempts to bring together what is known about the effectiveness of loneliness interventions, however the conclusions drawn have been partial, and often contradictory" (Jopling, 2015, p. 7). As a result, the campaign assembled an expert panel to hear about promising loneliness interventions happening in communities that may not have been captured in the published literature. While conceding that they found "a lack of high-quality evidence to demonstrate the impact of different interventions on loneliness," the members of the expert panel suggested that "evidence exists on a spectrum, and even where the evidence is of a lower quality it can be an important step in the development of a firmer understanding of what works" (p. 8). The expert panel identified a variety of approaches that held the most promise, grouping them into four types of interventions: foundation services, direct interventions, gateway services, and structural enablers. However, most of these approaches have little evidence to support their effectiveness.

Foundation Services

The campaign describes foundation services as the first steps "coming before and providing a way into the more commonly recognized loneliness interventions" (Jopling, 2015, p. 9) and focus on three main challenges surrounding the uptake and effectiveness of interventions. First, *reaching individuals* includes using data to identify individuals at high risk; training individuals in a community to recognize signs of loneliness, make referrals, and provide support; and linking interventions to health care. (See Chapter 7 for more on the role of the health care system.) Second, *understanding* the nature of an individual's loneliness and developing a personalized response includes guided discussions in which the individual's circumstances, needs, and wishes are identified. One key factor is the individual's trust in the person asking questions. Finally, *supporting lonely individuals* to access appropriate services includes providing links to a "trusted buddy or mentor" (Jopling, 2015). The expert panel felt the most effective approaches were framed as "holistic and person-centred services, aimed at promoting healthy and active ageing, building resilience and supporting independence" that could be tailored to address loneliness (Jopling, 2015, p. 12). The expert panel recognized the lack of a robust evidence base for the effectiveness of these approaches and suggested that these approaches warranted further study.

Direct Interventions

While the expert panel preferred more "holistic approaches," they also considered interventions that seek to address loneliness directly. These include "supporting individuals to reconnect with and/or maintain existing relationships, fostering and enabling new connections, and helping people to change their thinking about their social connections" (Jopling, 2015, p. 25). The report notes,

> It is clear the vast majority of loneliness interventions currently available seek to reduce loneliness by increasing the quantity and quality of relationships, and most do this by supporting individuals to develop new relationships. Most experts believed that these kinds of interventions were effective in tackling loneliness, but few held up specific examples as showing significant promise over others. Instead they argued that any and all such interventions could be helpful if they were chosen by the older person and well-suited to their needs (hence the importance of the foundation services). Many experts talked about the need for communities to offer a menu of such approaches. (Jopling, 2015, p. 10)

Experts varied in their opinions about whether group interventions or one-on-one approaches were more effective. The experts agreed that the most effective direct group-based interventions target a specific group, focus on a shared interest (or on education), and include the older individuals in the planning process. They also felt that some people had significant barriers to making connections, and so, in spite of the lack of evidence, they recognized the importance of one-on-one approaches such as "befriending."

Gateway Services

Gateway services are services such as transportation and technology that can affect social connection. In particular, the lack of access to such services could also impede the effectiveness of broader interventions. (See section later in this chapter on access to technology.)

Structural Enablers

Structural enablers are defined by the campaign as approaches that consider the environmental factors needed within communities to help reduce loneliness. These approaches are often used in conjunction with other interventions and include working with an asset-based community development approach (wherein the intervention identifies and takes advantages of community assets instead of identifying community needs), promoting volunteerism, and using age-friendly approaches (see more on age-friendly health systems later in this chapter).

TYPES OF INTERVENTIONS RELEVANT TO THE HEALTH CARE SYSTEM

Although the terms "treatment" and "intervention" are often used synonymously, they actually refer to different things. An individual suffering from an illness or disease receives *treatment* from a health care provider to mitigate the disease and its symptoms. *Interventions*, on the other hand, are designed to improve health status or encourage behavior change and are applied in the larger community by public health authorities (WHO, 2019b). While only a few treatments have been suggested to mitigate social isolation or loneliness, a variety of interventions targeting isolation and loneliness have been proposed.

Direct interventions are those that explicitly target social isolation, loneliness, or related social concepts. Direct interventions can fall into one of several categories: changing cognition, social skills training and psychoeducation, supported socialization, and wider community groups that create a broader sense of social integration (Mann et al., 2017). Outside of the health care system, these types of interventions often include one-on-one befriending approaches in which volunteers reach out through phone calls to individuals identified as being socially isolated or lonely. Within the health care system, this may include reaching out to individuals identified as being at risk for social isolation or loneliness in order to connect them to needed services. Alternatively, interventions may include convening groups of at-risk individuals, in part to provide opportunities for social interaction. However, these types of approaches do not necessarily help individuals develop high-quality relationships, and lonely people in particular may withdraw, for example, due to an unconscious predisposition or hypervigilance to social threat (Caciopppo et al., 2015a,b).

Indirect interventions are those that do not specifically aim to mitigate isolation or loneliness but may nonetheless have significant effects on an individual's perceived or objective isolation (Mann et al., 2017). For example, a physician may recommend hearing aids to assist an individual with impaired hearing; as a result, the individual may find it easier to interact in social environments and make connections with others, thereby reducing social isolation and loneliness. Similarly, participation in an exercise program for health may lead to reductions in social isolation or loneliness due to the social nature of the program rather than the exercise itself.

The following sections describe several types of interventions that aim to address social isolation or loneliness that are particularly relevant for the health care system.

Social Prescribing

No agreed-upon definition of social prescribing currently exists, though it is widely accepted that social prescribing helps patients access non-clinical sources of support, which are often provided by the community sector (Moffatt et al., 2017). Social prescribing has been defined as a "non-medical referral, or linking service, to help people identify their social needs and develop 'well-being' action plans to promote, establish, or re-establish integration and support in their communities, with the aim of improving personal well-being" (Carnes et al., 2017, p. 2). While community-based organizations have traditionally employed social prescribing as a way to help support individuals in their communities, social prescribing has been suggested as a way for health care practitioners to respond to isolation and loneliness in their patients. In her comments to this committee in 2018, Helen Stokes-Lampard, the chair of the Royal College of General Practitioners in the United Kingdom, described social prescribing as "a fancy name for what good doctors have always done, which is navigate our patients towards other resources outside of the health care sector that can help them."[4] Community-based organizations have long used this approach. For the purposes of this report, social prescribing will refer to the steps that health care providers can take to link patients with existing social services programs.

[4]Video presentation by Helen Stokes-Lampard to the committee. In Public Access Files for the Committee on the Health and Medical Dimensions of Social Isolation and Loneliness in Older Adults (received December 21, 2018).

Connecting people with volunteer organizations and community groups has the potential to affect health and well-being both directly (e.g., lowering stress) and indirectly (e.g., improving access to social services) and may be seen as a way of extending primary care (South et al., 2008). Social prescribing attempts to prevent worsening health by commissioning secondary services that can help alleviate social concerns that affect health (e.g., food or housing insecurity), thereby reducing the costly interventions provided in specialist or inpatient settings (Dayson and Bashir, 2014).

Various interventions to mitigate the negative effects of isolation and loneliness fall within the realm of the community sector. Community-based groups such as social welfare systems, community organizations, religious groups, and government groups may be natural partners for the health care system when it comes to addressing social isolation and loneliness. Because social prescribing is tailored to existing voluntary and community-sector-led programs, it is believed to result in better social and clinical outcomes for people with chronic conditions and their caretakers, a more cost-efficient way to use health and social care[5] resources, and a wider and more diverse and responsive local provider base (Dayson and Bashir, 2014). However, despite the promising nature of many community-based programs, this type of support often remains underused due to the weak or nonexistent link between health care practitioners and community-based services (South et al., 2008).

Different models of social prescribing interventions are presented in Box 9-2. Little evidence exists concerning the results of social prescribing interventions on social isolation and loneliness, and what evidence does exist is mixed (Moffatt et al., 2017). However, social prescribing interventions do have a number of promising features, including that they are long-term in nature, they address the existence of mental and physical comorbidities and social isolation simultaneously, they target specific groups (e.g., women, caretakers, or people with diabetes), they involve affected individuals in the intervention design process, and they address related socioeconomic issues (Centre for Policy on Ageing, 2014; Moffatt et al., 2017; Polley et al., 2016; see Figure 9-1).

One social prescribing tool tested in the United Kingdom, the Patient-Led Assessment for Network Support (PLANS), attempted to consolidate up-to-date information about health-relevant local resources into one website for people living with chronic health conditions (Blickem et al., 2013). The conceptual basis of PLANS was the notion that the needs of people with chronic health conditions cannot be adequately met through small targeted interventions that are not integrated into everyday life. The website included a self-assessment questionnaire, the results of which provided users with a tailored set of social and health resources available in the community. The resources were grouped into the areas of providing relevant health information, well-being (time spent doing meaningful and enjoyable things),

[5] Social care refers to "services that address health-related social risk factors and social needs" (NASEM, 2019, p. 1).

BOX 9-2
Models of Social Prescribing (SP)

Model 1: Information service
This service is an information-only service, with advertising and directory access to SP in a primary care practice.

Model 2: Information service and telephone line
This service advertises SP on leaflets and notice boards in the primary care practice. Based on this information, patients can self-initiate a telephone discussion with a worker.

Model 3: Primary care referral
Primary health care professionals assess patients during consultation and refer them to SP services if appropriate (e.g., if patients have nonclinical issues and require psychosocial support). Referrals to SP services are opportunistic.

Model 4: Practice-based general care worker
Primary care patients can be referred by health workers or self-refer to an SP link worker. Clinics are held in the general practice surgery so that it can act as a "one stop shop."

Model 5: Practice-based specialist referral worker
A specialist worker works from primary care practice, and patients can be referred through primary care referral or self-referral. Direct advice and specific services, such as Citizens Advice, may be offered, as well as referral or signposting onward.

Model 6: Non–primary care–based referral worker
Patients are referred to an external referral center by primary care practice staff, offering one-to-one facilitation, for example, and outreach service or set in the community.

SOURCE: Pescheny et al., 2018.

practical support (help with every day, independent living), and services related to diet and exercise (Blickem et al., 2013).

Another example of a social prescribing system was piloted in Rotherham, United Kingdom, from 2012 to 2014, with the aim of increasing the capacity of general practitioners to meet the non-clinical needs of patients with long-term conditions. The pilot employed a team of voluntary and community sector advisors who received referrals from general practitioners, completed an assessment of referred individuals to identify their needs, and then linked

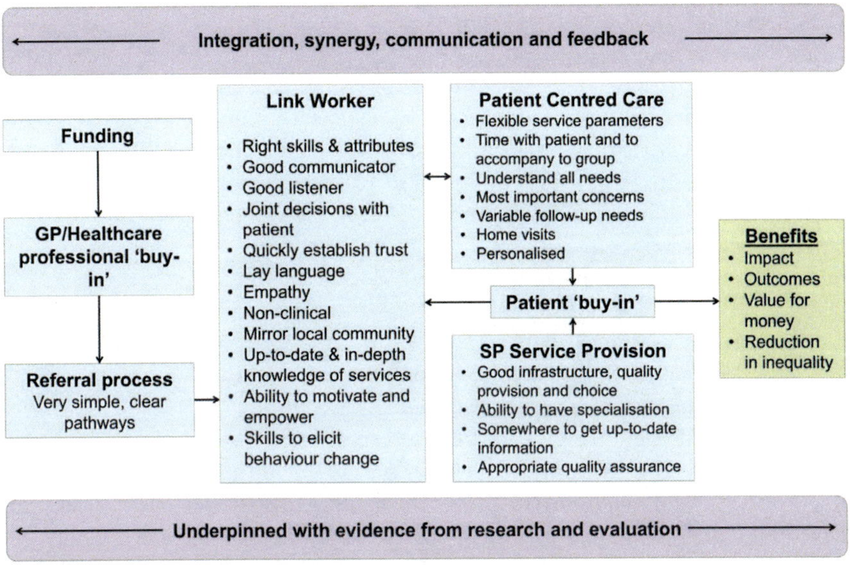

FIGURE 9-1 Key ingredients of social prescribing.
NOTE: GP = general practitioner; SP = social prescribing.
SOURCE: Polley et al., 2016.

individuals with appropriate social services. Referrals were made to a variety of social service providers, and the services addressing isolation or loneliness included befriending services, group activity programs, home visits, and group therapy sessions. An analysis of the pilot found that among the patients who received social prescribing services, inpatient admissions were reduced as much as 21 percent and accident and emergency attendance were reduced by as much as 20 percent (Dayson and Bashir, 2014). However, the sample size and length of the pilot were both small, so these results were not statistically significant.

Support Groups and Group Membership

In general, peer support groups, such as those for individuals with a common illness or condition, have proved to be of value. For social isolation and loneliness, group interventions may be aimed directly at those who are socially isolated or lonely. One approach is to provide guidance for improving social skills (Masi et al., 2011). For example, a "friendship enrichment program" in the Netherlands (that included training in skills relevant to friendship), which was aimed at women aged 55 and older, resulted in 63 percent of the participants reporting having made new friends through social and education activities (compared to 33 percent among women who did not participate in the program, but were interested in improving their friendships) (Martina and Stevens, 2007). However, the execution of social skills may be complicated by issues of performance anxiety

(Knowles et al., 2015). Support groups may also be directed at people who share common underlying causes of social isolation and loneliness, such as bereavement or widowhood (Chow et al., 2018; Stewart et al., 2001).

On the other hand, the reduction of social isolation or loneliness may result from an individual's participation in group activities aimed at other purposes, such as education, volunteerism, or health promotion activities. For example, a study of SilverSneakers®,[6] a fitness program for older adults, found that "membership directly increased physical activity and self-rated health, directly decreased social isolation, and indirectly decreased loneliness" (Brady et al., 2020, p. 301). A study of the "hidden elderly" in Hong Kong (defined as "older adults who are socially isolated and refuse social participation") found that participation in a tai chi qigong program resulted in improvement in loneliness (as measured by the de Jong Gierveld Loneliness Scale).[7] Key elements of the program included the training of community elders to act as "health ambassadors" of the project; these individuals lived near the hidden elderly and helped to create a sense of neighborhood and peer-to-peer relationships. A clinical trial, Leveraging Exercise to Age in Place (LEAP),[8] is now under way to evaluate the impact of a participation in a community exercise program on social isolation. The LEAP study plans to evaluate changes in the Duke Social Support Index at 26 weeks after enrollment. However, a recent AHRQ rapid review (discussed earlier in this chapter) states

> Physical activity interventions to reduce social isolation showed the most promise at improving the health of older adults; however, effects were inconsistent and short-term. (Veazie et al., 2019, p. ii)

Cognitive Behavioral Therapy and Mindfulness

The ways in which humans think and perceive involve both conscious and unconscious mechanisms. As a result, loneliness can generate a vicious cycle in which lonely people withdraw further because they perceive social interactions as negative or unfriendly. Hawkley et al. (2007) found that lonely individuals perceive greater negativity in social interactions than do non-lonely individuals and that lonely individuals perform more poorly on tests of executive functioning than non-lonely individuals (Cacioppo and Hawkley, 2009). Loneliness is also associated with hypervigilance for social threat[9] (Cacioppo et al., 2015b). Taken together, biased

---

[6] For more information on SilverSneakers®, see www.silversneakers.com (accessed November 14, 2019).

[7] See https://www.ncbi.nlm.nih.gov/pmc/articles/PMC5221552 (accessed November 14, 2019).

[8] See https://clinicaltrials.gov/ct2/show/NCT03624049 (accessed November 14, 2019).

[9] Hypervigilance to social threats is "an assumption in line with the evolutionary model of loneliness that indicates feeling socially isolated (or on the social perimeter) leads to increased attention and surveillance of the social world and an unwitting focus on self-preservation" (Cacioppo et al., 2016, p. 138).

perceptions and hypervigilance toward negativity may cause lonely individuals to unconsciously withdraw from social connections, even though they may consciously desire to connect with others. This reaction creates problems in particular when lonely individuals attempt to connect with others but perceive the interactions negatively and become discouraged, leading to a vicious cycle of loneliness and withdrawal.

Cognitive Behavioral Therapy

Cognitive behavioral therapy (CBT) is a type of psychotherapy that is used to help patients deal with a variety of issues ranging from more serious mental health disorders such as depression and posttraumatic stress disorder to day-to-day stressors and anxieties (Mayo Clinic, 2019). The goal of CBT is to teach individuals to identify their own faulty perceptions and irrational beliefs in order to approach and respond to challenging or stressful situations in a more clearheaded and effective way (McWhirter, 1990). By challenging automatic and negative thought patterns, CBT may be useful in helping lonely individuals reframe the way they think about their relationships, their assumptions about others' views, or their expectations of success at overcoming loneliness (Mann et al., 2017). CBT has been found effective in addressing social anxiety disorder, insomnia, and unipolar depression (Butler et al., 2006; Edinger et al., 2001; Gress et al., 2008; Heimberg, 2002; Koszycki et al., 2007).

Few CBT-based interventions for loneliness or isolation have been tested in RCTs, and those that have been tested through RCTs have found mixed results. Mann and colleagues (2017) identified 10 published RCTs on cognitive approaches to improving loneliness or related concepts (e.g., social support, social network, social isolation) in people with mental health problems. Of the interventions considered, most therapies showed no effect on loneliness; however, two online CBT interventions for individuals suffering from depression were found to be successful at decreasing depressed mood and loneliness at 12-month follow-up (Saulsberry et al., 2013). While there is limited evidence of the effectiveness of CBT in mitigating social isolation and loneliness, many consider CBT to be a promising path forward (Mann et al., 2017).

Interpersonal Psychotherapy

CBT and interpersonal psychotherapy are both recognized as being "empirically-based psychotherapeutic interventions for mood disorders," and "both are diagnosis-targeted, time-limited, present-focused treatments that encourage the patient to regain control of mood and functioning" (Markowitz and Weissman, 2004, p. 136). Interpersonal psychotherapy was originally developed as a treatment for depression (Cuijpers et al., 2011; De Mello et al., 2005). Interpersonal psychotherapy differs from CBT in that its focus is on maladaptive thinking specifically related to interpersonal relationships.

Interpersonal psychotherapy for depression focuses on two principles: viewing depression as a medical illness (not the fault of the patient) and making the connection between mood and triggering life events, such as bereavement (Markowitz and Weissman, 2004). While interpersonal therapy has not been extensively studied as an intervention specifically for social isolation or loneliness, its focus on maladaptive thinking and interpersonal relationships could be an approach to explore.

Mindfulness

Mindfulness, a way of being in which an individual maintains openness, patience, and acceptance while focusing on life situations in a non-judgmental way, has also been suggested as a way to mitigate the negative effects of isolation and loneliness (Gilmartin et al., 2017). Lindsay and colleagues (2019) conducted an RCT in which smartphone-based training was used to train participants in mindfulness techniques of awareness and acceptance for 2 weeks. The study found that individuals who received mindfulness training reported a 22 percent reduction in daily loneliness compared with the control group; thus, mindfulness training may be a promising way to mitigate the subjective risk factors associated with loneliness.

Pharmaceutical Interventions

Currently, nearly all interventions that have been proposed to treat isolation and loneliness are behavioral or psychological in nature. However, the interventions that focus solely on increasing the time spent socializing or increasing the number of social contacts may be greatly hindered by lonely individuals' negatively biased perceptions and tendency toward interacting defensively with others. To boost the possible success of behavioral interventions, adjunctive treatments or therapies that target the biological underpinnings of biased cognition have been suggested as a potential tool. Adjunctive therapy is a form of treatment used in tandem with a primary treatment with the goal of assisting the primary therapy (NCI, 2011). In theory, pharmaceuticals could be used to minimize some of the negative behavioral effects of social isolation and loneliness (e.g., anxiety, fear), allowing individuals to maximize the satisfaction gained from their social interactions and building relationships with others, which in turn may increase the success of behavioral therapies (e.g., CBT). However, consideration is needed for whether decreasing symptoms of loneliness, for example, might mitigate motivation to increase human connection, and thereby lead to increased isolation.

Research in animal models suggests that behavioral or psychological interventions for isolation and loneliness may benefit from adjunctive biological treatments that target the underlying neurobiology. This includes the potential use of selective serotonin reuptake inhibitors (e.g., fluoxetine), neurosteroids (e.g., allopregnenolone), or oxytocin (Cacioppo et al., 2015b). Fluoxetine has been associated with improving behaviors related to anxiety and fear (Cacioppo et al., 2015b; Mayo-Wilson et al., 2014; Pinna, 2010). In animal models, isolation of the animals has been associated with a decrease in the concentration in the brain of pregnenolone (Serra et al., 2000), a hormone that has been associated with memory enhancement (Vallée et al., 2001). In humans pregnenolone has been shown to improve depressive symptoms in individuals with bipolar disorder (Brown et al., 2014), though evidence of its effects on memory is contradictory (Vallée et al., 2001). The use of pregnenolone for loneliness is currently in a phase II clinical trial (NIH, 2016). Oxytocin is associated with social affiliation, and its use in animal models suggests it could mitigate the harmful effects of social isolation (Carter et al., 2008; Grippo et al., 2009, 2012; Young et al., 2014). The use of oxytocin in humans has been suggested to promote positive social behaviors, but the evidence for its use is mixed, and more research is needed about which individuals might benefit the most (Bartz et al., 2011; Cacioppo et al., 2015b).

Interventions That Target Social Determinants of Health Broadly

Social determinants of health are often interconnected, and therefore social isolation and loneliness may be addressed through efforts to address the social determinants of health more holistically. For example, many Medicaid programs are moving toward screening for social determinants of health and connecting individuals to needed supports (Manatt Health, 2019). An example of a program targeting the social determinants of health broadly is AIRnyc. This community-based organization uses community health workers to link patients to services in order to address social determinants related to diabetes prevention and management, asthma, hypertension, aging in place, behavioral health, maternal health, and substance use disorder at the individual and household levels.[10] (See Chapter 7 for more on the role of the health care system in addressing the social determinants of health. See later in this chapter for more on financing interventions for social isolation and loneliness through existing programs directed at the social determinants of health.)

Centene, one of the nation's largest Medicaid managed care organizations, serves more than 14.5 million managed care members across 32 states. The organization has committed itself to providing "access to high-quality health care, innovative programs, and a wide range of health solutions that help families and individuals get well, stay well, and be well" (Centene, 2019). Centene is in the process of developing new strategies to address the social determinants of health broadly, which could include social isolation and loneliness, through efforts to address factors known to be at the core of the health and well-being of individuals. Centene envisions these long-term efforts as a way to create sustainable funding for programs that will address issues such as linguistic and cultural differences between the social sector (e.g., community benefit organizations) and the health

[10] For more information, see https://www.air-nyc.org (accessed August 3, 2019).

sector (e.g., hospitals and payers organizations). Centene envisions a scalable program with broad impact that is guided by a standard set of protocols, procedures, and analytics that can be individualized to different markets. There has not yet been a formal evaluation of this program.

Interventions That Target Social Isolation and Loneliness in the Health Care System

A handful of trial interventions specifically targeting social isolation or loneliness within the health care system have been developed, though few of these have been empirically proven to work. CareMore Health is an integrated health plan and care delivery system for Medicare and Medicaid patients. In 2017 it created the Togetherness Program, which is composed of three inter-related approaches for helping people found to be isolated: Phone Pal, a phone-based interaction; a home-based visiting program; and leveraging existing care centers as social hubs with a community health worker embedded in the space. Individuals can opt into the Togetherness Program during their initial HealthyStart visit or can be referred to the program by physicians in the CareMore system.[11] Early results suggest that the Togetherness Program has decreased emergency room use among enrolled patients by 3.3 percent compared to baseline; additionally, hospital admissions per thousand members are 20.8 percent lower among program participants than in the control group (Business Wire, 2018). CareMore appointed a chief togetherness officer who manages the program and fosters internal and external partnerships related to the topic (Jain and Samitt, 2018).

UnitedHealthcare, a large health insurance company, launched the Navigate4Me program in fall 2017 for individuals enrolled in its Medicare Advantage plans who live with complex health issues such as diabetes, congestive heart failure, or multiple chronic conditions (UnitedHealth Group, 2018). The program offers health navigators who support and guide individuals through the complicated health care system, providing both clinical and administrative assistance (such as answering health questions and resolving billing issues) in addition to addressing the social determinants of health (e.g., by connecting individuals with reliable transportation or housing assistance). UnitedHealth Group reports early positive results, with a 14 percent reduction in hospitalizations and a 9 percent reduction in emergency room visits for people with congestive heart failure (UnitedHealth Group, 2018). In 2018, eligibility for the program was expanded and specifically made available to individuals at risk for social isolation.

Kaiser Permanente, an integrated managed care consortium, launched Thrive Local in 2019. This program created a new social health network in Oregon and southwest Washington State with the aim of creating connections between health care providers and social services agencies. To best address the social needs of its members, Thrive Local will be built locally in partnership with nonprofit and

[11] Presentation by Dr. Sachin Jain to the committee on April 25, 2019.

government agencies, with the goal of including other health systems and health centers (Kaiser Permanente, 2019). Thrive Local will be integrated into Kaiser's electronic health record as a way of tracking social needs and referrals to social providers (Johnson, 2019).

Other health insurance companies are beginning to identify social isolation and loneliness as problems that need to be addressed in their broader health campaigns. Humana's Bold Goal[12] is a population health strategy that specifically addresses the social determinants of health, including loneliness and social isolation, in order to improve health status. As part of this, Humana created a Loneliness Toolkit (Humana, 2018) for consumers that addresses such issues as health care needs, staying engaged, and supporting loved ones who may be isolated or lonely. Humana also developed a one-page guide (Humana, 2019) for physicians, which focuses on defining social isolation and loneliness, highlighting their major health impacts, presenting the three-item UCLA Loneliness Scale, and advising physicians on potential referrals and resources. Other health insurance companies are leveraging existing health promotion programs to combat isolation and loneliness. In May 2018, Cigna released the results from a survey assessing the impact of loneliness in the United States; the president and chief executive officer, David Cordani, said of the data: "[W]e're seeing a lack of human connection, which ultimately leads to a lack of vitality" (Cigna, 2018). Cigna is using existing programs, such as its Health Advisor Program, Health Information Line, and Employee Assistance Program, in order to address loneliness in the company's employee and patient populations (Cigna, 2018).

Interventions That Target Specific Risk Factors

Another approach to addressing social isolation and loneliness in the health care system is to identify specific underlying risk factors (particularly health-related risk factors) and to address those issues as appropriate within the health care system. Interventions that fail to target the underlying causes of isolation and loneliness are likely to be less successful.

For example, as mentioned in Chapter 4, untreated hearing loss is associated with social isolation and loneliness (Chen, 1994; Mick et al., 2014, 2018; Pronk et al., 2013; Sung et al., 2016; Weinstein and Ventry, 1982). Several studies suggest that treating hearing loss with hearing aids or cochlear implants may mitigate the effects of hearing loss on loneliness (Contrera et al., 2017; Weinstein et al., 2016).

Other interventions that target specific risk factors focus on enhancing cognition (Winningham and Pike, 2007); enhancing physical mobility or exercise (Brady et al., 2020; Ollonqvist et al., 2012; Tse et al., 2014; Wallace et al., 2014; Zijlstra et al., 2009); and dealing with bereavement or widowhood (Chow et al., 2018; Stewart et al., 2001). (See Chapter 7 for more on the role of the health care system in identifying and addressing the underlying causes of social isolation and loneliness.)

[12] For more information, see https://populationhealth.humana.com (accessed August 5, 2019).

COALITIONS AND PARTNERSHIPS TO ADDRESS SOCIAL ISOLATION AND LONELINESS

The 2019 National Academies consensus study report *Integrating Social Care into the Delivery of Health Care* identified assistance, alignment, and advocacy as key activities to facilitate the integration of health care and social care (NASEM, 2019). *Assistance* activities "reduce social risk by providing assistance in connecting patients with relevant social care resources" (p. 44). *Alignment* activities are "undertaken by health care systems to understand existing social care assets in the community, organize them in such a way as to encourage synergy among the various activities, and invest in and deploy them to prevent emerging social needs and improve health outcomes" (p. 46). *Advocacy* activities involve health care organizations partnering with social care organizations "to promote policies that facilitate the creation and redeployment of assets or resources in order to improve health outcomes and prevent emergence of unmet social needs" (p. 47). Furthermore, the National Academies committee that produced the report noted that in such activities, "health care organizations leverage their political, social, and economic capital within a community or local environment to encourage and enable health care and social care organizations to partner and pool resources, such as services and information, to achieve greater net benefit" (p. 47). Cross-sector coalitions and partnerships are two strategies for increasing assistance, alignment, and advocacy. For the purposes of this current report, the committee identified the formation of coalitions and partnerships to share best practices as among the key strategies (or even interventions themselves) underlying the identification and implementation of effective interventions for social isolation and loneliness in older adults. Several coalitions and partnerships have been formed specifically in response to the growing public recognition of the health impacts of social isolation and loneliness. The sections below highlight a few examples.

Oregon Healthy Aging Summit

The Oregon Healthy Aging Summit was a collaborative effort "to develop a roadmap and accelerate action to promote the healthy aging of older adults in Oregon"[13] by bringing together policy makers, providers, patients, and researchers to address issues related to social isolation. The summit sought to represent many diverse groups who may have specialized needs such as people of different races or sexual orientation or individuals living in less populous or rural locales. The summit was structured around the AHRQ rapid evidence review (described earlier in this chapter), with the review acting as a framework for summit presentations and discussions.

[13] Guise, J. M. 2018. PowerPoint presentation to committee—*Addressing social isolation to improve the health of older adults: A rapid review and summit.* In Public Access Files for the Committee on the Health and Medical Dimensions of Social Isolation and Loneliness in Older Adults (received December 21, 2018).

Several different programs targeting social isolation were discussed, including those related to physical activities, social support, arts and recreation, and access to health services. Some of the major priorities outlined by summit participants were:

- The development of an information system to connect health systems and community resources.
- The co-creation of measures and implementation strategies and the evaluation of programs using the same definitions and measures.
- The development and maintenance of a person-centered approach that promotes equity.

Post-summit activities included setting up a shared email (healthaging@ohsu.edu), establishing and expanding connections, collecting and distributing information on resources, and planning subsequent meetings with health system leaders to discuss sharing data and social services locator services.

Los Angeles Social Isolation and Loneliness Impact Coalition

The Los Angeles Social Isolation and Loneliness Impact Coalition was created through a collaborative arrangement between the Motion Picture and Television Fund (MPTF) and the AARP Foundation with the goal of addressing the health and financial impacts of social isolation and loneliness in older adults. The coalition seeks to build on and promote existing community-wide efforts focused on addressing social isolation and loneliness and creating partnerships and sustainable social interventions that can be expanded nationally. MPTF initiated a volunteer-operated call center called A Daily Call Sheet that facilitates communication with very isolated or low-income individuals, many of whom have chronic illnesses. In describing the work of the coalition to the committee, Maureen Feldman, the director of Social Isolation Impact Project in Los Angeles and the director and the founding chair of the Los Angeles Social Isolation and Loneliness Impact Coalition explained that to date, [roughly] 10,000 social calls have been made through this program to active industry members, retirees, and relatives of industry members. While the coalition is not specifically focused on the role of the health care system, coalition member and collaborative efforts have been broad and include

- annual summits on social isolation and loneliness with participation from for-profit and not-for-profit businesses, academic institutions, and faith-based organizations;
- the creation of a call program toolkit to help establish new social outreach programs and to train volunteers;
- the initiation of ongoing data collection and analysis protocols;
- the implementation of new friendly call programs;

- the training of local police on social isolation issues and resources for homeless individuals;
- connecting people in need with key resources; and
- providing access to economical graduate education to older adults.

According to Feldman, a survey of coalition members in 2018 revealed that the top reasons for joining the coalition included developing partnerships (87 percent), sharing of best practices (80 percent), and learning about the latest research (70 percent). In describing the work of the coalition, Feldman explained, "Together we will find ways to effectively collaborate and create meaningful change."

AARP Foundation Connect2Affect

As noted in Chapter 8, the AARP Foundation has partnered with the Gerontological Society of America, Give an Hour, n4a, and UnitedHealthcare to share information about successful interventions and the latest academic research on social isolation (AARP Foundation, 2019). The Connect2Affect website includes an option for individuals to share resources related to new research or best practices. Like the Campaign to End Loneliness' Learning Network (see Chapter 8), this repository largely represents an effort to share resources and does not primarily conduct evidence-based assessments of interventions on their own.

TECHNOLOGICAL INTERVENTIONS

Information technology (IT) can provide a platform for the delivery of targeted individual or group interventions. A variety of technologies have been tested as ways to reduce social isolation and loneliness in older adults (Chipps et al., 2017; Khosravi et al., 2016). Table 9-6 provides an overview of potential IT solutions with different functionalities, the types of technologies used, and specific examples of their use to address social isolation and loneliness. (This chapter will focus on the use of technology for interventions. See Chapters 6 and 7 for a discussion on the use of technology for assessment.)

With the growth of artificial intelligence (AI), social robots and conversational agents are often viewed as effective tools for social engagement in gerontology. Virtual reality is another platform that is expected to help older adults with social engagement. More traditional and widely available tools, such as social media groups and video conferencing, are frequently integrated into behavioral or supportive interventions for isolated older adults. With any of these technological approaches, challenges related to user friendliness remain.

Internet Use

The potential of the Internet to connect older adults has been examined since the early days of online communities. While new tools are being introduced to

TABLE 9-6 Types of Information Technology Tools to Address Older Adults' Social Isolation and Loneliness

Function	Technology	Example(s)
Assessment (mining data to identify or predict patterns of social isolation and loneliness)	Passive home-based monitoring sensors	Motion sensors and door/window sensors capture time spent inside versus outside the home, the number of visitors, the amount of time spent in the presence of others
	Tracking of usage patterns of online and phone tools	Tracking time spent interacting on social media platforms, time spent on the phone, number of phone calls and video calls initiated and received
	Wearable sensors	Activity and sleep tracking facilitated by a wrist-worn watch provides data for one's life-space (as a series of concentric areas radiating from the room where one sleeps and extending to the residential setting, neighborhood, community, and beyond)
Intervention	Social media "virtual communities"	Engagement in peer-support groups (for example, Facebook "secret groups" to exchange information and seek emotional support)
	Virtual reality	Virtual reality (VR) systems including hardware (a VR headset) and software (with virtual reality content specifically designed for older adults with the goal of providing reminiscence therapy elements with familiar experiences or engagement with new stimulations)
	Social robots/ conversational agents	Use of conversational agents with artificial intelligence functions to engage users in dialogue either for general companionship or for meeting specific goals (reminders, health or safety assessment)
	Video-mediated "friendly visits"	Use of video conferencing software such as Skype or FaceTime or commercially available software for volunteers or other staff to conduct regular "friendly visits"

increase social engagement, the inability of older adults to use them may exacerbate their isolation. Older adults who are not familiar with new media platforms seem more likely to become isolated from groups or cohorts that use emerging technologies for communication (Melenhorst et al., 2001). White et al. (2002) facilitated Internet access for 100 older adult volunteers from four congregate housing sites and two nursing facilities over a 5-month period. The volunteers were randomly assigned to receive Internet training or to a waitlist control group. Results showed a trend toward lower loneliness and depression among those who received training, but this was not statistically significant.

Cotten and colleagues (2013) examined the usage of information technologies among older adults in assisted and independent living communities in Alabama and found that Internet use was associated with lower levels of loneliness. Similar findings were reported by Russell et al. (2008) in a study surveying older Australian Internet users: Internet use facilitated access to bonding capital (maintaining close ties) and also bridging capital (connections across social networks). Also in Australia, in a later online survey study of older adults, greater use of the Internet as a communication tool was associated with a lower level of social loneliness; however, greater use of the Internet to find new people was associated with a higher level of emotional loneliness (Sum et al., 2008).

In 2010 Hogeboom and colleagues used the Health and Retirement Survey (HRS) to examine associations between Internet use and social networks among 2,284 adults over 50 years of age. Frequency of contact with friends, frequency of contact with family, and attendance at organizational meetings (not including religious services) were found to have a significant positive association with Internet use. These survey findings suggested that Internet use can strengthen social networks for older adults.

Internet use has also been found to be beneficial in the context of social isolation and loneliness for homebound older adults. The CHIPS (Computers for Homebound and Isolated Persons) Program sought to create an online community for individuals who were homebound and to connect seniors with others in similar circumstances (Bradley and Poppen, 2003). A 1-year follow-up showed that the participants' level of satisfaction in the amount of contact with others increased significantly.

Tsai and Tsai (2011) used video conferencing software to connect nursing home residents with remote family members during a 3-month intervention deployed in 16 nursing homes in Taiwan. The program had a long-term effect in alleviating depressive symptoms and loneliness for nursing home residents, and it also improved long-term emotional social support and short-term appraisal support.

Czaja and colleagues (2018) noted the importance for older adults of having "meaningful access" (p. 476) to the Internet and computer-mediated strategies for social support. They reported that access to the Personal Reminder Information and Social Management (PRISM) computer system yielded lower levels of social isolation and less perceived loneliness in older adults after 6 months. Although the differences between the PRISM group and the control group were not maintained after 12 months, the PRISM group still showed improvements in social isolation and loneliness compared to baseline. The investigators noted that technological interventions such as PRISM would not supplant human interaction, but might supplement other strategies.

Social Media Use

The Pew Research Center (2018) estimates that older adults are the fastest-growing group of individuals to adopt and use social media sites. Social media use can be differentiated into active and passive use. *Active use* refers to "activities that facilitate direct exchanges with others," whereas *passive use* pertains to the "monitoring of other people's lives without engaging in direct exchanges with others" (Verduyn et al., 2017, p. 281). However, different segments of the older adult population may be using social media in different ways or have different levels of comfort with its use. For example, older adults seem to use Facebook less actively than younger adults (Hayes et al., 2015).

A 2012 Pew Report identified three factors that contribute to social media use among older adults: receiving social support, reconnecting with peers in their age groups, and bridging generational gaps (Zickuhr and Madden, 2012). Jung et al. (2017) conducted in-depth interviews to identify why older adults use or avoid Facebook. Six main motivators were identified: the desire to keep in touch, sharing photos, social surveillance, responding to family member requests, convenience in communication, and curiosity. The main reasons given for avoiding Facebook included privacy considerations, technology limitations, the triviality of the communication, time commitment, and frustration with the platform features.

Ang and Chen (2018) found that online social participation has the potential to alleviate the negative effects of pain on mental well-being, indicating that online social participation could supplement attempts to facilitate social engagement in later life, in particular for those whose social activities may be affected by the pain they experience. Grieve and colleagues (2013) concluded that offline social connectedness and Facebook connectedness were separate constructs. Furthermore, by studying 274 older adult Facebook users, they found that using Facebook could provide the opportunities for developing and maintaining social connectedness in the online environment and showed that lower depression and anxiety and greater life satisfaction were associated with Facebook connectedness. A simple association between social network site usage and loneliness may not, however, be automatically assumed among community-dwelling older adults. Aarts et al. (2015) surveyed 626 adults aged 60 years or older in the Netherlands to investigate the relationship between social sites usage and loneliness and found that, in general, social network sites usage appeared unrelated to loneliness.

Social Robots and Conversational Agents

A *social robot* is defined as an artificial agent (often embodied with anthropomorphic or zoomorphic features) that interacts with humans by following the social norms and behaviors attached to its role (Broekens et al., 2009; Taipale et al., 2015). Social robots have been developed and tested for their potential to meet the mental health needs of older adults through interactions involving information exchange (Broadbent et al., 2014). Pu and colleagues (2019), in their meta-analysis of RCTs examining the effectiveness of social robots for older adults, reported that social robot interactions have the potential to "improve engagement, interaction, and stress indicators, as well as reduce loneliness and the use of medications among older adults" (p. e37). One of the most common and frequently examined social robots is PARO, a robotic baby harp seal, which has been tested in various settings with older adults with and without cognitive limitations (Jøranson et al., 2016; Liang et al., 2017; Robinson et al., 2013). Other examples include a robotic dog named AIBO (Banks et al., 2008), a humanoid communication robot called NAO (Soler et al., 2015), a humanoid robot designed to communicate and behave like a 3-year-old boy (Tanaka et al., 2012), and health care robots IrobiQ and Cafero (Broadbent et al., 2014).

Broader in concept than social robots, *conversational agents* are "systems that mimic human conversation using text or spoken language" (Laranjo et al., 2018, p. 1248). Conversational technologies involve the use of intuitive, natural language on the part of both the user and the system. This is in contrast to systems that require input that is formulated to be interpreted by a computer system (e.g., computer terminals) or technologies that require selection and interactions through the manipulation of graphical elements (e.g., point and click via mouse). Conversational technologies are envisioned to be more intuitive to use, easier to learn, and more resistant to communication breakdowns than non-conversational technologies (Cassell et al., 1999). Voice-based personal assistants such as the Amazon Alexa and Google Home are commercial examples of technologies that attempt to make use of conversational interaction.

Agents and *agent-based systems* refer to technologies that are capable of autonomous action. These systems can act without the direct involvement of humans, can initiate action in response to a certain set of conditions in their environment, and can interact with other agents and humans (Jennings and Wooldridge, 1998). A classic example of an agent is an automated online travel assistant that supports users in locating, selecting, and booking travel plans (e.g., Schiaffino and Amandi, 2009).

Embodied conversational agents (ECAs) leverage the use of parts of the body, such as hands, the face, or a tonal shift via vocal cords, to regulate conversation and contribute content (Cassell et al., 1999). For example, an ECA might express confusion through facial features in order to prompt a user to repeat or rephrase a sentence or clap to show enthusiasm or appreciation of a point. ECAs range in appearance from cartoonlike to highly realistic and possess the ability to engage in verbal and non-verbal conversation in a human-like manner (Cassell, 2001). The three key components of a typical ECA are (1) an interface through which information is collected from users, (2) a visual representation or interface through which the agent communicates with users, and (3) an algorithm or software that allows it to reason like a human (Cassell, 2001; Provoost et al., 2017).

ECAs have been investigated primarily in the areas of gaming and health care. In health care, ECAs have been used in patient education (e.g., nurse agents to explain medical documents to patients), clinician training (e.g., training mental health professionals), and the delivery of behavioral interventions (e.g., interventions targeting behavior change), including serious games and physical activity (Bickmore et al., 2009, 2010; Carpenter et al., 2012; Johnson et al., 2016; Kanaoka and Mutlu, 2015; Lisetti et al., 2013). Some work has examined the use of conversational agents specifically for older adults. Bickmore et al. (2013) demonstrated that ECAs were effective in significantly increasing physical activity levels in older adults when compared to a group of pedometer users. Vardoulakis et al. (2012) conducted a study with an agent (using the so-called "Wizard of Oz" methodology for which the older adult interacts with a computer controlled by another human) and found that older adults obtained a sense of companionship and support from the agent and were interested in discussing a wide range of topics. Yaghoubzadeh et al. (2013) used participatory design to create and demonstrate the feasibility of a virtual agent to assist with daily activities of older adults. Their study showed that older adults were able to engage and interact successfully with the agent (Yaghoubzadeh et al., 2013). In addition, ECAs have also been shown to be beneficial for health management. For example, Looije et al. (2010) showed that a virtual assistant was rated more highly than real persons, particularly for conveying empathy. The ability to express empathy is a social behavior that can significantly aid in persuasive efforts to facilitate healthy behaviors (Looije et al., 2010). Some ECAs have been developed for individuals with conditions that increase in prevelance with aging, such as dementia (Sakai et al., 2012). The conversational agents in these studies have taken on various appearances, from human-like (Bickmore et al., 2013) to animal characters (Looije et al., 2010).

ETHICAL AND PRACTICAL CONSIDERATIONS FOR INTERVENTION

When interventions for social isolation and loneliness are designed, various ethical and practical consideration arise, including (but not limited to) how levels of social isolation and loneliness are assessed (see Chapter 6), who implements the intervention, which settings are appropriate for an intervention, and what the intervention entails or how it functions. While many interventions considered in this chapter are relatively low-tech, technology-based interventions have been gaining in popularity. Various ethical considerations related to using technology with older adults have been studied, particularly around robotic care (Sharkey and Sharkey, 2012; Sorell and Draper, 2014), smart home technologies (Chung et al., 2016), and telehealth (Demiris et al., 2006, 2009). While newly introduced technologies can have a positive impact on health of older adults, potential harms also need to be considered, particularly in the areas of privacy, informed consent, and autonomy (Chung et al., 2016; Demiris et al., 2009). A recent review of the literature found that 67 percent of the current intelligent assistive technologies (IATs) in dementia care (e.g., handheld devices, mobility aids, smart home sensors, robots) were designed without considering their ethical implications (Ienca et al., 2018). Moreover, among those IATs developed with attention to ethics at the design level, there was great variation in the kinds of ethical considerations that had been addressed. For example, privacy considerations had been addressed in only 5 percent of the examined technologies.

In evaluating the potential of any intervention to prevent or mitigate social isolation and loneliness, either as a single intervention or in combination with other interventions, questions of accessibility, acceptability, cost, and the feasibility need to be addressed. This section explores potential ethical and practical concerns related to both technological and non-technological interventions.

Accessibility

Accessibility refers to ensuring that services and technologies are usable by people with disabilities, either by design or by the addition of adaptive software or hardware. Given that visual, motor, and hearing changes are common with aging, making technology accessible to older adults may include such things as making digital displays accessible to people with vision loss (e.g., providing options to increase font size) and accounting for motor changes such as tremors (Hanson, 2001; Kaeberlein and Martin, 2015; Saxon et al., 2015). However, ECAs and social robots as well as other new technologies (e.g., voice based personal assistants such as Amazon's Alexa) are adopting voice as an interaction mechanism. The use of one's voice may be a more accessible interface for people who have low vision, but, on the other hand, it may present issues for people who are deaf or hard of hearing. Adjusting the volume of audio output of technology is a way that people often compensate for age-related hearing loss (Pacala and Yueh, 2012), but the conversational aspect of these new technologies means that new dynamics need to be investigated in regard to accessibility (e.g., turn-taking in conversation when one party has hearing loss). Cognitive accessibility also needs to be considered in regard to voice-based interactions with ECAs or robots because of the normal cognitive changes that occur with aging as well as the increased incidence of dementia.

Research on technology for aging has expanded to encompass factors affecting other types of accessibility, including structural, financial, and personal barriers (Chung et al., 2016; Demiris et al., 2006, 2009). Although technology adoption by older adults is increasing (Pew Research Center, 2017), a large proportion of older adults remain without access to technology, such as the Internet and hardware (e.g., tablets), that are needed for use of these ECAs. In addition, disparities due to differences in socioeconomic status affect older adults' technology use and access to technology (Smith et al., 2015). Financial accessibility will likely be an issue because the ECA services that are emerging for older adults—particularly those that involve a "human in the loop"—often involve recurring monthly payments.

Another potential factor affecting accessibility is literacy. Preliminary studies show that many ECAs can be used by individuals with lower literacy levels (Bickmore et al., 2009, 2010). These studies show that ECAs are not bound by time constraints like providers, and they are able to convey information clearly and multiple times, making them easy to comprehend by patients (Bickmore et al., 2009, 2010).

Privacy and Data Protection

With the rise of consumer-facing technologies, discussions of privacy and confidentiality are evolving. Existing norms and legislation related to health information are being reconsidered and extended to include new devices oriented toward patients. Specific issues related to ECAs or social robots include the protection, storage, and transmission of audio and video data (Demiris et al., 2006). ECAs that interface with health care providers need to meet the standards set by the Health Insurance Portability and Accountability Act.[14] Consumers usually use passwords to protect information and accounts. Passwords that require the memorization of a string of characters may not be the ideal solution for many people, particularly for older adults with cognitive impairment, or in cases when multiple people, including caregivers, may interface with the technology. In this scenario, privacy issues intersect with accessibility concerns. Given that ECAs in the home use audio and sometimes video data, they pose privacy risks not only to people using them, but to others who enter the space where they are deployed. Another potential privacy risk relates to the transmission of data by social robots and ECAs to family members or health care providers concerning the health conditions and activities of older adults, who may not want that information shared.

Autonomy

Autonomy represents the freedom of an individual to make decisions regarding their own life in accordance with their own goals, values, and preferences. Autonomy is an essential guiding principle for interventions and a key ethical issue in the care of older adults. However, respecting the autonomy of older adults may present challenges when the older person does not have full decision-making capacity, or when other family members are involved in the older adult's care.[15] A 2019 study by AARP found that "76 percent of Americans age 50 and older say they prefer to remain in their current residence and 77 percent would like to live in their community as long as possible."[16] Many new technologies, including ECAs, are designed to support older adults in living independently. Regardless,

---

[14] Health Insurance Portability and Accountability Act, Public Law 191. 104th Congress. August 21, 1996.

[15] See https://journalofethics.ama-assn.org/article/autonomy-and-quality-life-elderly-patients/2008-06 (accessed November 4, 2019).

[16] See https://www.aarp.org/research/topics/community/info-2018/2018-home-community-preference.html (accessed November 4, 2019).

concerns may arise for the use of these types of technologies, leading to lost autonomy and personal liberty (Bickmore, 2005; Garner et al., 2016). However, the loss of independence and autonomy may not be the most important ethical factor to consider when it comes to particular populations, such as frail older adults (Zwijsen et al., 2011). Though the majority of published literature has not yet addressed the ethical implications of social robots or ECAs, there are some articles that have begun to outline some of the potential considerations (Bickmore, 2005; Bickmore et al., 2005). For example, Bickmore et al. (2005) discussed issues concerning an agent deceiving users into thinking it is a person, agents reducing expressivity, and the autonomy of users. Garner and colleagues (2016) conducted group discussions with various stakeholders to understand the concerns and reservations related to using a virtual carer system for older adults.

Informed Consent

For all types of interventions, informed consent is perhaps the ethical issue that has received the most attention in research. However, technological approaches confer unique challenges for the informed consent process. Some approaches stress the importance of ongoing consent and the ability to rescind consent (Neill, 2003). These approaches, however, assume that an individual is continuously able to assess risk and what is in his or her own best interests.

For technological interventions, researchers are beginning to argue that conventional ways of obtaining informed consent are not sufficient for research (Vitak et al., 2017). Some of these concerns arise because of the persistence and vastness of data created, stored, and transmitted by new technologies, which can lead to possible future uses that were unspecified at the time of consent (Vitak et al., 2017). Data collected by ECAs might be seen as valuable for researchers who study aging, and there is a need to understand how informed consent can best be obtained for older adults with these new technologies. Furthermore, in the case of ECAs, social relationships may be built over time. Users may develop trust in virtual agents that may affect their ability to assess risks. Trust—and misplaced trust—are informed consent–related issues found in many settings involving research or interventions (de Melo-Martín and Ho, 2008), but they become particularly complicated when trust is developed between participants and the system that is deployed. Trust developing between an individual and a device could mean that an older adult reveals more personal information than would otherwise be the case because of the perceived lower interpersonal risk of sharing and a failure to realize that in some cases this information may become accessible to third parties or other stakeholder groups.

Additional informed consent concerns that are specific to social robots or ECAs include the high level of digital literacy needed to understand the mechanisms of the technology. Moreover, users may need to understand AI, networks, and data transmision in order to fully apprehend the risks associated with ECAs.

Data literacy in this case becomes a great challenge because users need to understand how their data are collected, who can access them, and what the potential risks may be. Informed consent with ECAs, as with other technologies, is further complicated when individuals are experiencing cognitive impairment and dementia—conditions that increase in prevalence as people age. Ideally, an individual's capacity to consent is determined on a case-by-case basis with attention paid to the magnitude of the potential harm of the research or intervention and to the participant's understanding of the risks (Appelbaum, 2007); however, both of these factors are difficult to assess with the new technologies.

Finally, consideration may be needed regarding informed consent for the use of IT beyond research, such as a new technology introduced for patient care in the home (e.g., video cameras).

Exacerbating Rather Than Reducing Isolation

For older adults, particular attention will need to be paid to the impact of interventions that substitute for human contact. For example, attachment to companion animals has been shown to be associated with changes in psychological health (Raina et al., 1999). A key concern for technological interventions is that the same tools intended to address isolation and loneliness could lead to further isolation by ultimately substituting for human contact (Chung et al., 2016; Sharkey and Sharkey, 2012; Sparrow and Sparrow, 2006). This issue may be a particular concern with social robots and ECAs, given that these technologies rely on social interactions and building relationships. Pilot studies with ECAs have demonstrated that older adults can engage and interact with ECAs and thus may potentially develop relationships with these devices (Bickmore et al., 2005; Tsiourti et al., 2014). Methods that have been suggested to reduce isolation and dependence include periodically checking on a person's dependence and having time limits for the usage of the system (Garner et al., 2016). This approach becomes difficult to implement, however, when the effectiveness of the ECA may rely on a continuous connection and relationship built over time. As IT tools become formally integrated into traditional health services in order to reduce cost and human resources, it will be important to assess whether virtual or AI-based interactions meant to replace human observers or interaction partners lead to a lower quality of engagement and an increased sense of loneliness, at least for some older adults. Another challenge is attachment. ECAs and other technologies developed for older adults may have high costs, sometimes with services attached that require continuous payment, and the participants may have to stop using devices because of such constraints as the research study period, financial resources, and travel.

Additionally, as mentioned in Chapter 7, there may be stigma associated with being labelled as socially isolated or lonely. Such stigma might risk causing the individuals to be blamed for being isolated or feeling lonely instead of viewing these problems as being due to a variety of factors at the level of the individual, community, and society. As a result, individuals suffering from social isolation or loneliness may not want to identify as such for the purposes of receiving an intervention, thereby exacerbating their isolation or loneliness.

Perceptions of Safety and Functionality

Although interventions such as new technologies are often developed to support safety for older adults, unintended consequences may arise. For example, a power cord attached to a technology could pose a falling risk. ECAs, however, may be more likely to be on mobile platforms and therefore pose less of a hazard. Perceptions of functionality also might lead to potential safety issues (Yusif et al., 2016). Given the social element of the devices, people might expect devices to be able to fill social safety roles, such as alerting others in case of emergencies—even when this is beyond the technical capabilities of the device or not implemented for fear of adverse events and litigation. Additionally, individuals might come to depend on functionalities such as medication reminders, and if a device malfunctioned or a company shut down, it could leave older adults without the support they had come to rely on (Hensel et al., 2006).

Infantilization of Older Adults

The introduction of social robots or ECAs for older adults in some cases introduces concerns for the infantilization of these individuals (i.e., creating a behavioral pattern in which the older adult is treated in a child-like manner). This may be especially true when there is a perception that "toys" or "robotic pets" are ways to engage and entertain isolated or lonely older adults (Birks et al., 2016; Salari and Rich, 2001). Infantilization needs to be acknowledged and addressed by system designers both in the design and selection of features for the hardware and software systems and in the integration of existing knowledge bases for AI solutions. Because knowledge bases are informed by existing data and assumptions, ageism and other biases may be reflected in the way a system is designed to interact with an older adult.

Disparities in Access to Interventions

Older adults may have disparities in their ability to access a variety of interventions. For example, an individual who lives in a rural area may not have any local programs or an individual who has a functional limitation in mobility may be unable to access programs that exist even in their own communities. Limitations in access may be particularly acute when it comes to technological interventions. The concept of a digital divide has been of growing concern as the use of technology by health care consumers has increased. Questions of equity and "digital inclusion" (Powell and Deetjen, 2019, p. 1) have evolved from issues of simple access to infrastructure and equipment to include access to the knowledge and skills needed to use technology and now to a consideration of who benefits the most and in what ways (Ball et al., 2017; Powell and Deetjen, 2019). The following sections focus on disparities in access to technological interventions.

Differences Between Rural and Urban Environments

Early concerns regarding access to technology were primarily related to the availability of broadband Internet access for people in rural areas and low-income populations in urban areas (van Deursen and van Dijk, 2019). Although broadband is more widely available than in the past and the use of smartphones is now ubiquitous, the question still merits attention, in part because of variations across geographic areas, costs, ease of use, and acceptability to older adults. While access to Web-based and technology-enabled connections has increased and such connections have been described as "a basic utility for social inclusion" (van Deursen and van Dijk, 2019, p. 355), geographic disparities still exist, and issues have surfaced related to knowledge, skills, and costs over time. As of 2018, 39 percent of people living in rural areas in the United States did not have access to broadband in their homes, compared with 4 percent of people in urban areas (Stover, 2018). People living in rural areas often have a limited choice of broadband providers and may experience lower broadband speeds than in urban areas. Wired Internet connectivity is more costly in rural areas because of the lower population density and the need for longer wiring; additionally, wireless technology, particularly on mobile phones, can be costly, and download speeds can vary across carriers (Stover, 2018).

Access to broadband alone does not address access to the necessary hardware, software, peripherals, licenses, and subscription fees (van Deursen and van Dijk, 2019). The resource limitations experienced by some high-risk populations can worsen inequalities in access to technologically mediated supports to address social isolation and loneliness.

Rural residents are increasingly using mobile technologies, such as smartphones, rather than broadband as a means of accessing the Internet (Pew Research Center, 2019b; Stover, 2018). According to a survey conducted by the Pew Research Center in 2019, 71 percent of rural residents owned smartphones, compared with 83 percent of urban residents (Pew Research Center, 2019b). Similarly, 53 percent of older adults owned smartphones compared with 96 percent of young adults aged 18–29 and 79 percent of adults aged 50–64. These findings suggest that older adults living in rural areas do not have the same ubiquitous access to mobile technologies as do those who are younger and living in urban areas.

Age

Age has been specifically identified as a factor in the digital divide (Wu et al., 2015). In a study of adults in the Netherlands, where the Internet saturation is 98 percent, the investigators found that age was negatively related to access to multiple devices and peripherals (e.g., printers, scanners, additional screens, hard drives, docking stations) and also negatively related to total cost of maintenance expenses (van Deursen and van Dijk, 2019). This suggests that even in a technologically advanced society, older adults have fewer devices and peripherals, thereby limiting the types and extent of social connections that are possible using technology.

Pearl (2014) reported on the use of three technologies by members of Kaiser Permanente Northern California: Internet, mobile technologies, and video platforms. He found that 51.2 percent of members over the age of 70 had enrolled in the Kaiser Permanent website, compared with 71.6 percent of members aged 30–70 (Pearl, 2014). This suggests that older adults might be less likely to use technologically mediated strategies than young and middle-aged adults. Although a majority of adults over age 65 are using the Internet (73 percent in 2019), the rate is far lower than in younger age groups (88 percent of adults aged 50–64 and 97 percent of those aged 30–49 years) (Hong and Cho, 2017; Statista, 2020). In an analysis of survey data originally collected at three points in time by the Health Information National Trends Survey of the National Cancer Institute, Hong and Cho (2017) found that older adults were increasingly accessing the Internet. Older adults' use of Internet resources was primarily for obtaining health information and communicating with their physicians. The study found that education and income were related to Internet use, while rural-versus-urban residence was not. The authors concluded that although the "digital divide" was narrowing, it remained substantial for those who were older, less well educated, and with lower incomes. This suggests that the social determinants of health create barriers to older adults' access to technologies and that reducing these barriers could be helpful in efforts to reduce social isolation and loneliness. Adults aged 75 and older were less likely than adults aged 65–74 to use the Internet. Hong and Cho stated that "improved access to the Internet may enable older adults' access to health information, but it may not necessarily lead to the adoption of various aspects of HRIU (health-related Internet use), such as connecting with people online" (Hong and Cho, 2017, pp. 860–861).

Another perspective on the digital divide concerns how and when electronic technologies are used and how different age groups perceive them. Focus groups conducted by Ball et al. (2017) indicated that older adults were offended by the use of electronic technologies when family members or others were physically in their presence, but appreciated their use when apart. Thus, electronic technology use could worsen feelings of social isolation from those in direct contact with older adults but serve as a tool to enhance social connection when at a distance.

Older adults' use of certain technologies may depend strongly on their comfort and familiarity with the devices. As a result, training older adults in the use of the technology may encourage more seniors to use various devices. For example, Older Adults Technology Services[17] trains older adults in community settings in computer skills, including the use of email, the management of medical information, and the building of community networks.

Underserved Populations and the Social Determinants of Health

In a literature review of the impact of sociodemographic factors on the use of eHealth, Reiners et al. (2019) concluded that older adults and individuals with lower incomes were generally less likely to use eHealth. It also appeared that people with less education were less likely to use eHealth. Literacy skills are key to some uses of eHealth. This review suggested that limited access to the appropriate equipment and a lack of the skills needed to use the equipment contributed to older adults' lower levels of use of eHealth. These authors recommended tailoring eHealth strategies to the needs of individuals, providing education and support for the use of eHealth, and involving caregivers when possible. When older adults live alone, they may be less likely to use electronic strategies because of a lack of support. In a systematic review of studies of eHealth literacy among underserved U.S. populations, Chesser et al. (2015) noted that few of the studies they reviewed were conducted with rural populations.

Mitchell and colleagues (2019) evaluated data from the 2014 HRS and found that older adults from racial and ethnic minorities, including Hispanics and African Americans, used health-related technology less frequently than whites. Although differences were not found across racial and ethnic groups in younger ages, by age 62 differences began to emerge. The authors speculated that language may contribute to the differences seen in older Hispanic adults, and they noted no differences were found in the use of specific technologies, such as "e-mails, text messaging and mobile applications for health" (p. 11), suggesting that targeting the type of technology for its acceptability to the population may be an appropriate strategy.

Older Adults with Disabilities

In a review of the literature, Vázquez et al. (2018) found that the few studies that addressed the use of eHealth by older adults with intellectual disabilities indicated that eHealth was used by this population primarily as support for independent living, telehealth, and communication. The authors recommended using universal design in eHealth to increase the ease of use and also considering

[17] For more information, see https://www.oats.org (accessed October 16, 2019).

the use of strategies such as games and virtual reality. Gell and colleagues (2015) found that older adults with disabilities that led to functional limitations were significantly less likely to use the Internet than those without such limitations. This was particularly true for those individuals who needed help with activities of daily living or mobility outside the home and those with vision or memory impairments. Older adults with other issues, including pain and breathing problems, were more likely to use technology. The investigators noted this may have been because the ease of getting help using technology outweighed the difficulties of trying to do so in other non-technological ways for these specific impairments.

Infrastructure Issues

Pearl (2014) found that reimbursement issues detracted from physicians' willingness to use technology for virtual visits. Fee-for-service reimbursement systems do not always cover such visits, and issues persist concerning the amount of coverage and managing provider licensure issues across state lines. While newer approaches to care coordination and patient self-management may support using technology to reduce social isolation and loneliness, key infrastructure issues related to reimbursements and regulations may need to be resolved to allow for full adoption.

FINANCING OF INTERVENTIONS

Most of the interventions reviewed earlier in this chapter draw heavily on volunteers and patched together funding from various small grants and donations or are technological innovations that may base their marketing models on the sharing of data by users. While many of these programs had some positive impacts on participants, a volunteer-based model is difficult to grow or maintain on a large scale. Instead, more formal funding mechanisms are needed. The choice of funding source will depend in part on the type of intervention, the cost, and the population being served. However, because there is little scientific evidence to date on the cost and benefits of various interventions addressing social isolation and loneliness in general, and for interventions in health care settings in particular, the committee presents a discussion of funding options in a more general sense, providing a general assessment of possible paths forward.

As noted in Chapter 3, social isolation and loneliness have negative effects on health, but at the same time health limitations (e.g., auditory or mobility problems) result in significantly higher risks of social isolation and loneliness. Given these strong ties, a natural avenue for the implementation and funding of interventions is through the health care and health insurance systems. Furthermore, the 2019 National Academies consensus study report *Integrating Social Care into the Delivery of Health Care* describes the negative correlation between spending on social care and total health care costs that exists across countries and across states (NASEM, 2019). This correlation suggests that, in addition to improving the lives of individuals at risk for social isolation and loneliness, investment in this area may prove cost-effective.

Given the committee's charge to focus its attention on older Americans and the groups most at risk of social isolation and loneliness, this section begins with the potential role of the public Medicare and Medicaid program. Medicare is the primary health insurance provider for those aged 65 or older as well as for those eligible for Social Security Disability Insurance, while those older or disabled individuals with few resources have access to Medicaid. Given their target populations, these programs are well positioned to lead the way in identifying individuals at risk and in providing mechanisms to mitigate the impacts of social isolation and loneliness. Medicare is a federally run program and, as such, changes in this program directed toward social isolation and loneliness can have an impact on a large number of individuals. In 2018 there were approximately 60 million individuals enrolled in Medicare (CMS, 2019a). In contrast, Medicaid programs are run at the state level with funding from both states and the federal government. The state-level administration allows for individual states to tailor coverage to their populations and also allows for the piloting of different programs across states to provide data on numerous interventions at the same time. The total population covered by Medicaid is far larger than that covered by Medicare (approximately 75 million in 2018) (CMS, 2019a), but children make up the largest subset of beneficiaries, so the adult population covered by Medicaid is similar to that covered by Medicare.

The committee suggests three avenues along which the health care system—and particularly Medicare and Medicaid—may address these issues. The first of these avenues is through the use of traditional medical interventions targeting specific underlying health-related causes of social isolation or loneliness. The second is by financing interventions that target social isolation and loneliness, either directly or indirectly. Finally, financing may be considered for public health efforts to increase awareness of the health and medical impacts of social isolation and loneliness, both for reducing the stigma associated with social isolation and loneliness and for helping to identify those at risk. The following sections provide examples of approaches to funding interventions generally. However, the committee recognizes that relatively little is currently invested (particularly by Medicare and Medicaid) into these types of interventions, that many of the programs cited have not been evaluated for their impact specifically on social isolation and loneliness, and significant incentives will likely be needed in order for these approaches to gain traction.

Financing Interventions for Underlying Health-Related Causes

The first mechanism of financing to consider involves using traditional health care interventions that target the underlying cause of social isolation or loneliness. For example, when considering causes of social isolation and loneliness, physical barriers such as hearing or vision impairments or limitations on mobility loom large. Limitations like these make social connections more difficult and have been demonstrated to increase the likelihood of loneliness or isolation (see Chapter 4). Medicare currently covers some mobility devices when they are medically needed, but it does not cover hearing aids or low vision devices, although these items could potentially be included in an expanded definition of "durable medical equipment." In some states, Medicaid does cover hearing aids for those who qualify for benefits, but many states do not offer this coverage. Better coverage of hearing aids and other medically needed devices (e.g., wheelchairs, low-vision technologies) could potentially do much to help reduce the prevalence of social isolation and loneliness.[18]

Financing Interventions Targeting Social Isolation and Loneliness

Social isolation and loneliness might also be targeted by taking advantage of existing programs to assess or address the social determinants of health in general. The recent increase in recognition of the importance of these factors in affecting health outcomes has led to several states beginning to use their Medicaid programs to address such issues as food insecurity, homelessness, and domestic violence. Like social isolation and loneliness, these factors are strongly related to health outcomes, and improving social situations can lead to improvements in health. Although they are outside the typical scope of Medicaid programs and not required by the federal government, these types of outreach activities can be financed through Medicaid waivers that allow for pilot projects or through amendments to state Medicaid programs. While Medicaid programs have begun to address the social determinants of health among children and disabled beneficiaries, the committee has focused primarily on pilot projects that might inform outreach activities targeting older adults at risk of or experiencing social isolation and loneliness. A key component of these pilot projects is evaluation. As such, the research needed to learn about the effectiveness and best practices of these pilots, while still in its infancy, will at least begin to provide some answers in the coming years. However, a recent Government Accountability Office study found serious gaps in many demonstration projects that limited the ability to gauge the effectiveness of these programs (GAO-18-220).

Medicaid waiver programs (particularly the newest Section 1115 waivers) have been authorized by the Centers for Medicare & Medicaid Services (CMS) to allow Medicaid programs to adapt their services "to best meet their state's unique needs" such as by expanding coverage to specific groups, providing incentives for healthy behaviors, or improving behavioral health services (NCSL, 2019). As noted by Seema Verma, the CMS administrator,

> We know that behaviors and other determinants of health—like where we work, live, learn, and grow—are all factors in our overall health and wellbeing. As we

[18] H.R. 2050, introduced in 2017, called for a demonstration project for the inclusion of low-vision devices.

> seek to create a health care system that truly rewards value, we must consider the impact that factors beyond medical care have in driving up health costs. . . . As part of this demonstration, North Carolina will implement a groundbreaking program in select regions to pilot evidence-based interventions addressing issues like housing instability, transportation insecurity, food security, and interpersonal violence and toxic stress. (Verma, 2018)

Interventions of this type typically operate through accountable care organizations and managed care organizations and provide a number of services not normally associated with health insurance organizations. North Carolina has recently launched a pilot enhanced case management system to provide various social support services to Medicaid beneficiaries. The program includes services to help with housing, food security, and domestic violence. Examples include replacing carpet or an air conditioner for an individual with asthma and improving access to healthful food (NCDHHS, 2018). The One Care demonstration project operating through Medicare and Medicaid programs from the Commonwealth Care Alliance in Massachusetts provides a care partner to assist a patient with the social determinants of health as well as with traditional medical services. Loneliness is specifically listed as a targeted social determinant of health but the project is limited to adults younger than 65 (Commonwealth Care Alliance, 2018).

New York also has a broader program addressing the social determinants of health (NYSDOH, 2017, 2019). The New York program includes components that address economic security as well as housing and food security. Notable in the New York plan is that "social and community context" is called out as a key domain. Outreach in these areas can be provided through existing programs such as the Department for the Aging, Department of Health, Office for the Aging, senior centers, virtual senior centers, friendly visitor programs, caregiver support, and social adult day services. Similar pilot programs are operational in other states, and Medicaid managed care plans are similarly exploring ways to improve health outcomes by addressing the social determinants of health.

Medicaid waiver programs can be used as models for interventions specifically addressing social isolation and loneliness among low-income older adults and people with disabilities. An important step in reaching out with interventions along these lines is identifying those most at risk for social isolation and loneliness. Medicaid's existing coverage of home health care services provide a ready avenue to identify at least some of those at risk for social isolation and loneliness, as do other outreach programs such as Meals on Wheels or other state- and local-run programs.[19]

---

[19]Note that the Administration on Aging (AoA) operates in large part by providing funding to states and local communities to support programs addressing the well-being of older adults. A large portion of this funding goes to Meals on Wheels programs, which count on money from AoA for approximately one-third of its budget (Meals on Wheels America, 2017).

For older and disabled individuals who are not eligible for state Medicaid programs, Medicare affords similar opportunities to address social isolation and loneliness. While Medicare itself is a federal rather than state-run program, suggesting that interventions would need to be implemented more broadly, CMS recently finalized its policy to allow Medicare Advantage plans to expand benefits to cover interventions addressing the social determinants of health (CMS, 2019b), and this idea is already gaining traction with numerous private insurers (e.g., Anthem Inc., UnitedHealthcare, Kaiser Permanente) launching programs through their Medicare Advantage plans (Graham, 2019). While many of these programs focus on affordable housing, transportation, and food insecurity, the same models can be used to more aggressively target social isolation and loneliness. The idea behind these pilot projects is that by being more proactive in identifying and intervening for social isolation and loneliness or in reducing the risk, these interventions will act both to reduce total health care costs and increase well-being. Should these projects prove successful, one would imagine that private insurers serving the non-elderly and non-disabled population (i.e., those not covered by Medicare or Medicaid) would begin to consider similar interventions as cost savings mechanisms.

Outside the United States, the National Health Service in the United Kingdom has already created a system of social prescribing to encourage doctors to "prescribe" social activities and engagement. According to a recent evaluation, the most common sorts of interventions were "information and advice, community activity, physical activities, befriending and enabling" (Dayson and Bashir, 2014, p. i). The evaluation found substantial reduction in inpatient admissions, emergency department visits, and outpatient visits. It also found a substantial cost savings on the order of a 50 percent return on investment (see more on social prescribing earlier in this chapter). Similarly, the Australian government provides funding for a program in which volunteers visit low-income older adults (Sutherland Shire Council, 2018).

As described in Chapter 3, social isolation, particularly for an often less-mobile population, can have adverse outcomes on health. Increasing social activities and combating the isolation faced by many people with functional limitations and other disabilities is a key element in encouraging good overall health. The Health Plan of San Mateo found that addressing social isolation is a key to successfully transitioning individuals out of institutional care, particularly as many are leaving a very structured environment (HPSM, 2020). That organization is examining new types of peer supports and other related services to address isolation. The health plan contracts with an organization called Wider Circle,[20] which facilitates an activity-based social group led by peers to support individuals with day-to-day living tasks. Wider Circle also emphasizes physical activity and collects some

[20] For more information, see https://www.widercircle.com (accessed October 15, 2019).

data on health outcomes. The health plan acknowledged that extensive internal review are often required when these services are authorized, but because feedback received from members has been very positive, it will continue to provide these activities (Soper, 2017).

Financing Public Health Campaigns

Finally, financing needs to be considered for efforts at the society-wide level such as public health campaigns to increase awareness, remove stigma, and, more generally, enlist the public's help in reducing social isolation and loneliness. For example, the National Institutes of Health has promoted public health campaigns about smoking, physical activity, and heart disease (NIH, 2019). (See Chapter 8 for more on public health campaigns.) Publicity campaigns like these could encourage individuals to check in on neighbors or older family members. They could also reduce stigma and thus encourage lonely older adults to reach out for help themselves. By highlighting social isolation and loneliness, public health campaigns could help individuals approaching retirement and old age better plan for meaningful engagement and connections in the future. (See Chapter 10 for more on dissemination and implementation.)

REFRAMING INTERVENTION USING A PUBLIC HEALTH APPROACH

Because of the variety of ways that social isolation and loneliness affect health and well-being, there is no single treatment that can prevent or cure every instance of social isolation or loneliness. Instead, addressing these issues will necessarily involve a variety of different actors and an assortment of interventions focused on different demographics, risk factors, and health impacts. One way to address the problems of isolation and loneliness may be through using a public health framework while designing and implementing different interventions. As defined by the American Public Health Association, "public health promotes and protects the health of people and the communities where they live, learn, work, and play," which includes promoting wellness by encouraging healthy behaviors and assuring "the conditions in which people can be healthy." Furthermore, public health includes "spreading the word about ways to stay healthy and giving science-based solutions to problems" (APHA, 2019). A public health framework entails designing interventions to address one of three strategies: primary, secondary, and tertiary prevention.

The aim of *primary prevention* is to intervene before any health effects occur, such as by changing health behaviors or changing the built environment so that exposures to hazards are decreased (IWH, 2015). Strategies that focus on primary prevention typically include clinical preventive services (e.g., immunization or post-exposure prophylaxis for individuals exposed to a communicable disease), media campaigns raising public awareness about the link between certain behaviors and health outcomes (e.g., smoking and lung cancer, wearing seatbelts and automobile crash safety), and education aimed at personal health behaviors (e.g., oral and dental hygiene education) (WHO, 2019b). For social isolation and loneliness, primary prevention may include public health awareness campaigns and identifying individuals at high risk. Other approaches, while outside the scope of this committee's work, might include neighborhood and city planning for housing design and community spaces that would facilitate bringing people together (e.g., common spaces for gathering, sidewalks), facilitate interactions (e.g., opportunities for volunteering, intergenerational housing), and prevent isolation (e.g., more effective public transportation).[21]

Secondary prevention aims to reduce the impact of a disease or illness that has already occurred by, for example, using screening or assessment to identify the earliest stages of the condition. Some examples of secondary preventions strategies are regimens of daily low-dose aspirin for individuals who have suffered from heart attack or stroke; regular mammogram screening in order to detect early breast cancer; and regimens of antiretroviral medications for individuals who have human immunodeficiency virus. In the case of social connection, secondary prevention strategies are those that attempt to target or influence existing social isolation or loneliness that is felt acutely (in other words, a temporary state of loneliness or social isolation, perhaps due to a sentinel life event). This also includes the assessment for social isolation and loneliness, as discussed in Chapter 7.

Tertiary prevention involves managing a disease post-diagnosis in order to slow or soften the impact of the disease or to stop its progression (CDC, 2017). Examples of tertiary prevention include cardiac or stroke rehabilitation programs, chronic disease management programs for diabetes or depression, and support groups for people with cancer. In the case of social isolation and loneliness, tertiary prevention strategies attempt to address chronically experienced social isolation or loneliness (in other words, "trait" loneliness). Examples include the use of CBT (see earlier in this chapter).

One important consideration in the development of interventions for isolation and loneliness is *who* (i.e., which actor) is responsible for carrying out these actions. Different actors will be responsible for and involved in different types of interventions. Figure 9-2 suggests levels of responsibility for interventions in loneliness. (Note that these levels of responsibility correspond to the contextual factors of the committee's framework in Chapter 1.) The figure shows that primary prevention strategies such as public education campaigns and relevant research

[21] Fried, L. 2018. PowerPoint presentation to the committee—*Loneliness in older adults: Public health considerations.* In Public Access Files for the Committee on the Health and Medical Dimensions of Social Isolation and Loneliness in Older Adults (received December 21, 2018).

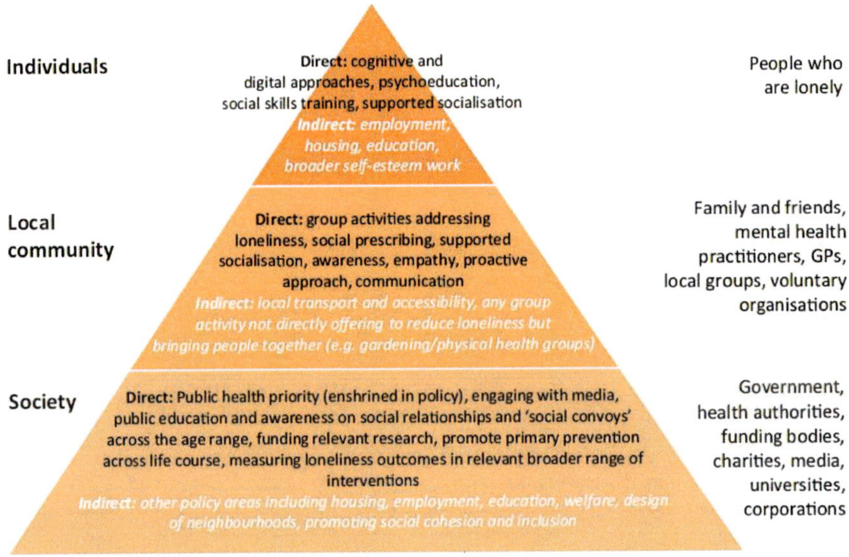

FIGURE 9-2 Levels of responsibility for interventions in loneliness.
NOTE: GP = general practitioner.
SOURCE: Mann et al., 2017.

funding are the responsibility of government health authorities and nonprofit organizations. Key partners here include organizations such as the U.S. Public Health Service, the Administration for Community Living, and area agencies on aging. Secondary prevention strategies are the responsibility of community actors such as general health care practitioners and local service groups. Those responsible for tertiary prevention strategies include affected individuals and their close associates or care team, including but not limited to family and friends (Mann et al., 2017). However, all of these actors will likely need to work together in concert to address the health and medical impacts of social isolation and loneliness using this public health approach. For example, the Trust for America's Health "is prioritizing the role of public health to improve the health and well-being of our nation's growing older adult population" by sharing "models of public health collaborations with the aging sector" (TFAH, 2020). In another example, age-friendly health systems (an initiative of The John A. Hartford Foundation and the Institute for Healthcare Improvement in partnership with the American Hospital Association and the Catholic Health Association of the United States) seek, in part, to "know and align care with each older adult's specific health outcome goals and care preferences" (IHI, 2020). Collaborations and partnerships such as these around public health and aging could consider their role in addressing social isolation and loneliness among older adults.

FINDINGS AND CONCLUSIONS

Interventions

- A variety of interventions have been proposed to address social isolation and loneliness. However, there is currently not enough evidence to identify the most effective interventions.
- The evidence base for interventions is limited by sample size and the length of follow-up.
- Few (if any) RCTs have been conducted on these interventions, and many interventions lack a theoretical basis.
- Features of successful interventions may include an educational approach to the intervention, the involvement of the individuals being targeted in the design of the intervention, and a strong theoretical basis for the approach of the intervention.
- Many intervention studies do not use a validated tool (as described in Chapter 6). Rather, these interventions are assessed using qualitative interviews, surveys, and internally designed measurement tools.
- Both direct and indirect interventions hold promise for ameliorating the negative health impacts of social isolation and loneliness. It is important that interventions target the underlying issue causing social isolation or loneliness, if the underlying cause is known (e.g., hearing loss or mobility limitations).
- The preservation of an individual's autonomy is an essential ethical principle that needs to be respected for all interventions.
- As new evidence develops, a centralized sharing of resources and best practices would benefit all stakeholders.

Technology

- A significant proportion of older adults are using technologies. With education and support, technology provides an important set of opportunities for the toolkit of strategies that can help prevent or mitigate social isolation and loneliness in older adults.
- Technologically mediated interventions might be helpful adjuncts to other interventions intended to prevent or mitigate social isolation and loneliness in older adults.
- Studies of the use of the Internet and, more specifically, social media by older adults introduce mixed findings; several studies show that online tools may increase connection and decrease isolation, while others have shown no links between Internet use and perceived isolation.
- The number of studies examining social robots for social isolation and loneliness has increased significantly in recent years, but there is insufficient evidence of their effectiveness.

- Conversational agents are designed to promote engagement and address loneliness, especially for older adults with mild cognitive impairment; the majority of the evaluations of conversational agents to date have focused on short-term feasibility and acceptability.
- The digital divide, especially the rural–urban digital divide, is a major moderator of the effectiveness of many interventions. Examples of the differences observed in the digital divide include familiarity; access to equipment, software, and fees; acceptability; ease of use with physical or emotional health problems or disabilities; and literacy.
- Special population groups (e.g., different age groups, people with different levels of literacy, people with different levels of income, people with varying functional status, and various racial, ethnic, and cultural groups) need to be considered when designing technological solutions to social isolation and loneliness for older adults.
- Clinician familiarity with technological strategies to improve health, including the prevention or treatment of social isolation and loneliness, is influenced by time, reimbursement strategies, and regulatory issues.
- As with other areas of health care, ethical and legal considerations especially must be explored when the technology is used in interventions for isolation and loneliness.

Financing of Interventions

- Current interventions are largely supported by volunteers, with much of the financial support coming from grants and donations. This is an unsustainable financing model.
- The availability of adequate resources to support and sustain interventions is key to their long-term success.
- Many efforts to develop newer approaches to the funding of interventions (largely for interventions directed at the social determinants of health in general) have not been evaluated for their impact on social isolation and loneliness specifically.
- The committee notes the following findings from the consensus study report *Integrating Social Care into the Delivery of Health Care* (NASEM, 2019):
    - Within existing definitions of health care, state Medicaid programs and their contracted managed care plans and accountable providers are innovating with . . . activities to pay for social care in health care settings using state plan amendment authority and the waiver process (p. 7).
    - There remains great variation among states in the level of social care activity; CMS provides only limited guidance about permissible social care activities and benefits (p. 7).
    - Medicare's new supplemental benefits guidance to Medicare Advantage plans . . . has created new opportunities to integrate social care into the health care of Medicare beneficiaries (p. 7).

- Patients enrolled in both Medicaid and Medicare have the highest social needs, but the division of their health care financing between state and federal agencies creates barriers to addressing those needs in a way that integrates social care (p. 9).
- Social service agencies and health care organizations have historically not worked together, and they are funded by different systems (p. 9).

NEXT STEPS AND RECOMMENDATIONS

The committee identified two key areas that need to be addressed related to interventions overall: strengthening community-based networks and resources and improving the overall evidence base.

Strengthening Ties to Community-Based Networks and Resources

Chapters 2 through 4 of this report show that social isolation and loneliness have wide-ranging health and medical impacts and are associated with a vast array of risk factors. Like other social determinants of health, social isolation and loneliness are community-wide problems and require coordinated solutions between the health care system and community-based social service providers. National, state, and local coalitions of public and private health care leaders, including minority-based community organizations, need to work collectively to develop strategies to address social isolation and loneliness in older adults. A report of the Campaign to End Loneliness recommended that service providers make connections with others in order to address the full range of needed supports and services, stating "Providers need to assess what contribution they make to the overall framework of loneliness interventions and build the necessary partnerships to deliver more effectively with other providers" (Jopling, 2015, p. 59).

As noted earlier, cross-sector coalitions and partnerships are two strategies for increasing assistance, alignment, and advocacy activities in order to integrate social care into health care. The committee concludes that such partnerships are similarly needed in order for the health care system to help address social isolation and loneliness in older adults. Therefore, the committee identifies the following goal and recommendations:

GOAL: Strengthen ties between the health care system and community-based networks and resources that address social isolation and loneliness in older adults.

RECOMMENDATION 9-1: Health care providers, organizations, and systems should partner with social service providers, including those serving vulnerable communities, in order to create effective team-based care (which includes services such as transportation and housing support) and

to promote the use of tailored community-based services to address social isolation and loneliness in older adults.

In particular, the committee notes that many health care organizations (e.g., hospitals) are required under federal law to submit community benefit reports. Efforts by such entities to partner with social service providers could be used as an example of their community benefit efforts. As an example of tailored community-based services, the 2019 National Academies consensus study report *Integrating Social Care into the Delivery of Health Care* cites examples of assistance and alignment as including the provision of transportation vouchers that can be used for ride-sharing services or public transit and the investment in community ride-sharing programs (NASEM, 2019). In the case of social isolation and loneliness, such services would allow individuals to travel to health care appointments and also to overcome individual transportation-related barriers to participation in local community events.

A variety of stakeholders, both within and outside the formal health care system, are testing new approaches to preventing, identifying, and intervening for social isolation or loneliness for older adults. The committee concluded that as new evidence develops, a centralized sharing of resources and best practices would benefit all stakeholders. The committee noted that the U.S. Department of Health and Human Services has funded resource centers aimed primarily at health and social care professionals on a variety of topics that are of wide interest for the care of older adults (HHS, 2019d). Existing centers include the National Falls Prevention Resource Center, the National Clearinghouse for Long-Term Care Information, the National Resource Center on Nutrition and Aging, and the National Resource Center on LGBT (Lesbian, Gay, Bisexual, and Transgender) Aging. These resource centers not only serve as centralized resources for information, but also may provide training and technical assistance (Meyer and Johnston, 2014). Therefore, the committee makes the following recommendation:

RECOMMENDATION 9-2: Given the public health impact of social isolation and loneliness, the U.S. Department of Health and Human Services should establish and fund a national resource center to centralize evidence, resources, training, and best practices on social isolation and loneliness, including those for older adults and for diverse and at-risk populations.

Improving the Evidence Base on Interventions

The committee found that the overall quality of the evidence for specific interventions for social isolation and loneliness in older adults, particularly for interventions related to health care providers, is mixed. Current research uses a variety of definitions, measures, outcomes, and length of follow-up. Furthermore, the population of older people aged 50 and older are heterogeneous in their personal characteristics, their specific needs, and the underlying causes of their social isolation and loneliness (if present). While there is some evidence for promising approaches, the committee concluded that researchers are only beginning to understand which specific approaches work best for which people and which risk factors. In particular, the committee emphasizes that as social isolation and loneliness are distinct concepts, different intervention approaches may be needed to address each of them.

As discussed in Chapter 7, the health care system has a key role to play in helping to improve the evidence base on effective interventions. To that end, a report from the Campaign to End Loneliness cautions:

> As long as there is a shortage of evidence of the impact of loneliness initiatives, there will always be an excuse not to fund this vital work. External evaluations are costly, but all organisations can build into their programmes the opportunity to gather data about their impact. By using recognized and accredited tools, even if only with a sample of service users, we can start to create a reservoir of comparable data, improving the evidence base and building a clearer picture of which initiatives work best and why. (Jopling, 2015, p. 59)

Furthermore, the report notes:

> There is a huge shortage of evidence of the impact of loneliness initiatives on minority communities, such as LGBT and BME [black, minority, and ethnic] older people, and older people who live in care homes. This is not necessarily because initiatives do not serve these communities, but because providers have not yet gathered the data that proves that they do, and we do not know enough to be able to work out which approaches work best. Providers need to make sure that the needs of these minority communities are built into service planning, and that efforts are made to evaluate the impact on these groups in particular. (Jopling, 2015, p. 59)

When it comes to specific technological interventions, many gaps in our understanding remain, particularly related to potential unintended harms and ethical concerns. Also, little is known about how current trends, such as the use of social media, will affect social isolation and loneliness in future generations of older adults.

In accordance with the committee's previously identified goal of developing a more robust evidence base on effective prevention, assessment, and intervention strategies for social isolation and loneliness in older adults, the committee identified three major aspects of the overall evidence base for effective clinical interventions that need to be addressed in order to determine best practices and approaches. First is to improve the breadth and overall quality of the evidence for interventions in clinical settings. The committee notes that along with recommendations for research in Chapters 2 and 3, the development of a more robust evidence base is key to identifying effective interventions that might be scaled rather than investing in random interventions. Second is to increase the overall funding for such studies. Third is to target research to major gaps in the current evidence base. Within this context, and as noted in Chapter 7, the committee emphasizes that the preservation of an individual's own decisions regarding his or her life (e.g., living arrangements, community participation) is essential as a guiding principle for all interventions. (See Chapter 10 for more on engaging with the recipients of interventions.)

RECOMMENDATION 9-3: Funders should prioritize research that builds a scientific foundation for clinical and public health interventions that reduce the health and medical impacts of social isolation and loneliness based on standard theoretical frameworks. Researchers and health care providers and systems that study interventions for social isolation or loneliness should consider the following key elements in the design and evaluation of any intervention in order to enhance the ability to compare across studies:

- **A theoretical framework that drives particular approaches**
- **Appropriate choice of measure**
- **Specific target population**
- **Scalability**
- **Sustainability**
- **Ways to encourage data sharing**

For the above recommendation, because of the variability in research designs to date, it is especially important for researchers to describe the theoretical frameworks driving their approaches in order to build a more coherent body of knowledge.

RECOMMENDATION 9-4: Major funders of health research, including the government (e.g., the National Institutes of Health, the Center for Medicare & Medicaid Innovation, and the Patient-Centered Outcomes Research Institute), foundations, and large health plans, should fund research on effective interventions in clinical settings to identify, prevent, and mitigate the effects of social isolation and loneliness in older adults.

RECOMMENDATION 9-5: Those who fund, develop, and operate programs to assess, prevent, and intervene in social isolation and loneliness should prioritize research on the following major gaps in the evidence base:

- **Tailored interventions based on a public health framework of primary, secondary, and tertiary prevention. In particular, researchers should examine improved measures to identify individuals who may be at high risk for social isolation or loneliness and primary interventions in order to target such individuals.**

- **Trends among current younger adults as they age (e.g., use of technology, economic trends) to gain knowledge that informs future approaches to addressing social isolation and loneliness.**
- **Flexibility in funding to allow for the pilot testing and evaluation of innovative funding mechanisms for interventions.**
- **Approaches for assessments of and interventions among understudied groups of older adults (e.g., low income, lesbian, gay, bisexual, transgender) and those who face unique barriers to health.**

RECOMMENDATION 9-6: System designers as well as those who are developing and deploying technology in interventions should ensure that technological innovations related to social isolation and loneliness are properly assessed and tested so as to understand their full range of benefits and potential adverse consequences in order to prevent harm, and they should work to understand and take into account contextual issues, such as broadband access and having sufficient knowledge and support for using the technology.

10

Dissemination and Implementation

The gap between discovery of public health knowledge and application in practice settings and policy development is due in part to ineffective dissemination.

—Brownson et al. (2018)

The dissemination and implementation of scientific evidence into regular and effective use is complex due to the multiplicity and capacity of health care systems and providers and the diversity of the target audiences. However, such efforts are imperative in order to improve the quality of care, patient outcomes, and population health. Several reports of the Institute of Medicine describe opportunities for the implementation of evidence to improve population health and health care delivery (IOM, 2009, 2011a,b, 2012, 2013, 2015). The gap between the existence of evidence-based practices and the application of such practices has been linked to poor health outcomes (Conway et al., 2012; Shever et al., 2011; Sving et al., 2012). Two main challenges exist for the dissemination and implementation of information related to the social isolation and loneliness of older adults. First, better dissemination is needed regarding the evidence of the health impacts of social isolation and loneliness. Second, the best practices of implementation science will need to be used in order to ensure that health care systems and providers are able to more quickly adopt evidence-based practices. This will be particularly important as the evidence base on the effectiveness of specific interventions for social isolation and loneliness improves.

DEFINITION OF TERMS

Multiple and inconsistent terms are used in the field of dissemination and implementation science (Rabin and Brownson, 2018). For purposes of this report, *evidence-based practice* is defined as the conscientious and judicious use of current best evidence in conjunction with clinical expertise, patient values, and circumstances to guide health care decisions (Straus et al., 2010; Titler, 2014). Ideally, when enough reliable research evidence is available, practice is guided by findings from research in conjunction with clinical expertise and patient values. In some cases, however, a sufficient research base may not be available, and health care decision making relies on other evidence sources, such as scientific principles, case reports, and outcomes of quality improvement projects.

Dissemination research in health is the scientific study of the targeted distribution of evidence-based information and intervention materials to specific public health or clinical practice audiences with the intent of spreading and sustaining knowledge use and evidence-based interventions (HHS, 2018). The mechanisms and approaches to packaging and conveying the evidence necessary to improve public health and community and clinical care services are dependent on the type of audience (users), how the messages are framed, and the local context in which users reside, work, and live. For example, successful dissemination of health information may occur differently, depending on whether the audience consists of consumers, caregivers, practitioners, policy makers, employers, administrators, or other multiple stakeholder groups.

Translation science, more recently known as *implementation science*, focuses on testing interventions to promote the integration of evidence-based practices in order to improve patient outcomes and population health and also to explicate what implementation strategies work for whom, in what settings, and why (Eccles and Mittman, 2006; HHS, 2018; Titler, 2010, 2014). Implementation research seeks to understand the practice behaviors of health care professionals, health care organizations, consumers, and policy makers in their respective contexts or settings (HHS, 2018).

Evidence-based practice and implementation science, though related, are not interchangeable terms. Evidence-based practice is the actual application of evidence in practice (the "doing of" evidence-based practice), whereas implementation science is the study of implementation interventions, factors, and contextual variables that affect knowledge uptake and use in practices and communities.

The translation research model (Titler and Everett, 2001; Titler et al., 2009, 2016; see Figure 10-1) is based on Rogers's (2003) diffusion of innovations framework in which the rate and extent of the adoption of evidence-based health care practices are influenced by the nature of the innovation (e.g., clinical topic for the evidence-based practice) and the manner in which the innovation is communicated to the users of the evidence-based practices within a social system. Successful implementation requires strategies to address each of these areas (Titler, 2010; Titler et al., 2016).

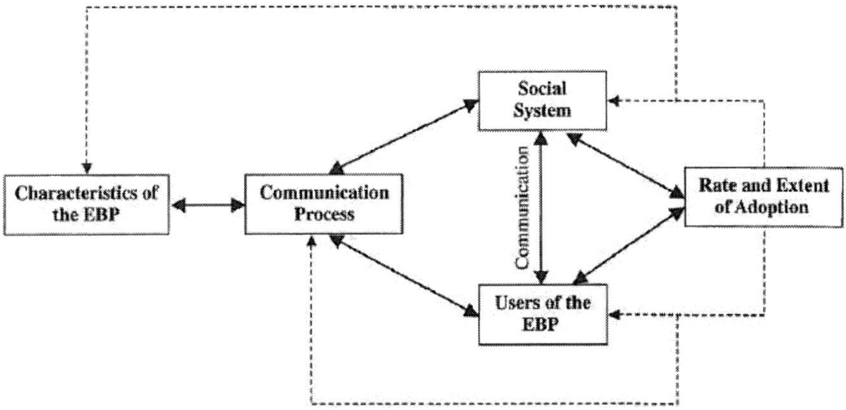

FIGURE 10-1 Translation research model.
NOTE: EBP = evidence-based practice.
SOURCE: Adapted from Titler et al., 2016.

An important principle to remember when planning for implementation is that the attributes of the evidence-based practice topic as perceived by users and stakeholders (e.g., ease of use, valued part of practice) are neither stable features nor sure determinants of their adoption. Rather, the interaction among the characteristics of the evidence-based practice topic, the intended users, and the context in which practices will be implemented all determine the rate and extent of adoption (Dogherty et al., 2012; Greenhalgh et al., 2005).

OVERVIEW OF IMPLEMENTATION STRATEGIES

To narrow the gaps between the known evidence and what is applied in routine health care, implementation scientists have prioritized the development, refinement, and testing of implementation strategies. *Implementation strategies* are methods or actions (i.e., interventions) to promote and facilitate the adoption, implementation, sustainment, and scale-up of evidence-based programs, practices, or models of care. Interventions can be discrete, involving one action or process (e.g., clinical reminders), or they can consist of two or more discrete strategies (Kirchner et al., 2018).

The challenges facing implementation include the inconsistent terminology used in naming and defining implementation strategies, the lack of an agreed-upon taxonomy, and the variations in how the implementation strategies are operationalized (e.g., who is targeted, who delivers it, temporality). The following sections describe implementation strategies that address each of the four components of the model illustrated in Figure 10-1.

ADDRESSING THE CHARACTERISTICS OF THE TOPIC

The complexity of a topic influences implementation. For example, evidence-based practices to decrease the social isolation and loneliness of older adults will likely include several actionable recommendations applicable across health care settings and the community (Andermann, 2016; Malani et al., 2019; Veazie et al., 2019). Several implementation strategies can be used to address the characteristics of the topic. For example, *quick reference guides* give targeted concise information in a manner to assist those implementing recommendations in performing specific tasks (Titler, 2018). A variety of quick reference guide formats are available, such as laminated checklists and decision-making algorithms. Quick reference guides concisely and accurately convey essential actions and information from the practice recommendations and are accessible at the point of care delivery (Anderson and Titler, 2019; Arditi et al., 2017; Pantoja et al., 2019). The design and content of quick reference guides will affect their use in practice and the subsequent implementation of evidence-based practices (Flodgren et al., 2016; Versloot et al., 2015; Wilson et al., 2016). As discussed in Chapter 9, Humana developed a one-page (two-sided) guide for physicians that focuses on defining social isolation and loneliness, highlighting the major health impacts of social isolation and loneliness, presenting the three-item UCLA Loneliness Scale, and advising physicians on potential referrals and resources (e.g., area agencies on aging, ride-sharing services, food resources) (Humana, 2019).

The empirical support for electronic clinical decision support interventions is mixed (IOM, 2011a). Reminders embedded in electronic health records have small to modest effects on clinician behavior and appear to be more effective when included as part of multi-faceted implementation strategies than when used alone (Anderson and Titler, 2019).

Conveying key messages about recommended practices at the point of care delivery is another way to foster the implementation of recommendations and is useful for reducing complexity. Distilling the recommendations to a few key points on visual displays can be very effective when the displays are designed appropriately. Examples include posters and infographics. Selecting the key message tools to promote implementation requires consideration of the knowledge of the end users, the context in which the tools will be used, and their design and usability (Flodgren et al., 2016; Grimshaw et al., 2012).

ADDRESSING USERS OF THE EVIDENCE-BASED INFORMATION

When designing implementation strategies that address the users of the evidence-based practices, it is essential to first delineate the targeted audiences or key stakeholders for the use of the information as well as the nature of the context in which they work or interact with the specified patient population. For example, interventions to decease social isolation may include social workers, psychologists, public policy makers, community health workers, and clinicians such as primary care physicians, physician assistants, nurse practitioners, mental health care providers, and physical therapists (among others). The interventions may target the general population to increase awareness about the issue (i.e., social isolation, loneliness) and considerations for addressing it.

Members of a group such as individuals within a health care system (e.g., nurses, physicians, community health workers) influence how quickly and widely evidence-based practices are adopted (Rogers, 2003). Implementation strategies that have demonstrated effectiveness in improving evidence-based practices of the users include performance gap assessment, audit and feedback, trying the evidence-based practice, engaging with the recipients of the evidence-based practices to address their values and preferences (e.g., shared decision making), and ongoing meetings to address barriers and acknowledge success (Fønhus et al., 2018; Greenhalgh et al., 2005; Hysong, 2009; Hysong et al., 2006, 2012; Ivers et al., 2012; Stacey et al., 2017; Titler and Anderson, 2019). These strategies are discussed in the following sections.

Performance Gap Assessment

Performance gap assessment is the provision of baseline or current practice indicators at the beginning of a practice change. It is used to engage clinicians in discussions about the current practice and about the formulation of strategies to promote alignment of their practices with evidence-based practices. As discussed in Chapter 7, many health care delivery systems are exploring practice-based strategies to identify and address the social determinants of health (including social isolation and loneliness); yet, clinicians may see such approaches as burdensome. As evidence-based practices for social isolation and loneliness emerge, performance gap assessment could provide the opportunity for clinicians to engage in the alignment of their practices for the implementation of these evidence-based practices.

Audit and Feedback

Audit and feedback is the ongoing auditing of performance indicators, aggregating data into reports, and discussing the findings with practitioners on a regular basis during the practice change (Hysong, 2009; Hysong et al., 2012; Ivers et al., 2012). This strategy helps clinicians see how their efforts to improve care and patient outcomes are progressing throughout the implementation process (Ivers et al., 2014).

Trying the Evidence-Based Practice

The users of evidence-based practices usually try the method for a period of time before fully adopting (Greenhalgh et al., 2005; Rogers, 2003). When an evidence-based practice is given a trial as part of an implementation, users have an opportunity to use the evidence-based practice, provide feedback to the implementation team, and modify the practice as necessary. This feedback loop will be key to Recommendation 7-1, the performance of assessments to identify social isolation or loneliness in older adults. As the committee noted, more needs to be learned about who should receive assessments, who should conduct the assessments, the ideal frequency of assessment, and appropriate referrals. Feedback garnered by the initiation of assessment in clinical settings will provide valuable data on how to best intervene.

Engaging with the Recipients of the Evidence-Based Practices

An important component of implementing evidence-based practices is engaging with the recipients of the practices to address their values and preferences. Putting the patient, family, and community at the center of health care decisions is a core component of implementing evidence-based practices. It is essential to address patient values, characteristics, and contextual factors that are important to them. This is similar to the finding in Chapter 9 that a common factor of many successful interventions for social isolation and loneliness is the active engagement of the older adult in the design of the intervention itself to ensure that the voice of the individual is at the center of interventions.

Furthermore, shared decision making is a process by which patients and health care workers partner to make informed health decisions that benefit the patients and are aligned with consumers' knowledge and values (Msowoya and Gephart, 2019). One approach to promoting shared decision making is the use of patient decision aides. Patient decision aides (also known as shared decision-making aides) are evidence-based documents or tools that support patients by making decisions explicit, providing information about options and associated benefits and harms, and helping to clarify congruence between decisions and personal values (Msowoya and Gephart, 2019; Stacey et al., 2017). These types of processes will be important, again, to ensure the autonomy of individuals who are identified as socially isolated or lonely. Participation in interventions, and personal preferences for lifestyle (e.g., living arrangements, community participation) need to be respected and honored in interventions.

When engaging patients, families, groups, and communities in health care decision making, it is important to be attuned to health literacy, health numeracy, and primary language. Health literacy, or the ability to understand written information about health, and health numeracy, the ability to understand quantitative data or information presented as numbers or graphs, are important for health care decision making. Thus it is necessary to ensure that patient materials and tools are in the patient's primary language and convey the appropriate meaning following translation (Msowoya and Gephart, 2019).

Meetings with Key Stakeholders

Another implementation strategy is to have regular meetings with key stakeholders and those implementing the evidence-based practices in order to track the process of implementation, provide guidance, address questions that arise, solve ongoing challenges, and share implementation strategies that are working (Titler et al., 2009, 2016).

COMMUNICATION STRATEGIES

Information and shared understanding move through communication channels, such as mass media, and interpersonal or interactive communication routes, such as the Internet and social media. Which of the various communication strategies one uses for implementation depends on the stage of implementation (see Figure 10-2), the audience targeted for communication, the nature of the information to be communicated, and the desired outcomes. For example, if the desired outcome is to increase awareness about the impact of social isolation on the health of community-dwelling older adults, implementers may consider using mass media delivered through the Internet by professional organizations and consumer groups. (See Chapter 8 for more on public health campaigns.) When selecting communication strategies, it is important to be clear about the types of audiences to be reached and the information sources they use. This section describes the following communication strategies to promote implementation:

- Mass media and social media
- Education
- Opinion leadership and change champions
- Educational outreach

Mass Media and Social Media

Mass media and social media can help to address the initial steps of implementation—knowledge and shared understanding. "Mass media" refers to various technologies that allow for the imparting of information in a directional message from one source to many people. The primary channels of mass media are television, radio, print materials, Internet sources, and digital technology (Bala et al., 2017; Carson-Chahhoud et al., 2017). The characteristics of a mass media communication that influence the amount of attention that the communication attracts include the seriousness of the issue being discussed, the human interest (as with a personal story), timeliness, and conflict and controversy (Brownson et al., 2018a). The use of mass media to align clinician professional practices with the evidence most likely increases awareness and persuasion early during implementation (Grimshaw et al., 2012).

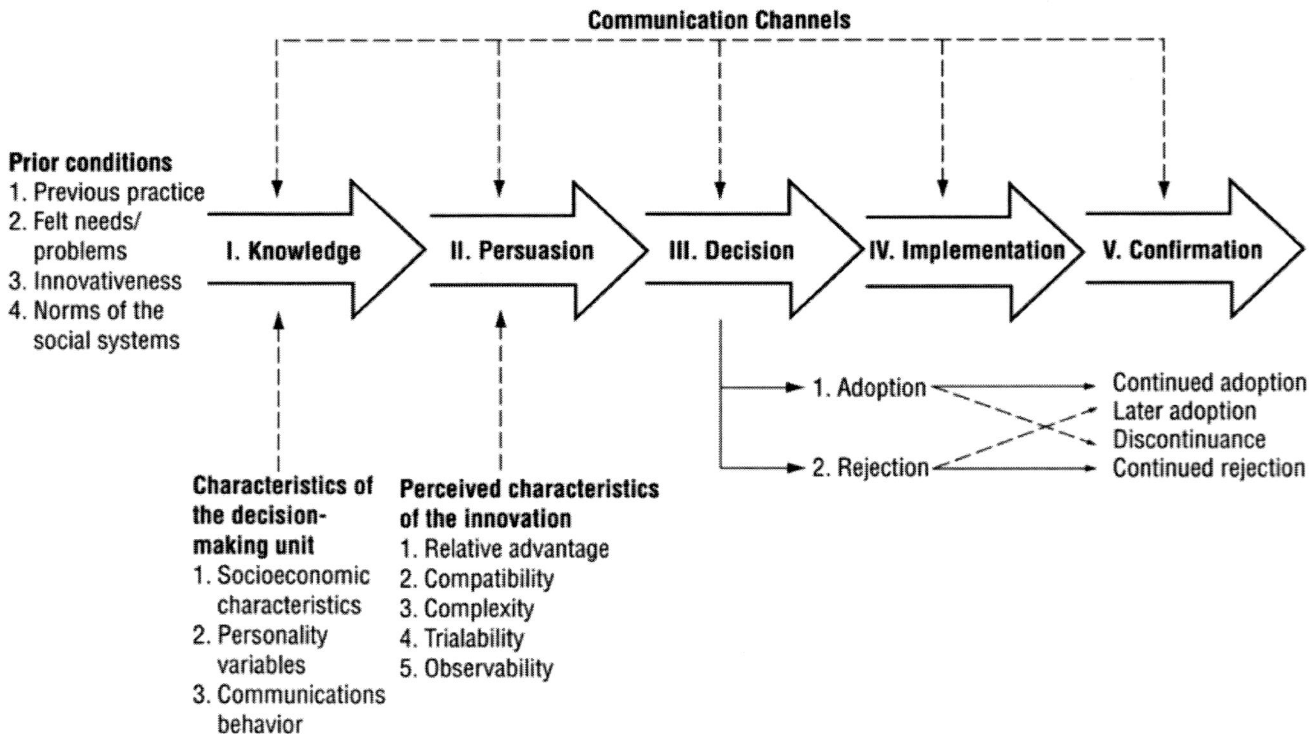

FIGURE 10-2 Stages of the decision-making process.
SOURCE: Rogers, 2003.

The definition of social media is broad and constantly changing, but social media can be thought of as a form of electronic communication using a variety of platforms through which users create online communities to share information, ideas, messages, and other content such as videos. Social media makes it possible for information and knowledge to be rapidly shared (Kirton, 2019; Roland, 2018; Ventola, 2014). The types of social media can be grouped by function (Djuricich, 2014; Kirton, 2019; Ventola, 2014), such as:

- Social networking—Facebook, Google Plus, Twitter
- Professional networking—LinkedIn
- Media sharing—YouTube, Flickr, Instagram
- Content production—blogs such as Tumblr and Blogger and microblogs such as Twitter
- Knowledge or information aggregation—Wikipedia

Although dissemination of evidence-based practice information through social media is significantly and positively associated with more downloads and citations of the evidence, it is unclear if the use of such dissemination pathways has a positive effect on practice behaviors (Brownson et al., 2018a; Puljak, 2016). Studies have demonstrated that the use of social media increases users' knowledge about evidence-based practices and, based on self-reports, the application of evidence in their practice (Dyson et al., 2017; Frisch et al., 2014; Maloney et al., 2015; Tunnecliff et al., 2017). Bernhardt et al. (2011) describe how social media can be leveraged to enhance the dissemination and implementation of research evidence. More research using rigorous designs is needed to fully explicate the impact of social media on improving the knowledge, skills, and application of evidence in health care.

When using social and mass media, the considerations about messaging include knowing the audience, defining the customer, specifying the message and framing it, and selecting the communication channels (Brownson et al., 2018a; Steensma et al., 2018). A challenge for the dissemination of information related to evidence-based practices is defining the customer. "Failure to properly identify customers is the undoing of many valuable innovations" (Steensma et al., 2018, p. 193). Defining the customer helps frame the message and identify the proper communication channels and social media platforms for reaching them. This is particularly relevant for social isolation and loneliness in that there are likely a variety of underlying causes that likely require very key messages and intervention approaches.

Education

As discussed in Chapter 8, educating the users of evidence-based practices is necessary but not sufficient in order to change practice, and didactic education alone does little to change practice behavior (Forsetlund et al., 2009; Giguère et al., 2012). There is moderate evidence that educational meetings that include both didactic and interactive learning are more effective in aligning professional practice behaviors with the evidence-based practices than didactic meetings alone or interactive learning alone (Forsetlund et al., 2009). Depending on the complexity of the evidence-based practices to be implemented, a variety of educational approaches can be considered, including train-the-trainer programs, high-fidelity simulation, and ongoing point-of-care coaching (Brownson et al., 2018a; Titler and Anderson, 2019). Many Web sources have packaged selected resources into implementation toolkits that include printed materials, training videos, and slide presentations. A toolkit could be developed for communities and health systems to facilitate the implementation of evidence-based practices to address social isolation and loneliness. For example, as discussed in Chapter 9, Humana created a Loneliness Toolkit (Humana, 2018) directed at consumers. The toolkit includes information on health-related issues (e.g., stress, substance abuse, vision and hearing impairment), staying engaged (e.g., transportation alternatives, housing options, use of social media), supporting loved ones (e.g., personal coping skills, caregiver support groups), and general community resources (e.g., area agencies on aging, ride-sharing services, support groups).

Opinion Leadership and Change Champions

Studies and systematic reviews have demonstrated that opinion leaders are effective in changing the behaviors of health care practitioners (Anderson and Titler, 2014; Cranley et al., 2019; Dagenais et al., 2015; Flodgren et al., 2011; McCormack et al., 2013; Van Eerd et al., 2016; Yousefi Nooraie et al., 2017), especially in combination with educational outreach or performance feedback. Opinion leaders are from the local peer group, viewed as a respected source of influence, considered by associates as technically competent, and trusted to judge the fit between the evidence-based practices and the local situation (Dobbins et al., 2009; Flodgren et al., 2011; Grimshaw et al., 2012). Opinion leadership is multifaceted and complex, with role functions varying by the circumstances, but few successful projects that have implemented evidence-based practices have managed without opinion leaders (Greenhalgh et al., 2005; McCormack et al., 2013). Opinion leaders among groups of older adults may encourage participation in interventions, most likely for community-based interventions.

Change champions are also helpful for implementing innovations (Dogherty et al., 2012; Rogers, 2003). They are practitioners within the local setting (e.g., clinic, patient care unit, public health agency) who are expert clinicians, are passionate about the evidence-based practice topic, are committed to improving the quality of care, and have a positive working relationship with other health professionals (Rogers, 2003). They circulate information, encourage peers to adopt the evidence-based practices, arrange demonstrations, and orient peers to the evidence-based practices (Titler et al., 2016). The scope of influence that change champions have is usually within a specific unit or team within an agency, whereas the influence of an opinion leader spans multiple units or teams across an agency. For example, if an evidence-based practice tool to assess social isolation is being implemented across multiple primary care practices in a health system, to implement the practice, one nurse and one physician opinion leader could work across the practice sites in collaboration with change champions who are located in each primary care setting. This will be key to the implementation of Recommendation 7-1 (assessing for social isolation and loneliness) wherein the committee concluded that an important aspect of selecting a tool for use in clinical settings is standardization, meaning that within a specific health care system or organization all clinicians would use the same tool or set of tools rather than resorting to different tools.

Educational Outreach

Multiple studies have demonstrated the effectiveness of educational outreach, also known as academic detailing, in improving the practice behaviors of clinicians (Avorn, 2010; IOM, 2011a; O'Brien et al., 2007; Titler et al., 2009, 2016; Wilson et al., 2016). Educational outreach involves interactive face-to-face education and dialogue with practitioners in their setting by an individual (usually a clinician) with expertise in a particular topic (e.g., the prevention of social isolation). Academic detailers are able to explain the research foundations of the evidence-based practices and respond convincingly to specific questions, concerns, or challenges that a practitioner might raise. Clinicians' perceptions of educational outreach as an implementation strategy are quite positive and perceived as helpful in overcoming implementation barriers (Wilson et al., 2016).

ADDRESSING THE SOCIAL CONTEXT

The social context for evidence-based practice implementation refers to the characteristics of the physical setting of implementation and the dynamic practice factors in which implementation processes occur (May et al., 2016; Shuman et al., 2018a; Squires et al., 2015). Context factors that affect implementation include

- Organizational capacity for evidence-based practice (Brownson et al., 2018b; Doran et al., 2012; Everett and Sitterding, 2011; French et al., 2009; Kueny et al., 2015; Stetler et al., 2009; Yamada et al., 2017),
- Leadership support (Aarons et al., 2014; Birken et al., 2016; Hauck et al., 2012; Jun et al., 2016; Richter et al., 2016; Riley et al., 2018; Shuman et al., 2018a; Wong and Giallonardo, 2013),

- Practice climates for use of evidence-based practices (Ehrhart et al., 2014; Jacobs et al., 2014; Shuman et al., 2018a; Yamada et al., 2017), and
- Evidence-based practices competencies of mid-level managers and supervisors (Gifford et al., 2007; Melnyk et al., 2014; Shuman et al., 2019).

The organizational capacity needed includes strong leadership, a clear strategic vision, good managerial relationships, visionary staff in key positions, a climate conducive to experimentation and risk taking, and effective systems for data capture and transforming data into information (Brownson et al., 2018b; Riley et al., 2018; Titler and Anderson, 2019). Elements of system readiness for assimilating evidence-based practices into care delivery include a tension for change, a fit of the evidence-based practices with the system, clear implications of adopting or not adopting the evidence-based practices, support and advocacy for the evidence-based practice topic (e.g., reducing the social isolation of community-dwelling older adults), the time and resources necessary for implementation, and the capacity to evaluate the impact of evidence-based practices on processes and outcomes of health care during and following implementation (Brownson et al., 2018b; Titler and Anderson, 2019).

When promoting the use of evidence-based practices, it is crucial to consider the context in which the potential users of the evidence will work because the settings for implementation are dynamic, and each setting carries its own set of contextual factors, such as the practice climate and leadership behaviors that influence the implementation and sustainability of the evidence-based practices (Riley et al., 2018; Titler and Anderson, 2019).

Implementation strategies that target the social context generally address infrastructure elements of the system (Riley et al., 2018). These strategies, described in the following sections, include

- Performing an environmental scan,
- Understanding the governance of the organization,
- Engaging with key leadership stakeholders,
- Addressing the standards of practice and documentation systems, and
- Promoting linkages among health systems and communities.

Environmental Scan

An environmental scan is a process that assesses internal strengths and challenges for a specific topic—in this case, the implementation of evidence-based practices. Environmental scans include the structure and function of the organization—how things are done within a system or community. One purpose of an environmental scan is to understand the mission, vision, and values of an organization and to articulate how the proposed evidence-based practices will contribute to meeting these organizational attributes. Those who lead the implementation of evidence-based practices to address social isolation and loneliness will need to articulate how these recommendations will contribute to comprehensive care for the older adults served by the particular health system. (See Chapter 7 for more on comprehensive care.)

Organizational Governance and Engaging with Key Leadership Stakeholders

Understanding the governance structure is necessary so that work can be integrated into existing structures. Selected members of the implementation team will need to meet with key leadership stakeholders representing each of the disciplines that will be users of the evidence-based practices. Given the wide variety of health care workers who will be required to fully address social isolation and loneliness (see Chapter 8), it will be important for such meetings to include representatives across the health care workforce.

Addressing Standards of Practice and Documentation Systems

Written standards of practice (e.g., policies, procedures, clinical pathways) and documentation systems need to support the use of the evidence-based practices (Titler, 2010). Clinical information systems may need to be revised in order to support practice changes; documentation systems that fail to readily support the new practice thwart change (IOM, 2011b). For example, having an electronic health record or medical record that is capable of capturing data on social isolation and loneliness will be key to the implementation of Recommendation 7-3, the inclusion of social isolation in the electronic health record or medical record.

Promoting Linkages Among Health Systems and Communities

Several models of care delivery and role specialization have emerged to provide continuity and linkages across levels and sites of care delivery and with communities. These models include case management, care coordination, patient navigation programs, and transitional models of care (Hirschman et al., 2015; IOM, 2011b; Lamb and Newhouse, 2018; NASEM, 2016c; Naylor et al., 2013). People working within these models of care are key stakeholders to engage in implementing evidence-based practices and to provide linkages with the community. A care coordinator or patient navigator may be among the first to know if community-dwelling older adults are suffering from social isolation and can help navigate referrals and follow-up for community services to address the issue (see Chapter 8). These professionals are also well positioned to communicate the importance of this issue broadly among the health care workforce. To realize the full impact of implementing evidence-based practices within health care settings, it is essential to have partnerships and linkages with communities and those outside the health sector (e.g., social services, law enforcement, urban planning and housing programs) (Brownson et al., 2018b; McMillen and Adams, 2018). To that end, Recommendation 9-1 calls for the integration of health care and social care in order to provide effective team-based care and promote the use of tailored community-based services to address social isolation and loneliness.

SUSTAINABILITY

As noted in Chapter 9, the sustainability of an intervention is a key element in the design and evaluation of that intervention. Sustainability refers to the degree to which the implemented evidence-based practices continue after implementation. Given the considerable effort and resources required to implement such practices, it is crucial to determine which improvements are sustained or decay following implementation. However, few studies have addressed the determinants of sustaining evidence-based practices following adoption (Stirman and Dearing, 2019). Experts agree, however, that planning for sustainability during development and delivery of implementation interventions contributes to sustainability and continued improvements (Ploeg et al., 2014; Shuman et al., 2018b; Stirman and Dearing, 2019; Tricco et al., 2016). The following principles are helpful to consider when planning implementation (Chambers et al., 2013; Colón-Emeric et al., 2016; Johnson et al., 2019; Lennox et al., 2018; Ploeg et al., 2014; Shuman et al., 2018b; Stirman and Dearing, 2019; Titler et al., 2009; Tricco et al., 2016).

1. Use implementation strategies that address the needs and context of the organization.
2. Address alignment with the organization's values, mission, and vision.
3. Integrate evidence-based programs or practices into existing staffing models and workflow.
4. Engage with key stakeholders early and often (stakeholder participation).
5. Include programs for training new staff and conducting annual competencies of all staff.
6. Plan for workforce turnover.
7. With use of non-professional health workers such as lay health workers, plan for mechanisms to support their ability to deliver the evidence-based practices.
8. Plan for and adapt to the dynamic contexts in which the evidence-based programs or interventions are implemented.
9. Set boundaries for potential adaptations, including impact on outcomes.
10. Include outcomes meaningful to the key stakeholders in evaluations, and share the findings.
11. Incorporate selected metrics into quality and performance improvement programs for ongoing monitoring.

CONCLUSION

Promoting and sustaining use of evidence-based practices and programs is a dynamic process that is influenced by the context or setting, the population served, and the attributes of what is being implemented. The science of implementation is growing with multiple challenges and opportunities in advancing this field of inquiry. As the evidence base for effective interventions in health care settings for social isolation and loneliness in older adults is improved (as discussed in previous chapters), consideration of best practices for dissemination and implementation of this information is needed both in the planning of the intervention to be tested as well as in consideration of any implementation plan.

References

AACN (American Association of Colleges of Nursing). 2006. *The essentials of doctoral education for advanced nursing practice.* Washington, DC: American Association of Colleges of Nursing.

AACN. 2008. *The essentials of baccalaureate education for professional nursing practice.* Washington, DC: American Association of Colleges of Nursing.

AACN. 2011. *The essentials of master's education in nursing.* Washington, DC: American Association of Colleges of Nursing.

AACN. 2016. *Advancing healthcare transformation: A new era for academic nursing.* http://www.aacnnursing.org/portals/42/publications/aacn-new-era-report.pdf (accessed June 27, 2019).

AACN. 2019. *Essentials task force.* https://www.aacnnursing.org/About-AACN/AACN-Governance/Committees-and-Task-Forces/Essentials (accessed December 19, 2019).

Aarons, G. A., M. G. Ehrhart, L. R. Farahnak, and M. Sklar. 2014. Aligning leadership across systems and organizations to develop a strategic climate for evidence-based practice implementation. *Annual Review of Public Health* 35:255–274.

AARP Foundation. 2019. *Connect 2 affect.* https://connect2affect.org (accessed August 11, 2019).

Aarts, S., S. T. M. Peek, and E. J. M. Wouters. 2015. The relation between social network site usage and loneliness and mental health in community-dwelling older adults. *International Journal of Geriatric Psychiatry* 30(9):942–949.

Aartsen, M. J., T. van Tilburg, C. H. M. Smits, and K. C. P. M. Knipscheer. 2004. A longitudinal study of the impact of physical and cognitive decline on the personal network in old age. *Journal of Social and Personal Relationships* 21(2):249–266.

ACGME (Accreditation Council for Graduate Medical Education). 2018. *Common program requirements (residency).* https://www.acgme.org/Portals/0/PFAssets/ProgramRequirements/CPRResidency2019.pdf (accessed November 7, 2019).

ACGME. 2019. *"The heart of what we do"—Dr. Vivek Murthy on rediscovering meaning in medicine.* https://www.acgme.org/Newsroom/Blog/Details/ArticleID/8071/The-Heart-of-What-We-Do-Dr-Vivek-Murthy-on-Rediscovering-Meaning-in-Medicine (accessed August 11, 2019).

ACHP (Alliance of Community Health Plans). 2018. *Accelerating adoption of evidence-based care: Payer–provider partnerships.* https://www.transforming-care.org/wp-content/uploads/2018/11/Accelerating-Adoption-of-Evidence-Based-Care-Splash-FINAL.pdf (accessed October 22, 2019).

Acierno, R., M. A. Hernandez, A. B. Amstadter, H. S. Resnick, K. Steve, W. Muzzy, and D. G. Kilpatrick. 2010. Prevalence and correlates of emotional, physical, sexual, and financial abuse and potential neglect in the United States: The National Elder Mistreatment Study. *American Journal of Public Health* 100(2):292–297.

ACL (Administration for Community Living). 2018. *2017 Profile of older Americans.* https://acl.gov/sites/default/files/Aging%20and%20Disability%20in%20America/2017OlderAmericansProfile.pdf (accessed February 4, 2019).

Adams, K. B. 2008. Specific effects of caring for a spouse with dementia: Differences in depressive symptoms between caregiver and non-caregiver spouses. *International Psychogeriatrics* 20(3):508–520.

AGHE (Association for Gerontology in Higher Education). 2014. *Gerontological competencies for undergraduate and graduate education.* Washington, DC: Association for Gerontology in Higher Education.

AGHE. 2019. *AGHE's mission.* https://www.aghe.org/about-us (accessed September 14, 2019).

Air, T., P. J. Tully, S. Sweeney, and J. Beltrame. 2016. Epidemiology of cardiovascular disease and depression. In B. T. Baune and P. J. Tully (eds.), *Cardiovascular diseases and depression: Treatment and prevention in psychocardiology.* Switzerland: Springer. Pp. 5–21.

Akerlind, I., and J. O. Hornquist. 1992. Loneliness and alcohol abuse: A review of evidences of an interplay. *Social Science & Medicine* 34(4):405–414.

Alberti, P. M., K. M. Sutton, L. A. Cooper, W. G. Lane, S. Stephens, and M. A. Gourdine. 2018. Communities, social justice, and academic health centers. *Academic Medicine* 93(1):20–24.

Alma, M. A., S. F. Van der Mei, W. N. Feitsma, J. W. Groothoff, T. G. Van Tilburg, and T. P. Suurmeijer. 2011. Loneliness and self-management abilities in the visually impaired elderly. *Journal of Aging & Health* 23(5):843–861.

Altfeld, S. J., G. E. Shier, M. Rooney, T. J. Johnson, R. L. Golden, K. Karavolos, E. Avery, and A. J. Perry. 2013. Effects of an enhanced discharge planning intervention for hospitalized older adults: A randomized trial. *Gerontologist* 53(3):430–440.

Alun, J., and B. Murphy. 2019. Loneliness, social isolation and cardiovascular risk. *British Journal of Cardiac Nursing* 14(10).

Alvarez, R., J. Ginsburg, J. Grabowski, S. Post, and W. Rosenberg. 2016. The social work role in reducing 30-day readmissions: The effectiveness of the bridge model of transitional care. *Journal of Gerontological Social Work* 59(3):222–227.

Amstadter, A. B., J. M. Cisler, J. L. McCauley, M. A. Hernandez, W. Muzzy, and R. Acierno. 2011. Do incident and perpetrator characteristics of elder mistreatment differ by gender of the victim? Results from the National Elder Mistreatment Study. *Journal of Elder Abuse & Neglect* 23(1):43–57.

Anda, R. F., V. J. Felitti, J. D. Bremner, J.D. Walker, C. Whitfield, B. D. Perry, S. R. Dube, and W. H. Giles. 2006. The enduring effects of abuse and related adverse experiences in childhood. A convergence of evidence from neurobiology and epidemiology. *European Archives of Psychiatry and Clinical Neuroscience* 256(3):174–186.

Andermann, A. 2016. Taking action on the social determinants of health in clinical practice: A framework for health professionals. *Canadian Medical Association Journal* 188(17-18):e474–e483.

Anderson, C., and M. G. Titler. 2014. Development and verification of an agent-based model of opinion leadership. *Implementation Science* 9:136.

Anderson, C., and M. G. Titler. 2019. Launching implementation. In G. LoBiondo-Wood, J. Haber, and M. G. Titler (eds.), *Evidence-based practice for nursing healthcare quality improvement.* Philadelphia, PA: Elsevier. Pp. 197–205.

Anderson, G. O., and C. E. Thayer. 2018. *Loneliness and social connections: A national survey of adults 45 and older.* Washington, DC: AARP Foundation.

Andersson, H., C. Lindholm, and B. Fossum. 2011. MRSA—Global threat and personal disaster: Patients' experiences. *International Nursing Review* 58(1):47–53.

Andreadou, E., M. Anagnostouli, V. Vasdekis, E. Kararizou, M. Rentzos, T. Kontaxis, and I. Evdokimidis. 2011. The impact of comorbidity and other clinical and sociodemographic factors on health-related quality of life in Greek patients with Parkinson's disease. *Aging & Mental Health* 15(7):913–921.

Andreasen, J., H. Lund, M. Aadahl, and E. E. Sorensen. 2015. The experience of daily life of acutely admitted frail elderly patients one week after discharge from the hospital. *International Journal of Qualitative Studies on Health and Well-Being* 10:27370.

Andrew, N., and S. Meeks. 2018. Fulfilled preferences, perceived control, life satisfaction, and loneliness in elderly long-term care residents. *Aging and Mental Health* 22(2):183–189.

Ang, S., and T. Y. Chen. 2018. Going online to stay connected: Online social participation buffers the relationship between pain and depression. *Journals of Gerontology, Series B: Psychological Sciences and Social Sciences* 74(6):1020–1031.

Ansryan, L. Z., H. U. Aronow, J. E. Borenstein, V. Mena, F. Haus, K. Palmer, E. Chan, J. W. Swanson, S. Mass, B. Rosen, G. D. Braunstein, and L. Burnes Bolton. 2018. Systems addressing frail elder care: Description of a successful model. *Journal of Nursing Administration* 48(1):11–17.

Antonuci, T. C., and H. Akiyama. 1987. An examination of sex differences in social support among older men and women. *Sex Roles* 17(11–12):737–749.

APHA (American Public Health Association). 2019. *What is public health?* https://www.apha.org/what-is-public-health (accessed November 10, 2019).

Appelbaum, P. S. 2007. Assessment of patients' competence to consent to treatment. *New England Journal of Medicine* 357(18):1834–1840.

Arditi, C., M. Rège-Walther, P. Durieux, and B. Burnand. 2017. Computer-generated reminders delivered on paper to healthcare professionals: Effects on professional practice and healthcare outcomes. *Cochrane Database of Systematic Reviews* 2017(7):CD001175.

Arizona Direct Care Initiative. 2011. *Principles of caregiving.* http://www.azdirectcare.org/uploads/All_AgingandPhysicalDisabilities2011.pdf (accessed June 27, 2019).

Asch, J. M., D. A. Asch, E. V. Klinger, J. Marks, N. Sadek, and R. M. Merchant. 2019. Google search histories of patients presenting to an emergency department: An observational study. *BMJ Open* 9(2):e024791.

Asian Scientist Newsroom. 2014. Tai Chi reduces stress and inflammation. https://www.asianscientist.com/2014/10/health/tai-chi-reduces-stress-inflammation (accessed December 19, 2019).

Austin, J., H. H. Dodge, T. Riley, P. G. Jacobs, S. Thielke, and J. Kaye. 2016. A smart-home system to unobtrusively and continuously assess loneliness in older adults. *IEEE Journal of Translational Engineering in Health and Medicine* 4:2800311.

Avorn, J. 2010. Transforming trial results into practice change: The final translational hurdle: Comment on "Impact of the ALLHAT/JNC7 Dissemination Project on thiazide-type diuretic use." *Archives of Internal Medicine* 170(10):858–860.

Ayalon, L., S. Shiovitz-Ezra, and I. Roziner. 2016. A cross-lagged model of the reciprocal associations of loneliness and memory functioning. *Psychology and Aging* 31(3):255–261.

Bala, M. M., L. Strzeszynski, and R. Topor-Madry. 2017. Mass media interventions for smoking cessation in adults. *Cochrane Database of Systematic Reviews* 2017(11):CD004704.

Ball, C., J. Francis, K.-T. Huang, T. Kadylak, S. R. Cotton, and R. V. Rikard. 2017. The physical–digital divide: Exploring the social gap between digital natives and physical natives. *Journal of Applied Gerontology* 38(8):1167–1184.

Banks, M. R., L. M. Willoughby, and W. A. Banks. 2008. Animal-assisted therapy and loneliness in nursing homes: Use of robotic versus living dogs. *Journal of the American Medical Directors Association* 9(3):173–177.

Bantry-White, E. 2018. Supporting ethical use of electronic monitoring for people living with dementia: Social work's role in assessment, decision-making, and review. *Journal of Gerontological Social Work* 61(3):261–279.

Barbosa, L. M., B. Monteiro, and S. G. Murta. 2016. Retirement adjustment predictors—A systematic review. *Work, Aging and Retirement* 2(2):262–280.

Barger, S. D., and B. N. Uchino. 2017. Racial and ethnic variation in the association of social integration with mortality: Ten-year prospective population-based US study. *Scientific Reports* 7:43874.

Barger, S. D., N. Messerli-Bürgy, and J. Barth. 2014. Social relationship correlates of major depressive disorder and depressive symptoms in Switzerland: Nationally representative cross sectional study. *BMC Public Health* 14(1):273.

Barrett, A. E., and C. Gumber. 2019. Feeling older and driving less: The effect of age identity on older adults' transition from driving. *Innovation in Aging* 3(1):1–8.

Barretta, D., D. Dantzler, and W. Kayson. 1995. Factors related to loneliness. *Psychological Reports* 76(3 Pt 1):827–830.

Barrington, C., D. K. H. Messias, and L. Weber. 2012. Implications of racial and ethnic relations for health and well-being in new Latino communities: A case study of West Columbia, South Carolina. *Latino Studies* 10(1-2):155–178.

Barth, J., S. Schneider, and R. von Kanel. 2010. Lack of social support in the etiology and the prognosis of coronary heart disease: A systematic review and meta-analysis. *Psychosomatic Medicine* 72(3):229–238.

Bartz, J. A., J. Zaki, N. Bolger, and K. N. Ochsner. 2011. Social effects of oxytocin in humans: Context and person matter. *Trends in Cognitive Sciences* 15(7):301–309.

Bassuk, S. S., T. A. Glass, and L. F. Berkman. 1999. Social disengagement and incident cognitive decline in community-dwelling elderly persons. *Annals of Internal Medicine* 131(3):165–173.

Bazemore, A., S. Petterson, L. E. Peterson, and R. L. Phillips, Jr. 2015. More comprehensive care among family physicians is associated with lower costs and fewer hospitalizations. *Annals of Family Medicine* 13(3):206–213.

Bazemore, A., A. V. Neale, P. Lupo, and D. Seehusen. 2018. Advancing the science of implementation in primary health care. *Journal of the American Board of Family Medicine* 31(3):307–311.

BCIA (Boston College Institute on Aging). 2019. BC Talks Aging. https://www.bc.edu/centers/ioa/videos.html (accessed November 26, 2019).

Beam, C. R., and E. M. Collins. 2019. Trajectories of depressive symptomatology and loneliness in older adult sexual minorities and heterosexual groups. *Clinical Gerontology* 42(2):172–184.

Beauchamp, T., and J. Childress. 2013. *Principles of bioethics, 7th ed.* New York: Oxford University Press.

Becher, K., M. Oelke, B. Grass-Kapanke, J. Flohr, E. A. Mueller, U. Papenkordt, B. Schulte-Frei, K. C. Steinwachs, S. Süss, and M. Wehling. 2013. Improving the health care of geriatric patients: Management of urinary incontinence: A position paper. *Zeitschrift fur Gerontologie und Geriatrie* 46(5):456–464.

Bekhet, A. K., and J. A. Zauszniewski. 2012. Mental health of elders in retirement communities: Is loneliness a key factor? *Archives of Psychiatric Nursing* 26(3):214–224.

Bekhet, A. K., J. A. Zauszniewski, and W. E. Nakhla. 2009. Reasons for relocation to retirement communities: A qualitative study. *Western Journal of Nursing Research* 31(4):462–479.

Beller, J., and A. Wagner. 2018a. Loneliness, social isolation, their synergistic interaction, and mortality. *Health Psychology* 37(9):808–813.

Beller, J., and A. Wagner. 2018b. Disentangling loneliness: Differential effects of subjective loneliness, network quality, network size, and living alone on physical, mental, and cognitive health. *Journal of Aging and Health* 30(4):521–539.

Benefield, L. E., and B. J. Holtzclaw. 2014. Aging in place: Merging desire with reality. *Nursing Clinics of North America* 49(2):123–131.

Benford, R. D., and D. A. Snow. 2000. Framing processes and social movements: An overview and assessment. *Annual Review of Sociology* 26:611–639.

Benito-León, J., E. D. Louis, and F. Bermejo-Pareja. 2009. Population-based case-control study of morale in Parkinson's disease. *European Journal of Neurology* 16(3):330–336.

Bennett, D. A., J. A. Schneider, Y. Tang, S. E. Arnold, and R. S. Wilson. 2006. The effect of social networks on the relation between Alzheimer's disease pathology and level of cognitive function in old people: A longitudinal cohort study. *Lancet Neurology* 5(5):406–412.

Berkman, L. F., and L. Breslow. 1983. *Health and ways on living: The Alameda county study.* New York: Oxford University Press.

Berkman, L., and T. A. Glass. 2000. Social integration, social networks, social support, and health. In L. Berkman and I. Kawachi (eds.), *Social epidemiology*. New York: Oxford University Press. Pp. 137–173.

Berkman, L. F., and S. L. Syme. 1979. Social networks, host resistance, and mortality: A nine-year follow-up study of Alameda county residents. *American Journal of Epidemiology* 109(2):186–204.

Berkman, L. F., T. Glass, I. Brissette, and T. E. Seeman. 2000. From social integration to health: Durkheim in the new millennium. *Social Science & Medicine* 51(6):843–857.

Bernhardt, J. M., D. Mays, and M. W. Kreuter. 2011. Dissemination 2.0: Closing the gap between knowledge and practice with new media and marketing. *Journal of Health Communication* 16(Suppl 1):32–44.

Bernier, S., S. Lapierre, and S. Desjardins. 2019. Social interactions among older adults who wish for death. *Clinical Gerontologist* 43(1):4–16.

Beutel, M. E., E. M. Klein, E. Brähler, I. Reiner, C. Jünger, M. Matthias, J. Wiltink, P. S. Wild, T. Münzel, K. J. Lackner, and A. N. Tibubos. 2017. Loneliness in the general population: Prevalence, determinants and relations to mental health. *BMC Psychiatry* 17(1):97.

Bickmore, T. W. 2005. *Ethical issues in using relational agents for older adults.* Paper presented at the AAAI Fall Symposium on Caring Machines: AI in Eldercare, Washington, DC.

Bickmore, T. W., L. Caruso, K. Clough-Gorr, and T. Heeren. 2005. "It's just like you talk to a friend": Relational agents for older adults. *Interacting with Computers* 17(6):711–735.

Bickmore, T. W., L. M. Pfeifer, and M. K. Paasche-Orlow. 2009. Using computer agents to explain medical documents to patients with low health literacy. *Patient Education and Counseling* 75(3):315–320.

Bickmore, T. W., L. M. Pfeifer, D. Byron, S. Forsythe, L. E. Henault, B. W. Jack, R. Silliman, and M. K. Paasche-Orlow. 2010. Usability of conversational agents by patients with inadequate health literacy: Evidence from two clinical trials. *Journal of Health Communication* 15(Suppl 2):197–210.

Bickmore, T. W., R. A. Silliman, K. Nelson, D. M. Cheng, M. Winter, L. Henault, and M. K. Paasche-Orlow. 2013. A randomized controlled trial of an automated exercise coach for older adults. *Journal of the American Geriatrics Society* 61(10):1676–1683.

Biddle, K. D., F. d'Oleire Uquillas, H. I. L. Jacobs, B. Zide, D. R. Kirn, D. M. Rentz, K. A. Johnson, R. A. Sperling, and N. J. Donovan. 2019. Social engagement and amyloid-beta-related cognitive decline in cognitively normal older adults. *American Journal of Geriatric Psychiatry* 27(11):1247–1256.

Birditt, K., and T. C. Antonucci. 2008. Life sustaining irritations? Relationship quality and mortality in the context of chronic illness. *Social Science & Medicine* 67(8):1291–1299.

Birken, S. A., L. D. DiMartino, M. A. Kirk, S.-Y. Lee, M. McClelland, and N. M. Albert. 2016. Elaborating on theory with middle managers' experience implementing healthcare innovations in practice. *Implementation Science* 11(1):2.

Birks, M., M. Bodak, J. Barlas, J. Harwood, and M. Pether. 2016. Robotic seals as therapeutic tools in an aged care facility: A qualitative study. *Journal of Aging Research* 2016:8569602.

Birmingham, W. C., and J. Holt-Lunstad. 2018. Social aggravation: Understanding the complex role of social relationships on stress and health-relevant physiology. *International Journal of Psychophysiology* 131:13–23.

Black, B. S., D. Johnston, P. V. Rabins, A. Morrison, C. Lyketsos, and Q. M. Samus. 2013. Unmet needs of community-residing persons with dementia and their informal caregivers: Findings from the Maximizing Independence at Home Study. *Journal of the American Geriatrics Society* 61(12):2087–2095.

Black, S. D. 1982. *Inequalities in health: The Black report.* New York: Penguin Books.

Blanquet, M., A. Debost-Legrand, L. Gerbaud, C. De La Celle, A. Brigand, L. Mioche, C. Sass, J. Hazart, and A. Aw. 2016. Metabolic syndrome and social deprivation: Results of a French observational multicentre survey. *Family Practice* 33(1):17–22.

Blickem, C., A. Kennedy, I. Vassilev, R. Morris, H. Brooks, P. Jariwala, T. Blakeman, and A. Rogers. 2013. Linking people with long-term health conditions to healthy community activities: Development of Patient-Led Assessment for Network Support (PLANS). *Health Expectations* 16(3):e48–e59.

BLS (Bureau of Labor Statistics). 2017. *Unpaid eldercare in the United States—2015–2016 summary.* https://www.bls.gov/news.release/elcare.nr0.htm (accessed July 5, 2019).

Blum, K., and D. W. Sherman. 2010. Understanding the experience of caregivers: A focus on transitions. *Seminars in Oncology Nursing* 26(4):243–258.

Blyth, F. M., and N. Noguchi. 2017. Chronic musculoskeletal pain and its impact on older people. *Best Practice and Research: Clinical Rheumatology* 31(2):160–168.

Boehlen, F., W. Herzog, R. Quinzler, W. E. Haefeli, I. Maatouk, D. Niehoff, K. U. Saum, H. Brenner, and B. Wild. 2015. Loneliness in the elderly is associated with the use of psychotropic drugs. *International Journal of Geriatric Psychiatry* 30(9):957–964.

Bookwala, J. 2005. The role of marital quality in physical health during the mature years. *Journal of Aging and Health* 17(1):85–104.

Borenstein, J., H. U. Aronow, L. B. Bolton, J. Choi, C. Bresee, and G. D. Braunstein. 2013. Early recognition of risk factors for adverse outcomes during hospitalization among Medicare patients: A prospective cohort study. *BMC Geriatrics* 13:72.

Borenstein, J., H. U. Aronow, L. B. Bolton, M. I. Dimalanta, E. Chan, K. Palmer, X. Zhang, B. Rosen, and G. D. Braunstein. 2016. Identification and team-based interprofessional management of hospitalized vulnerable older adults. *Nursing Outlook* 64(2):137–145.

Bos, H. M., L. Boschloo, R. A. Schoevers, and T. G. Sandfort. 2015. Depression and anxiety in patients with and without same-sex attraction: Differences in clinical expression, lifestyle factors, and vulnerability indicators. *Brain and Behavior* 5(9):e00363.

Boyle, P. A. 2019. The second act: Seeking best practices for encore worker management. *Gerontologist,* July 10 [Epub ahead of print].

Braak, H., and K. Del Tredici. 2012. Alzheimer's disease: Pathogenesis and prevention. *Alzheimer's & Dementia* 8(3):227–233.

Bradley, N. and W. Poppen, W. 2003. Assistive technology, computers and Internet may decrease sense of isolation for homebound elderly and disabled persons. *Technology and Disability* 15(1):19–25.

Brady, S., L. A. D'Ambrosio, A. Felts, E. Y. Rula, K. P. Kell, and J. F. Coughlin. 2020. Reducing isolation and loneliness through membership in a fitness program for older adults: Implications for health. *Journal of Applied Gerontology* 39(3):301–310.

Braithwaite, S. R., C. Giraud-Carrier, J. West, M. D. Barnes, and C. L. Hanson. 2016. Validating machine learning algorithms for Twitter data against established measures of suicidality. *JMIR Mental Health* 3(2):e21.

Bränström, R., and J. E. Pachankis. 2018. Sexual orientation disparities in the co-occurrence of substance use and psychological distress: A national population-based study (2008–2015). *Social Psychiatry and Psychiatric Epidemiology* 53(4):403–412.

Brindle, R. C., K. A. Duggan, M. R. Cribbet, C. E. Kline, R. T. Krafty, J. F. Thayer, S. R. Mulukutla, and M. H. Hall. 2018. Cardiovascular stress reactivity and carotid intima-media thickness: The buffering role of slow-wave sleep. *Psychosomatic Medicine* 80(3):301–306.

Brinkhues, S., N. H. T. M. Dukers-Muijrers, C. J. P. A. Hoebe, C. J. H. Van Der Kallen, P. C. Dagnelie, A. Koster, R. M. A. Henry, S. J. S. Sep, N. C. Schaper, C. D. A. Stehouwer, H. Bosma, P. H. M. Savelkoul, and M. T. Schram. 2017. Socially isolated individuals are more prone to have newly diagnosed and prevalent type 2 diabetes mellitus—The Maastricht study. *BMC Public Health* 17(1):955.

Broadbent, E., K. Peri, N. Kerse, C. Jayawardena, I. Kuo, C. Datta, and B. MacDonald. 2014. Robots in older people's homes to improve medication adherence and quality of life: A randomised crossover trial. In Beetz M., B. Johnston, and M.A. Williams (eds.), *Social Robotics.* ICSR 2014. Lecture Notes in Computer Science, vol. 8755. Cham, Switzerland: Springer.

Brody, J. E. 2017. The surprising effects of loneliness on health. *The New York Times.* December 11. https://www.nytimes.com/2017/12/11/well/mind/how-loneliness-affects-our-health.html (accessed November 20, 2019).

Broekens, J., M. Heerink, and H. Rosendal, H. 2009. Assistive social robots in elderly care: A review. *Gerontechnology* 8(2):94–103.

Brooks, H. L., K. Rushton, K. Lovell, P. Bee, L. Walker, L. Grant, and A. Rogers. 2018. The power of support from companion animals for people living with mental health problems: A systematic review and narrative synthesis of the evidence. *BMC Psychiatry* 18(1):31.

Brown, E. G., S. Gallagher, and A. M. Creaven. 2018. Loneliness and acute stress reactivity: A systematic review of psychophysiological studies. *Psychophysiology* 55(5):e13031.

Brown, E. S., J. Park, C. E. Marx, L. S. Hynan, C. Gardner, D. Davila, A. Nakamura, P. Sunderajan, A. Lo, and T. Holmes. 2014. A randomized, double-blind, placebo-controlled trial of pregnenolone for bipolar depression. *Neuropsychopharmacology* 39(12):2867–2873.

Brown, S. L., and I. F. Lin. 2012. The gray divorce revolution: Rising divorce among middle-aged and older adults, 1990–2010. *Journals of Gerontology, Series B: Psychological Sciences and Social Sciences* 67(6):731–741.

Brown, S. L., J. R. Bulanda, and G. R. Lee. 2012. Transitions into and out of cohabitation in later life. *Journal of Marriage and Family* 74(4):774–793.

Brownson, R. C., A. A. Eyler, J. K. Harris, J. B. Moore, and R. G. Tabak. 2018a. Getting the word out: New approaches for disseminating public health science. *Journal of Public Health Management and Practice* 24(2):102–111.

Brownson, R. C., J. E. Fielding, and L. W. Green. 2018b. Building capacity for evidence-based public health: Reconciling the pulls of practice and the push of research. *Annual Review of Public Health* 39:27–53.

Buchman, A. S., P. A. Boyle, R. S. Wilson, B. D. James, S. E. Leurgans, S. E. Arnold, and D. A. Bennett. 2010. Loneliness and the rate of motor decline in old age: The Rush Memory and Aging Project, a community-based cohort study. *BMC Geriatrics* 10:77.

Buhse, M. 2015. The elderly person with multiple sclerosis: Clinical implications for the increasing life-span. *Journal of Neuroscience Nursing* 47(6):333–339; quiz, E331.

Burholt, V., and T. Scharf. 2014. Poor health and loneliness in later life: The role of depressive symptoms, social resources, and rural environments. *Journals of Gerontology, Series B: Psychological Sciences and Social Sciences* 69(2):311–324.

Business Wire. 2018. *CareMore Health announces new outcomes data from first-of-its-kind Togetherness Program.* https://www.businesswire.com/news/home/20181218005059/en/CareMore-Health-Announces-New-Outcomes-Data-First-of-its-Kind (accessed December 1, 2019).

Butler, A. C., J. E. Chapman, E. M. Forman, and A. T. Beck. 2006. The empirical status of cognitive–behavioral therapy: A review of meta-analyses. *Clinical Psychology Review* 26(1):17–31.

Cacioppo, J. T., and L. C. Hawkley. 2009. Perceived social isolation and cognition. *Trends in Cognitive Sciences* 13(10):447–454.

Cacioppo, J. T., and W. Patrick. 2008. *Loneliness: Human nature and the need for social connection.* New York: W.W. Norton & Company.

Cacioppo, J. T., L. C. Hawkley, L. E. Crawford, J. M. Ernst, M. H. Burleson, R. B. Kowalewski, W. B. Malarkey, E. Van Cauter, and G. G. Berntson. 2002. Loneliness and health: Potential mechanisms. *Psychosomatic Medicine* 64(3):407–417.

Cacioppo, J. T., L. C. Hawkley, and R. A. Thisted. 2010. Perceived social isolation makes me sad: 5-year cross-lagged analyses of loneliness and depressive symptomatology in the Chicago Health, Aging, and Social Relations Study. *Psychology and Aging* 25(2):453–463.

Cacioppo, J. T., S. Cacioppo, J. P. Capitanio, and S. W. Cole. 2015a. The neuroendocrinology of social isolation. *Annual Review of Psychology* 66:733–767.

Cacioppo, S., J. P. Capitanio, and J. T. Cacioppo. 2014. Toward a neurology of loneliness. *Psychological Bulletin* 140(6):1464–1504.

Cacioppo, S., A. J. Grippo, S. London, L. Goossens, and J. T. Cacioppo. 2015b. Loneliness: Clinical import and interventions. *Perspectives on Psychological Science* 10(2):238–249.

Cacioppo, S., M. Bangee, S. Balogh, C. Cardenas-Iniguez, P. Qualter, and J. T. Cacioppo. 2016. Loneliness and implicit attention to social threat: A high-performance electrical neuroimaging study. *Cognitive Neuroscience* 7(1-4):138–159.

Cahill, S., and A. M. Diaz-Ponce. 2011. "I hate having nobody here. I'd like to know where they all are": Can qualitative research detect differences in quality of life among nursing home residents with different levels of cognitive impairment? *Aging & Mental Health* 15(5):562–572.

Calati, R., C. Ferrari, M. Brittner, O. Oasi, E. Olié, A. F. Carvalho, and P. Courtet. 2019. Suicidal thoughts and behaviors and social isolation: A narrative review of the literature. *Journal of Affective Disorders* 245:653–667.

Campaign to End Loneliness. 2019a. *Measuring your impact on loneliness in later life*. https://www.campaigntoendloneliness.org/wp-content/uploads/Loneliness-Measurement-Guidance1-1.pdf (accessed November 14, 2019).

Campaign to End Loneliness. 2019b. *About the campaign*. https://www.campaigntoendloneliness.org/about-the-campaign (accessed August 12, 2019).

Campaign to End Loneliness. 2019c. *The Campaign to End Loneliness Learning Network*. https://www.campaigntoendloneliness.org/campaigns/learning-network (accessed August 12, 2019).

Canham, S. L., P. M. Mauro, C. N. Kaufmann, and A. Sixsmith. 2016. Association of alcohol use and loneliness frequency among middle-aged and older adult drinkers. *Journal of Aging and Health* 28(2):267–284.

Canli, T., L. Yu, X. Yu, H. Zhao, D. Fleischman, R. S. Wilson, P. L. De Jager, and D. A. Bennett. 2018. Loneliness 5 years ante-mortem is associated with disease-related differential gene expression in postmortem dorsolateral prefrontal cortex. *Translational Psychiatry* 8(1):2.

Cantarero-Prieto, D., M. Pascual-Saez, and C. Blázquez-Fernández. 2018. Social isolation and multiple chronic diseases after age 50: A European macro-regional analysis. *PLOS ONE* 13(10):e0205062.

Caputo, J. 2019. Crowded nests: Parent-adult child coresidence transitions and parental mental health following the great recession. *Journal of Health and Social Behavior* 60(2):204–221.

Carnes, D., R. Sohanpal, C. Frostick, S. Hull, R. Mathur, G. Netuveli, J. Tong, P. Hutt, and M. Bertotti. 2017. The impact of a social prescribing service on patients in primary care: A mixed methods evaluation. *BMC Health Services Research* 17(1):835.

Carpenter, C., L. Osterberg, and G. Sutcliffe. 2012. *SAMHT—Suicidal avatars for mental health training*. Paper presented at the Proceedings of the 25th International Florida Artificial Intelligence Research Society Conference, FLAIRS-25.

Carr, D. 2009. Who's to blame? Perceived responsibility for spousal death and psychological distress among older widowed persons. *Journal of Health and Social Behavior* 50(3):359–375.

Carr, D. C., S. Urena, and M. G. Taylor. 2018. Adjustment to widowhood and loneliness among older men: The influence of military service. *Gerontologist* 58(6):1085–1095.

Carson-Chahhoud, K. V., F. Ameer, K. Sayehmiri, K. Hnin, J. E. M. van Agteren, F. Sayehmiri, M. P. Brinn, A. J. Esterman, A. B. Chang, and B. J. Smith. 2017. Mass media interventions for preventing smoking in young people. *Cochrane Database of Systematic Reviews* 2017(6):CD001006.

Carter, C. S., A. J. Grippo, H. Pournajafi-Nazarloo, M. G. Ruscio, and S. W. Porges. 2008. Oxytocin, vasopressin and sociality. *Progress in Brain Research* 170:331–336.

Caspi, A., H. Harrington, T. E. Moffitt, B. J. Milne, and R. Poulton. 2006. Socially isolated children 20 years later: Risk of cardiovascular disease. *Archives of Pediatric & Adolescent Medicine* 160(8):805–811.

Cassel, J. 1976. The contribution of the social environment to host resistance: The fourth Wade Hampton Frost Lecture. *American Journal of Epidemiology* 104(2):107–123.

Cassell, J. 2001. Embodied conversational agents: Representation and intellegence in user interfaces. *Artificial Intellegence Magazine* 22(4):67–83.

Cassell, J., T. Bickmore, M. N. Billinghurst, L. W. Campbell, K. Chang, H. Vilhjálmsson, and H. Yan. 1999. Embodiment in conversational interfaces: Rea. *Proceedings of the SIGCHI Conference on Human Factors in Computing Systems*. Pp. 520–527.

Castelino, F., M. Prabhu, M. S. Pai, A. Kamath, A. K. Mohapatra, and E. S. Devi. 2018. Lived experiences of patients with chronic obstructive pulmonary diseases (COPD)–Qualitative review. *Indian Journal of Public Health Research and Development* 9(4):262–265.

Cattan, M., M. White, J. Bond, and A. Learmouth. 2005. Preventing social isolation and loneliness among older people: A systematic review of health promotion interventions. *Ageing & Society* 25(1):41–67.

CDC (Centers for Disease Control and Prevention). 2001. *Ten great public health achievements: United States, 1900–1999.* https://www.cdc.gov/mmwr/preview/mmwrhtml/mm4850bx.htm (accessed June 27, 2019).

CDC. 2017. *Picture of America: Prevention.* https://www.cdc.gov/pictureofamerica/pdfs/Picture_of_America_Prevention.pdf (accessed November 10, 2019).

CDC. 2019. *About chronic diseases.* https://www.cdc.gov/chronicdisease/about/index.htm (accessed July 26, 2019).

Centene. 2019. *Who we are.* https://www.centene.com/who-we-are.html (accessed November 4, 2019).

Centre for Policy on Ageing. 2014. *Rapid review: Loneliness—Evidence of the effectiveness of interventions.* http://www.cpa.org.uk/information/reviews/CPA-Rapid-Review-Loneliness.pdf (accessed February 11, 2019).

Chambers, D. A., R. E. Glasgow, and K. C. Stange. 2013. The dynamic sustainability framework: Addressing the paradox of sustainment amid ongoing change. *Implementation Science* 8(1):117.

Chan, A. W., D. S. Yu, and K. C. Choi. 2017. Effects of tai chi qigong on psychosocial well-being among hidden elderly, using elderly neighborhood volunteer approach: A pilot randomized controlled trial. *Clinical Interventions in Aging* 12:85–96.

Chang, Q., C. H. Chan, and P. S. F. Yip. 2017. A meta-analytic review on social relationships and suicidal ideation among older adults. *Social Science and Medicine* 191:65–76.

Chappell, N. L., and M. Badger. 1989. Social isolation and well-being. *Journal of Gerontology* 44(5):S169–S176.

Chatters, L. M., H. O. Taylor, E. J. Nicklett, and R. J. Taylor. 2018. Correlates of objective social isolation from family and friends among older adults. *Healthcare* 6(1):6010024.

Che, X., R. Cash, S. K. Ng, P. Fitzgerald, and B. M. Fitzgibbon. 2018. A systematic review of the processes underlying the main and the buffering effect of social support on the experience of pain. *Clinical Journal of Pain* 34(11):1061–1076.

Chen, H. L. 1994. Hearing in the elderly: Relation of hearing loss, loneliness, and self-esteem. *Journal of Gerontological Nursing* 20(6):22–28.

Chesser, A., A. Burke, J. Reyes, and T. Tohrberg. 2015. Navigating the digital divide: A systematic review of eHealth literacy in underserved populations in the United States. *Informatics for Health and Social Care* 41(1):1–19.

Cheung, G., S. Edwards, and F. Sundram. 2017. Death wishes among older people assessed for home support and long-term aged residential care. *International Journal of Geriatric Psychiatry* 32(12):1371–1380.

Chihuri, S., T. J. Mielenz, C. J. DiMaggio, M. E. Betz, C. DiGuiseppi, V. C. Jones, and G. Li. 2016. Driving cessation and health outcomes in older adults. *Journal of the American Geriatrics Society* 64(2):332–341.

Chipps, J., M. A. Jarvis, and S. Ramlall. 2017. The effectiveness of e-Interventions on reducing social isolation in older persons: A systematic review of systematic reviews. *Journal of Telemedicine and Telecare* 23(10):817–827.

Choi, H., and N. F. Marks. 2011. Socioeconomic status, marital status continuity and change, marital conflict, and mortality. *Journal of Aging & Health* 23(4):714–742.

Choi, H., M. R. Irwin, and H. J. Cho. 2015. Impact of social isolation on behavioral health in elderly: Systematic review. *World Journal of Psychiatry* 5(4):432–438.

Choi, N. G., and D. M. DiNitto. 2015. Role of new diagnosis, social isolation, and depression in older adults' smoking cessation. *Gerontologist* 55(5):793–801.

Chow, A. Y. M., M. Caserta, D. Lund, M. H. P. Suen, D. Xiu, I. K. N. Chan, and K. S. M. Chu. 2018. Dual-Process Bereavement Group Intervention (DPBGI) for widowed older adults. *Gerontologist* 59(5):983–994.

Christakis, N. A., and P. D. Allison. 2006. Mortality after the hospitalization of a spouse. *New England Journal of Medicine* 354(7):719–730.

Christakis, N. A., and J. H. Fowler. 2008. The collective dynamics of smoking in a large social network. *New England Journal of Medicine* 358(21):2249–2258.

Christiansen, J., F. B. Larsen, and M. Lasgaard. 2016. Do stress, health behavior, and sleep mediate the association between loneliness and adverse health conditions among older people? *Social Science and Medicine* 152:80–86.

Chumaeva, N., M. Hintsanen, T. Hintsa, N. Ravaja, M. Juonala, O. T. Raitakari, and L. Keltikangas-Jarvinen. 2010. Early atherosclerosis and cardiac autonomic responses to mental stress: A population-based study of the moderating influence of impaired endothelial function. *BMC Cardiovascular Disorders* 10:16.

Chung, J., G. Demiris, and H. J. Thompson. 2016. Ethical considerations regarding the use of smart home technologies for older adults: An integrative review. *Annual Review of Nursing Research* 34(1):155–181.

Cichero, J. A., and K. W. Altman. 2012. Definition, prevalence and burden of oropharyngeal dysphagia: A serious problem among older adults worldwide and the impact on prognosis and hospital resources. *Nestle Nutrition Institute Workshop Series* 72:1–11.

Cigna. 2018. *New Cigna study reveals loneliness at epidemic levels in America.* https://www.cigna.com/newsroom/news-releases/2018/new-cigna-study-reveals-loneliness-at-epidemic-levels-in-america (accessed August 13, 2019).

Cigna/Ipsos. 2018. Cigna U.S. loneliness index. https://www.cigna.com/assets/docs/newsroom/loneliness-survey-2018-full-report.pdf (accessed December 11, 2019).

CMS (Centers for Medicare & Medicaid Services). 2014. *CMS Final competency set: CMS direct service workforce core competencies.* https://www.medicaid.gov/sites/default/files/2019-12/dsw-core-competencies-final-set-2014.pdf (accessed December 19, 2019).

CMS. 2019a. *CMS fast facts.* https://www.cms.gov/fastfacts (accessed November 25, 2019).

CMS. 2019b. *CMS finalizes Medicare Advantage and Part D payment and policy updates to maximize competition and coverage.* https://www.cms.gov/newsroom/press-releases/cms-finalizes-medicare-advantage-and-part-d-payment-and-policy-updates-maximize-competition-and (accessed November 10, 2019).

Cobb, S. 1976. Presidential address—1976. Social support as a moderator of life stress. *Psychosomatic Medicine* 38(5):300–314.

Cohen, S. 1988. Psychosocial models of the role of social support in the etiology of physical disease. *Health Psychology* 7(3):269–297.

Cohen, S., and T. A. Wills. 1985. Stress, social support, and the buffering hypothesis. *Psychological Bulletin* 98(2):310–357.

Cohen, S., W. J. Doyle, D. P. Skoner, B. S. Rabin, and J. M. Gwaltney, Jr. 1997. Social ties and susceptibility to the common cold. *JAMA* 277(24):1940–1944.

Cohen, S., B. H. Gottlieb, and L. G. Underwood. 2000. Social relationships and health. In S. Cohen, L. G. Underwood, and B. H. Gottlieb (eds.), *Social support measurement and intervention: A guide for health and social scientists.* New York: Oxford University Press. Pp. 3–25.

Cohen, S., W. J. Doyle, R. Turner, C. M. Alper, and D. P. Skoner. 2003. Sociability and susceptibility to the common cold. *Psychological Science* 14(5):389–395.

Cohen-Mansfield, J. 2001. Nonpharmacologic interventions for inappropriate behaviors in dementia: A review, summary, and critique. *American Journal of Geriatric Psychiatry* 9(4):361–381.

Cohen-Mansfield, J., and A. Libin. 2005. Verbal and physical non-aggressive agitated behaviors in elderly persons with dementia: Robustness of syndromes. *Journal of Psychiatric Research* 39(3):325–332.

Cohen-Mansfield, J., and R. Perach. 2015. Interventions for alleviating loneliness among older persons: A critical review. *American Journal of Health Promotion* 29(3):e109–e125.

Cohen-Mansfield, J., M. Dakheel-Ali, M. S. Marx, K. Thein, and N. G. Regier. 2015. Which unmet needs contribute to behavior problems in persons with advanced dementia? *Psychiatry Research* 228(1):59–64.

Cohen-Mansfield, J., H. Hazan, Y. Lerman, and V. Shalom. 2016. Correlates and predictors of loneliness in older-adults: A review of quantitative results informed by qualitative insights. *International Psychogeriatrics* 28(4):557–576.

Cohen-Mansfield, J., T. Hai, and M. Comishen. 2017. Group engagement in persons with dementia: The concept and its measurement. *Psychiatry Research* 251:237–243.

Cole, S. W., L. C. Hawkley, J. M. Arevalo, C. Y. Sung, R. M. Rose, and J. T. Cacioppo. 2007. Social regulation of gene expression in human leukocytes. *Genome Biology* 8(9):R189.

Cole, S. W., L. C. Hawkley, J. M. Arevalo, and J. T. Cacioppo. 2011. Transcript origin analysis identifies antigen-presenting cells as primary targets of socially regulated gene expression in leukocytes. *Proceedings of the National Academy of Sciences* 108(7):3080–3085.

Cole, S. W., J. P. Capitanio, K. Chun, J. M. Arevalo, J. Ma, and J. T. Cacioppo. 2015a. Myeloid differentiation architecture of leukocyte transcriptome dynamics in perceived social isolation. *Proceedings of the National Academy of Sciences* 112(49):15142–15147.

Cole, S. W., M. E. Levine, J. M. Arevalo, J. Ma, D. R. Weir, and E. M. Crimmins. 2015b. Loneliness, eudaimonia, and the human conserved transcriptional response to adversity. *Psychoneuroendocrinology* 62:11–17.

Colón-Emeric, C., M. Toles, M. P. Cary, Jr., M. Batchelor-Murphy, T. Yap, Y. Song, R. Hall, A. Anderson, A. Burd, and R. A. Anderson. 2016. Sustaining complex interventions in long-term care: A qualitative study of direct care staff and managers. *Implementation Science* 11:94.

Commonwealth Care Alliance. 2018. Commonwealth Care Alliance one care. https://www.commonwealthfund.org/publications/international-innovation/2018/nov/commonwealth-care-alliance-one-care (accessed December 12, 2019).

Communications Network. 2008. *Are we there yet?* https://www.comnetwork.org/resources/a-guide-to-evaluating-foundationnonprofit-communications (accessed September 27, 2019).

Contrera, K. J., Y. K. Sung, J. Betz, L. Li, and F. R. Lin. 2017. Change in loneliness after intervention with cochlear implants or hearing aids. *Laryngoscope* 127(8):1885–1889.

Conway, L. J., M. Pogorzelska, E. Larson, and P. W. Stone. 2012. Adoption of policies to prevent catheter-associated urinary tract infections in United States intensive care units. *American Journal of Infection Control* 40(8):705–710.

Cook, S. L. 2015. Redirection: An extension of career during retirement. *The Gerontologist* 55(3): 360–373.

Copen, C. E., K. Daniels, J. Vespa, and W. D. Mosher. 2012. First marriages in the United States: Data from the 2006–2010 National Survey of Family Growth. *National Health Statistics Report* 49:1–21.

Coppersmith G. A., C. T. Harman, M. H. Dredze. 2014. Measuring post traumatic stress disorder in Twitter. In *Proceedings of the 8th International Conference on Weblogs and Social Media, ICWSM 2014*. Palo Alto, CA: AAAI Press. Pp. 579–582.

Cornwell, B., L. P. Schumm, and E. O. Laumann. 2008. The social connectedness of older adults: A national profile. *American Sociological Review* 73(2):185–203.

Cornwell, E. Y., and L. J. Waite. 2009. Social disconnectedness, perceived isolation, and health among older adults. *Journal of Health and Social Behavior* 50(1):31–48.

Cotten, S. R., W. A. Anderson, and B. M. McCullough. 2013. Impact of internet use on loneliness and contact with others among older adults: Cross-sectional analysis. *Journal of Medical Internet Research* 15(2):e39.

Coyle, C. E., and E. Dugan. 2012. Social isolation, loneliness, and health among older adults. *Journal of Aging and Health* 24(8):1346–1363.

Coyle, C. E., B. A. Steinman, and J. Chen. 2017. Visual acuity and self-reported vision status: Their associations with social isolation in older adults. *Journal of Aging and Health* 29(1):128–148.

Cranley, L. A., J. M. Keefe, D. Taylor, G. Thompson, A. M. Beacom, J. E. Squires, C. A. Estabrooks, J. W. Dearing, P. G. Norton, and W. B. Berta. 2019. Understanding professional advice networks in long-term care: An outside-inside view of best practice pathways for diffusion. *Implementation Science* 14(1):10.

Creswell, J. D., M. R. Irwin, L. J. Burklund, M. D. Lieberman, J. M. Arevalo, J. Ma, E. C. Breen, and S. W. Cole. 2012. Mindfulness-based stress reduction training reduces loneliness and pro-inflammatory gene expression in older adults: A small randomized controlled trial. *Brain, Behavior, and Immunity* 26(7):1095–1101.

Crisp, D. A., T. D. Windsor, P. Butterworth, and K. J. Anstey. 2013. What are older adults seeking? Factors encouraging or discouraging retirement village living. *Australasian Journal on Ageing* 32(3):163–170.

Crittenden, C. N., S. D. Pressman, S. Cohen, D. Janicki-Deverts, B. W. Smith, and T. E. Seeman. 2014. Social integration and pulmonary function in the elderly. *Health Psychology* 33(6):535–543.

Crooks, V. C., J. Lubben, D. B. Petitti, D. Little, and V. Chiu. 2008. Social network, cognitive function, and dementia incidence among elderly women. *American Journal of Public Health* 98(7):1221–1227.

CSDH (Commission on Social Determinants of Health). 2008. *Closing the gap in a generation: Health equity through action on the social determinants of health.* Geneva, Switzerland: World Health Organization.

CSWE (Council on Social Work Education). 2015. *Educational policies and accreditation standards.* https://www.cswe.org/getattachment/Accreditation/Standards-and-Policies/2015-EPAS/2015EPASandGlossary.pdf.aspx (accessed September 19, 2019).

CSWE. 2019. *Geriatric social work competency scale II with life-long leadership skills: Social work practice behaviors in the field of aging.* https://www.cswe.org/getattachment/Centers-Initiatives/CSWE-Gero-Ed-Center/Teaching-Tools/Gero-Competencies/GeriatricSocialWorkCompetencyScaleII-LifelongLeadershipSkills.pdf.aspx (accessed September 19, 2019).

CTA (Consumer Technology Association). 2018. *What is artificial intelligence? A practical guide to understanding the definition, meaning and importance of cognitive technologies and their adoption in industry.* Arlington, VA: Consumer Technology Association.

Cudjoe, T. K. M., D. L. Roth, S. L. Szanton, J. L. Wolff, C. M. Boyd, and R. J. Thorpe, Jr. 2020. The epidemiology of social isolation: National Health and Aging Trends Study. *Journals of Gerontology. Series B: Psychological Sciences and Social Sciences* 75(1):107–113.

Cuffee, Y., C. Ogedegbe, N. J. Williams, G. Ogedegbe, and A. Schoenthaler. 2014. Psychosocial risk factors for hypertension: An update of the literature. *Current Hypertension Reports* 16(10):483.

Cuijpers, P., A. S. Geraedts, P. van Oppen, G. Andersson, J. C. Markowitz, and A. van Straten. 2011. Interpersonal psychotherapy for depression: A meta-analysis. *American Journal of Psychiatry* 168(6):581–592.

Cundiff, J. M., and T. W. Smith. 2017. Social status, everyday interpersonal processes, and coronary heart disease: A social psychophysiological view. *Social and Personality Psychology Compass* 11(4):e12310.

Cupitt, S. 2013. *The Campaign to End Loneliness evaluation: Health and wellbeing boards' uptake of campaign messages.* https://campaigntoendloneliness.org/wp-content/uploads/downloads/2013/06/Health-and-wellbeing-boards-uptake-of-Campaign-messages.pdf (accessed June 27, 2019).

Curtin, A., D. C. Martins, C. Gillsjö, and D. Schwartz-Barcott. 2017. Ageing out of place: The meaning of home among Hispanic older persons living in the United States. *International Journal of Older People Nursing* 12(3):e12150.

Czaja, S. J., W. R. Boot, N. Charness, W. A. Rogers, and J. Sharit. 2018. Improving social support for older adults through technology: Findings from the PRISM randomized controlled trial. *Gerontologist* 58(3):467–477.

Dagenais, C., M. C. Laurendeau, and M. Briand-Lamarche. 2015. Knowledge brokering in public health: A critical analysis of the results of a qualitative evaluation. *Evaluation and Program Planning* 53(2015):10–17.

Danese, A., T. E. Moffitt, H. Harrington, B. J. Milne, G. Polanczyk, C. M. Pariante, R. Poulton, and A. Caspi. 2009. Adverse childhood experiences and adult risk factors for age-related disease: Depression, inflammation, and clustering of metabolic risk markers. *Archives of Pediatric & Adolescent Medicine* 163(12):1135–1143.

Das, A. 2013. How does race get "under the skin"? Inflammation, weathering, and metabolic problems in late life. *Social Science & Medicine* 77:75–83.

Davidson, S., and P. Rossall. 2015. *Evidence review: Loneliness in later life.* https://www.ageuk.org.uk/globalassets/age-uk/documents/reports-and-publications/reports-and-briefings/health—wellbeing/rb_june15_lonelines_in_later_life_evidence_review.pdf (accessed February 11, 2019).

Davis, A., C. M. McMahon, K. M. Pichora-Fuller, S. Russ, F. Lin, B. O. Olusanya, S. Chadha, and K. L. Tremblay. 2016. Aging and hearing health: The life-course approach. *Gerontologist* 56(Suppl 2): S256–S267.

Dayson, C., and N. Bashir. 2014. *The social and economic impact of the Rotherham Social Prescribing Pilot: Main evaluation report.* Sheffield, UK: Sheffield Hallam University Centre for Regional Economic and Social Research.

de Jong Gierveld, J. 2004. Remarriage, unmarried cohabitation, living apart together: Partner relationships following bereavement or divorce. *Journal of Marriage and Family* 66:234–243.

de Jong Gierveld, J., and F. Kamphuis. 1985. The development of a Rasch-type loneliness scale. *Applied Psychological Measurement* 9(3):289–299.

de Jong Gierveld, J., and T. Van Tilburg. 2006. A 6-item scale for overall, emotional, and social loneliness: Confirmatory tests on survey data. *Research on Aging* 28(5):582–598.

De Marchis, E., M. Knox, D. Hessler, R. Willard-Grace, J. N. Olayiwola, L. E. Peterson, K. Grumbach, and L. M. Gottlieb. 2019a. Physician burnout and higher clinic capacity to address patients' social needs. *Journal of the American Board of Family Medicine* 32(1):69–78.

De Marchis, E. H., D. Hessler, C. Fichtenberg, N. Adler, E. Byhoff, A. J. Cohen, K. M. Doran, S. Ettinger de Cuba, E. W. Fleegler, C. C. Lewis, S. T. Lindau, E. L. Tung, A. G. Huebschmann, A. A. Prather, M. Raven, N. Gavin, S. Jepson, W. Johnson, E. Ochoa, Jr., A. L. Olson, M. Sandel, R. S. Sheward, and L. M. Gottlieb. 2019b. Part I: A quantitative study of social risk screening acceptability in patients and caregivers. *American Journal of Preventive Medicine* 57(6 Suppl 1):S25–S37.

De Mello, M. F., J. de Jesus Mari, J. Bacaltchuk, H. Verdeli, and R. Neugebauer. 2005. A systematic review of research findings on the efficacy of interpersonal therapy for depressive disorders. *European Archives of Psychiatry and Clinical Neuroscience* 255(2):75–82.

de Melo-Martín, I., and A. Ho. 2008. Beyond informed consent: The therapeutic misconception and trust. *Journal of Medical Ethics* 34(3):202–205.

De Vogli, R., T. Chandola, and M. G. Marmot. 2007. Negative aspects of close relationships and heart disease. *Archives of Internal Medicine* 167(18):1951–1957.

Deckx, L., M. van den Akker, and F. Buntinx. 2014. Risk factors for loneliness in patients with cancer: A systematic literature review and meta-analysis. *European Journal of Oncology Nursing* 18(5):466–477.

DeMilto, L., and M. Nakashian. 2016. *Using social determinants of health data to improve health care and health: A learning report.* Princeton, NJ: Robert Wood Johnson Foundation.

Demiris, G., D. P. Oliver, and K. L. Courtney. 2006. Ethical considerations for the utilization of telehealth technologies in home and hospice care by the nursing profession. *Nursing Administration Quarterly* 30(1):56–66.

Demiris, G., A. Z. Doorenbos, and C. Towle. 2009. Ethical considerations regarding the use of technology for older adults. The case of telehealth. *Research in Gerontological Nursing* 2(2):128–136.

Desmarais, P., K. L. Lanctôt, M. Masellis, S. E. Black, and N. Herrmann. 2018. Social inappropriateness in neurodegenerative disorders. *International Psychogeriatrics* 30(2):197–207.

Dhruva, A., K. Lee, S. M. Paul, C. West, L. Dunn, M. Dodd, B. E. Aouizerat, B. Cooper, P. Swift, and C. Miaskowski. 2012. Sleep–wake circadian activity rhythms and fatigue in family caregivers of oncology patients. *Cancer Nursing* 35(1):70–81.

Diaz, R. M., G. Ayala, E. Bein, J. Henne, and B. V. Marin. 2001. The impact of homophobia, poverty, and racism on the mental health of gay and bisexual Latino men: Findings from 3 U.S. cities. *American Journal of Public Health* 91(6):927–932.

Dickens, A.P., S. H. Richards, C. J. Greaves, and J. L. Campbell. 2011. Interventions targeting social isolation in older people: A systematic review. *BMC Public Health* 11:647.

DiJulio, B., L. Hamel, C. Muñana, and M. Brodie. 2018. *Loneliness and social isolation in the United States, the United Kingdom, and Japan: An international survey.* Kaiser Family Foundation. http://files.kff.org/attachment/Report-Loneliness-and-Social-Isolation-in-the-United-States-the-United-Kingdom-and-Japan-An-International-Survey (accessed November 20, 2019).

DiMatteo, M. R. 2004. Social support and patient adherence to medical treatment: A meta-analysis. *Health Psychology* 23(2):207–218.

DiMatteo, M. R., H. S. Lepper, and T. W. Croghan. 2000. Depression is a risk factor for noncompliance with medical treatment: Meta-analysis of the effects of anxiety and depression on patient adherence. *Archives of Internal Medicine* 160(14):2101–2107.

Diniz, B. S., M. A. Butters, S. M. Albert, M. A. Dew, and C. F. Reynolds, 3rd. 2013. Late-life depression and risk of vascular dementia and Alzheimer's disease: Systematic review and meta-analysis of community-based cohort studies. *British Journal of Psychiatry* 202(5):329–335.

Ditah, I. C., P. Devaki, B. Njei, C. O. Jaiyeoba, C. M. Ditah, O. Ewelukwa, and H. N. Luma. 2013. Sa2028 Epidemiology of fecal incontinence in U.S. adults from 2005 to 2010: Prevalence, trends, and risk factors. *Gastroenterology* 144(5):S-363.

Ditzen, B., and M. Heinrichs. 2014. Psychobiology of social support: The social dimension of stress buffering. *Restorative Neurology and Neuroscience* 32(1):149–162.

Djuricich, A. M. 2014. Social media, evidence-based tweeting, and JCEHP. *Journal of Continuing Education in the Health Professions* 34(4):202–204.

Doane, L. D., and E. K. Adam. 2010. Loneliness and cortisol: Momentary, day-to-day, and trait associations. *Psychoneuroendocrinology* 35(3):430–441.

Dobbins, M., S. E. Hanna, D. Ciliska, S. Manske, R. Cameron, S. L. Mercer, L. O'Mara, K. DeCorby, and P. Robeson. 2009. A randomized controlled trial evaluating the impact of knowledge translation and exchange strategies. *Implementation Science* 4(1):61–77.

Dogherty, E. J., M. B. Harrison, C. Baker, and I. D. Graham. 2012. Following a natural experiment of guideline adaptation and early implementation: A mixed-methods study of facilitation. *Implementation Science* 7:9.

d'Oleire Uquillas, F., H. I. L. Jacobs, K. D. Biddle, M. Properzi, B. Hanseeuw, A. P. Schultz, D. M. Rentz, K. A. Johnson, R. A. Sperling, and N. J. Donovan. 2018. Regional tau pathology and loneliness in cognitively normal older adults. *Translational Psychiatry* 8(1):282.

Domènech-Abella, J., E. Lara, M. Rubio-Valera, B. Olaya, M. V. Moneta, L. A. Rico-Uribe, J. L. Ayuso-Mateos, J. Mundó, and J. M. Haro. 2017. Loneliness and depression in the elderly: The role of social network. *Social Psychiatry and Psychiatric Epidemiology* 52(4):381–390.

Domènech-Abella, J., J. Mundo, J. M. Haro, and M. Rubio-Valera. 2019. Anxiety, depression, loneliness and social network in the elderly: Longitudinal associations from the Irish Longitudinal Study on Ageing (TILDA). *Journal of Affective Disorders* 246:82–88.

Donaldson, T., J. K. Earl, and A. M. Muratore. 2010. Extending the integrated model of retirement adjustment: Incorporating mastery and retirement planning. *Journal of Vocational Behavior* 77:279–289.

Dong, X., and R. Chen. 2017. Gender differences in the experience of loneliness in U.S. Chinese older adults. *Journal of Women & Aging* 29(2):115–125.

Donisi, V., F. Tedeschi, M. Percudani, A. Fiorillo, L. Confalonieri, C. De Rosa, D. Salazzari, M. Tansella, G. Thornicroft, and F. Amaddeo. 2013. Prediction of community mental health service utilization by individual and ecological level socio-economic factors. *Psychiatry Research* 209(3):691–698.

Donovan, N. J., O. I. Okereke, P. Vannini, R. E. Amariglio, D. M. Rentz, G. A. Marshall, K. A. Johnson, and R. A Sperling. 2016. Association of higher cortical amyloid burden with loneliness in cognitively normal older adults. *JAMA Psychiatry* 73(12):1230–1237.

Donovan, N. J., Q. Wu, D. M. Rentz, R. A. Sperling, G. A. Marshall, and M. M. Glymour. 2017. Loneliness, depression and cognitive function in older U.S. adults. *International Journal of Geriatric Psychiatry* 32(5):564–573.

Doran, D., B. R. Haynes, C. A. Estabrooks, A. Kushniruk, A. Dubrowski, I. Bajnok, L. M. Hall, M. Li, J. Carryer, D. Jedras, and Y. Q. Bai. 2012. The role of organizational context and individual nurse characteristics in explaining variation in use of information technologies in evidence based practice. *Implementation Science* 7:122.

Douthit, N., S. Kiv, T. Dwolatzky, and S. Biswas. 2015. Exposing some important barriers to health care access in the rural USA. *Public Health* 129(6):611–620.

Drageset, J., G. E. Eide, M. Kirkevold, and A. H. Ranhoff. 2013. Emotional loneliness is associated with mortality among mentally intact nursing home residents with and without cancer: A five-year follow-up study. *Journal of Clinical Nursing* 22(1–2):106–114.

Dyson, M. P., A. S. Newton, K. Shave, R. M. Featherstone, D. Thomson, A. Wingert, R. M. Fernandes, and L. Hartling. 2017. Social media for the dissemination of Cochrane child health evidence: Evaluation study. *Journal of Medical Internet Research* 19(9):e308.

Eaton, C. K. 2018. Social workers, nurses, or both: Who is primarily responsible for hospital discharge planning with older adults? *Social Work in Health Care* 57(10):851–863.

Eccles, M. P., and B. S. Mittman. 2006. Welcome to implementation science. *Implementation Science* 1(1):1–3.

Edge, C. E., A. M. Cooper, and M. Coffey. 2017. Barriers and facilitators to extended working lives in Europe: A gender focus. *Public Health Reviews* 38:2.

Edinger, J. D., W. K. Wohlgemuth, R. A. Radtke, G. R. Marsh, and R. E. Quillian. 2001. Cognitive behavioral therapy for treatment of chronic primary insomnia: A randomized controlled trial. *JAMA* 285(14):1856–1864.

Edwards, J. D., M. Lunsman, M. Perkins, G. W. Rebok, and D. L. Roth. 2009. Driving cessation and health trajectories in older adults. *Journals of Gerontology, Series A: Biological Sciences and Medical Sciences* 64(12):1290–1295.

Ehrhart, M. G., G. A. Aarons, and L. R. Farahnak. 2014. Assessing the organizational context for EBP implementation: The development and validity testing of the Implementation Climate Scale (ICS). *Implementation Science* 9(1):157.

Eichstaedt J. C., R. J. Smith, R. M. Merchant, L. H. Ungar, P. Crutchley, D. Preo iuc-Pietro, D. A. Asch, and H. A. Schwartz. 2018. Facebook language predicts depression in medical records. *Proceedings of the National Academy of Sciences* 115(44):11203–11208.

Eisenberger, N. I., M. Moieni, T. K. Inagaki, K. A. Muscatell, and M. R. Irwin. 2017. In sickness and in health: The co-regulation of inflammation and social behavior. *Neuropsychopharmacology* 42(1):242–253.

Ekwall, A. K., B. Sivberg, and I. R. Hallberg. 2005. Loneliness as a predictor of quality of life among older caregivers. *Journal of Advanced Nursing* 49(1):23–32.

Ellwardt, L., T. G. Van Tilburg, and M. J. Aartsen. 2015. The mix matters: Complex personal networks relate to higher cognitive functioning in old age. *Social Science & Medicine* 125:107–115.

Eloniemi-Sulkava, U., T. Rahkonen, M. Suihkonen, P. Halonen, M. Hentinen, and R. Sulkava. 2002. Emotional reactions and life changes of caregivers of demented patients when home caregiving ends. *Aging & Mental Health* 6(4):343–349.

Englander, R., T. Cameron, A. J. Ballard, J. Dodge, J. Bull, and C. A. Aschenbrener. 2013. Toward a common taxonomy of competence domains for the health professions and competencies for physicians. *Academic Medicine* 88(8):1088–1094.

Ertel, K. A., M. M. Glymour, and L. F. Berkman. 2008. Effects of social integration on preserving memory function in a nationally representative U.S. elderly population. *American Journal of Public Health* 98(7):1215–1220.

Eubanks, V. 2018. *Automating inequality: How high-tech tools profile, police, and punish the poor.* New York: St. Martin's Press.

Evans, I. E. M., D. J. Llewellyn, F. E. Matthews, R. T. Woods, C. Brayne, and L. Clare. 2018. Social isolation, cognitive reserve, and cognition in older people with depression and anxiety. *Aging & Mental Health* 23(12):1691–1700.

Evans, I. E. M., D. J. Llewellyn, F. E. Matthews, R. T. Woods, C. Brayne, and L. Clare. 2019. Living alone and cognitive function in later life. *Archives of Gerontology and Geriatrics* 81:222–233.

Everett, L. Q., and M. C. Sitterding. 2011. Transformational leadership required to design and sustain evidence-based practice: A system exemplar. *Western Journal of Nursing Research* 33(3):398–426.

EWA (Eldercare Workforce Alliance). 2019. *#TogetherWeCare Campaign.* https://eldercareworkforce.org/resources/togetherwecare (accessed June 27, 2019).

Falk Dahl, C. A., and A. A. Dahl. 2010. Lifestyle and social network in individuals with high level of social phobia/anxiety symptoms: A community-based study. *Social Psychiatry & Psychiatric Epidemiology* 45(3):309–317.

Farrell, T. W., E. Widera, L. Rosenberg, C. D. Rubin, A. D. Naik, U. Braun, A. Torke, I. Li, C. Vitale, and J. Shega. 2017. AGS position statement: Making medical treatment decisions for unbefriended older adults. *Journal of the American Geriatric Society* 65(1):14–15.

FHWA (Federal Highway Administration). 2017. *Distribution of licensed drivers—2016*. https://www.fhwa.dot.gov/policyinformation/statistics/2016/dl20.cfm (accessed September 17, 2019).

Finch, T. L., C. Bamford, V. Deary, N. Sabin, and S. W. Parry. 2014. Making sense of a cognitive behavioural therapy intervention for fear of falling: Qualitative study of intervention development. *BMC Health Services Research* 14:436.

Findlay, R. A. 2003. Interventions to reduce social isolation amongst older people: Where is the evidence? *Ageing & Society* 23(5):647–658.

Finlay, J. M., and L. C. Kobayashi. 2018. Social isolation and loneliness in later life: A parallel convergent mixed-methods case study of older adults and their residential contexts in the Minneapolis metropolitan area, USA. *Social Science and Medicine* 208:25–33.

Fiori, K. L., T. C. Antonucci, and K. S. Cortina. 2006. Social network typologies and mental health among older adults. *Journals of Gerontology, Series B: Psychological Sciences and Social Sciences* 61(1):P25–P32.

Fleisch Marcus, A., A. H. Illescas, B. C. Hohl, and A. A. Llanos. 2017. Relationships between social isolation, neighborhood poverty, and cancer mortality in a population-based study of U.S. adults. *PLOS ONE* 12(3):e0173370.

Flexner, A. 1910. *Medical education in the United States and Canada: A report to The Carnegie Foundation for the Advancement of Teaching*. Boston, MA: D.B. Updike, The Merrymount Press.

Flintner, M., and K. Bamrick. 2017. *Training the next generation: Residency and fellowship programs for nurse practitioners in community health centers*. Middletown, CT: Community Health Center, Inc., and the Weitzman Institute.

Flodgren, G., E. Parmelli, G. Doumit, M. Gattellari, M. A. O'Brien, J. Grimshaw, and M. P. Eccles. 2011. Local opinion leaders: Effects on professional practice and health care outcomes. *Cochrane Database of Systematic Reviews* 2011(8):CD000125.

Flodgren, G., A. M. Hall, L. Goulding, M. P. Eccles, J. M. Grimshaw, G. C. Leng, and S. Shepperd. 2016. Tools developed and disseminated by guideline producers to promote the uptake of their guidelines. *Cochrane Database of Systematic Reviews* 2016(8):CD010669.

Flowers, L., A. Houser, C. Noel-Miller, J. Shaw, J. Bhattacharya, L. Schoemaker, and M. Farid. 2014. *Medicare spends more on socially isolated older adults*. https://www.aarp.org/content/dam/aarp/ppi/2017/10/medicare-spends-more-on-socially-isolated-older-adults.pdf (accessed November 12, 2019).

Flønhus, M. S., T. K. Dalsbø, M. Johansen, A. Fretheim, H. Skirbekk, and S. A. Flottorp. 2018. Patient-mediated interventions to improve professional practice. *Cochrane Database of Systematic Reviews* 2018(9):CD012472.

Forsetlund, L., A. Bjørndal, A. Rashidian, G. Jamtvedt, M. A. O'Brien, F. Wolf, D. Davis, J. Odgaard-Jensen, and A. D. Oxman. 2009. Continuing education meetings and workshops: Effects on professional practice and health care outcomes. *Cochrane Database of Systematic Reviews* 2009(2):CD003030.

Fouad, M. N., T. A. Wynn, R. Scribner, Y.-M. M. Schoenberger, D. Antoine-Lavigne, S. Eady, W. A. Anderson, and L. B. Bateman. 2017. Impacting the social determinants of health through a regional academic–community partnership: The experience of the Mid-South Transdisciplinary Collaborative Center for Health Disparities Research. *Ethnicity & Disease* 27(Suppl 1):277–286.

FrameWorks Institute. 2019. *Aging*. https://frameworksinstitute.org/reframing-aging.html (accessed September 27, 2019).

Frank, D. 2018. *1 in 3 U.S. adults are lonely, survey shows*. AARP. https://www.aarp.org/home-family/friends-family/info-2018/loneliness-survey.html (accessed July 27, 2019).

Fredriksen-Goldsen, K. I., C. A. Emlet, H. J. Kim, A. Muraco, E. A. Erosheva, J. Goldsen, and C. P. Hoy-Ellis. 2013. The physical and mental health of lesbian, gay male, and bisexual (LGB) older adults: The role of key health indicators and risk and protective factors. *Gerontologist* 53(4):664–675.

French, B., L. H. Thomas, P. Baker, C. R. Burton, L. Pennington, and H. Roddam. 2009. What can management theories offer evidence-based practice? A comparative analysis of measurement tools for organisational context. *Implementation Science* 4:28.

Fried, E. I., C. Bockting, R. Arjadi, D. Borsboom, M. Amshoff, A. O. Cramer, S. Epskamp, F. Tuerlinckx, D. Carr, and M. Stroebe. 2015. From loss to loneliness: The relationship between bereavement and depressive symptoms. *Journal of Abnormal Psychology* 124(2):256–265.

Fried, L. P., C. M. Tangen, J. Walston, A. B. Newman, C. Hirsch, J. Gottdiener, T. Seeman, R. Tracy, W. J. Kop, G. Burke, and M. A. McBurnie. 2001. Frailty in older adults: Evidence for a phenotype. *Journals of Gerontology, Series A: Biological Sciences and Medical Sciences* 56(3):M146–M156.

Friedberg, M. W., M. B. Rosenthal, R. M. Werner, K. G. Volpp, and E. C. Schneider. 2015. Effects of a medical home and shared savings intervention on quality and utilization of care. *JAMA Internal Medicine* 175(8):1362–1368.

Friedman, H. S., J. S. Tucker, J. E. Schwartz, C. Tomlinson-Keasey, L. R. Martin, D. L. Wingard, and M. H. Criqui. 1995. Psychosocial and behavioral predictors of longevity. The aging and death of the "termites". *American Psychologist* 50(2):69–78.

Friedman, N. L., and M. P. Banegas. 2018. Toward addressing social determinants of health: A health care system strategy. *Permanente Journal* 22:18–095.

Friedmann, E., and C. A. Krause-Parello. 2018. Companion animals and human health: Benefits, challenges, and the road ahead for human–animal interaction. *Revue Scientifique et Technique* 37(1):71–82.

Frisch, N., P. Atherton, E. Borycki, G. Mickelson, J. Cordeiro, H. Novak Lauscher, and A. Black. 2014. Growing a professional network to over 3,000 members in less than 4 years: Evaluation of InspireNet, British Columbia's virtual nursing health services research network. *Journal of Medical Internet Research* 16(2):e49.

Fulmer, T. 2007. How to try this: Fulmer SPICES. *American Journal of Nursing* 107(10):40–49.

Fulmer, T., G. Paveza, C. VandeWeerd, S. Fairchild, L. Guadagno, M. Bolton-Blatt, and R. Norman. 2005. Dyadic vulnerability and risk profiling for elder neglect. *Gerontologist* 45(4):525–534.

Fultz, N. H., and A. R. Herzog. 2001. Self-reported social and emotional impact of urinary incontinence. *Journal of the American Geriatrics Society* 49(7):892–899.

Galambos, C. 2017a. Frail elderly syndrome. In L. J. Carpenito (ed.), *Nursing diagnosis: Application to clinical practice, 15th ed.* Philadelphia: WoltersKluwer/Lippencott Williams, and Wilkins. Pp. 294–297.

Galambos, C. 2017b. Risk for frail elderly syndrome. In L. J. Carpenito (ed.), *Nursing diagnosis: Application to clinical practice, 15th ed.* Philadelphia: WoltersKluwer/Lippencott Williams, and Wilkins. Pp. 297–301.

Galambos, C., R. R. Greene, N. P. Knopf, and H. Cohen. 2018. *Foundations of social work practice in the field of aging: A competency-based approach, 2nd ed.* Washington, DC: NASW Press.

Gale, C. R., L. Westbury, and C. Cooper. 2018. Social isolation and loneliness as risk factors for the progression of frailty: The English Longitudinal Study of Ageing. *Age and Ageing* 47(3):392–397.

Gallicchio, L., S. C. Hoffman, and K. J. Helzlsouer. 2007. The relationship between gender, social support, and health-related quality of life in a community-based study in Washington County, Maryland. *Quality of Life Research* 16(5):777–786.

Gallo, L. C., A. L. Fortmann, S. C. Roesch, E. Barrett-Connor, J. P. Elder, K. E. de los Monteros, S. Shivpuri, P. J. Mills, G. A. Talavera, and K. A. Matthews. 2012. Socioeconomic status, psychosocial resources and risk, and cardiometabolic risk in Mexican-American women. *Health Psychology* 31(3):334–342.

Gardiner, C., G. Geldenhuys, and M. Gott. 2018. Interventions to reduce social isolation and loneliness among older people: An integrative review. *Health and Social Care in the Community* 26(2):147–157.

Garg, A., R. Boynton-Jarrett, and P. H. Dworkin. 2016. Avoiding the unintended consequences of screening for social determinants of health. *JAMA* 316(8):813–814.

Garland, K., E. Beer, B. Eppingstall, and D. W. O'Connor. 2007. A comparison of two treatments of agitated behavior in nursing home residents with dementia: Simulated family presence and preferred music. *American Journal of Geriatric Psychiatry* 15(6):514–521.

Garner, T. A., W. A. Powell, and V. Carr. 2016. Virtual carers for the elderly: A case study review of ethical responsibilities. *Digital Health* 2:1–14.

Gaut, G., M. Steyvers, Z. E. Imel, D. C. Atkins, and P. Smyth. 2017. Content coding of psychotherapy transcripts using labeled topic models. *IEEE Journal of Biomedical and Health Informatics* 21(2):476–487.

Geda, Y. E., L. S. Schneider, L. N. Gitlin, D. S. Miller, G. S. Smith, J. Bell, J. Evans, M. Lee, A. Porsteinsson, K. L. Lanctôt, P. B. Rosenberg, D. L. Sultzer, P. T. Francis, H. Brodaty, P. P. Padala, C. U. Onyike, L. A. Ortiz, S. Ancoli-Israel, D. L. Bliwise, J. L. Martin, M. V. Vitiello, K. Yaffe, P. C. Zee, N. Herrmann, R. A. Sweet, C. Ballard, N. A. Khin, C. Alfaro, P. S. Murray, S. Schultz, and C. G. Lyketsos. 2013. Neuropsychiatric symptoms in Alzheimer's disease: Past progress and anticipation of the future. *Alzheimers and Dementia* 9(5):602–608.

Gee, N. R., and M. K. Mueller. 2019. A systematic review of research on pet ownership and animal interactions among older adults. *Anthrozoös* 32(2):183–207.

Gell, N. M., D. E. Rosenberg, G. Demiris, A. Z. LaCroix, and K. V. Patel. 2015. Patterns of technology use among older adults with and without disabilities. *Gerontologist* 55(3):412–421.

Gerst-Emerson, K., and J. Jayawardhana. 2015. Loneliness as a public health issue: The impact of loneliness on health care utilization among older adults. *American Journal of Public Health* 105(5):1013–1019.

Gerst-Emerson, K., T. E. Shovali, and K. S. Markides. 2014. Loneliness among very old Mexican Americans: Findings from the Hispanic established populations epidemiologic studies of the elderly. *Archives of Gerontology & Geriatrics* 59(1):145–149.

Gianaros, P. J., M. E. Bleil, M. F. Muldoon, J. R. Jennings, K. Sutton-Tyrrell, J. M. McCaffery, and S. B. Manuck. 2002. Is cardiovascular reactivity associated with atherosclerosis among hypertensives? *Hypertension* 40(5):742–747.

Gifford, W., B. Davies, N. Edwards, P. Griffin, and V. Lybanon. 2007. Managerial leadership for nurses' use of research evidence: An integrative review of the literature. *Worldviews on Evidence-Based Nursing* 4(3):126–145.

Giguère, A, F. Légaré, J. Grimshaw, S. Turcotte, M. Fiander, A. Grudniewicz, S. Makosso-Kallyth, F. M. Wolf, A. P. Farmer, and M. P. Gagnon. 2012. Printed educational materials: Effects on professional practice and health care outcomes. *Cochrane Database of Systematic Reviews* 2012(10):CD004398.

Gilbey, A., and K. Tani. 2015. Companion animals and loneliness: A systematic review of quantitative studies. *Anthrozoos* 28(2):181–197.

Gilmartin, H., A. Goyal, M. C. Hamati, J. Mann, S. Saint, and V. Chopra. 2017. Brief mindfulness practices for healthcare providers—A systematic literature review. *American Journal of Medicine* 130(10):1219.e1–1219.e17.

Glass, A. P., and J. Skinner. 2013. Retirement communities: We know what they are . . . or do we? *Journal of Housing for the Elderly* 27:1–6.

Glass, A. P., and R. S. Vander Plaats. 2013. A conceptual model for aging better together intentionally. *Journal of Aging Studies* 27(4):428–442.

Glass, T. A., and G. L. Maddox. 1992. The quality and quantity of social support: Stroke recovery as psycho-social transition. *Social Science & Medicine* 34(11):1249–1261.

Glozier, N., G. H. Tofler, D. M. Colquhoun, S. J. Bunker, D. M. Clarke, D. L. Hare, I. B. Hickie, J. Tatoulis, D. R. Thompson, A. Wilson, and M. G. Branagan. 2013. Psychosocial risk factors for coronary heart disease. *Medical Journal of Australia* 199(3):179–180.

Godin, J., O. Theou, K. Black, S. A. McNeil, and M. K. Andrew. 2019. Long-term care admissions following hospitalization: The role of social vulnerability. *Healthcare* 7(91).

Gold, R., E. Cottrell, A. Bunce, M. Middendorf, C. Hollombe, S. Cowburn, P. Mahr, and G. Melgar. 2017. Developing electronic health record (EHR) strategies related to health center patients' social determinants of health. *Journal of the American Board of Family Medicine* 30(4):428–447.

Golden, J., R. M. Conroy, I. Bruce, A. Denihan, E. Greene, M. Kirby, and B. A. Lawlor. 2009. Loneliness, social support networks, mood and wellbeing in community-dwelling elderly. *International Journal of Geriatric Psychiatry* 24(7):694–700.

Goll, J. C., G. Charlesworth, K. Scior, and J. Stott. 2015. Barriers to social participation among lonely older adults: The influence of social fears and identity. *PLOS ONE* 10(2):e0116664.

Golub, S. A., J. C. Tomassilli, D. W. Pantalone, M. Brennan, S. E. Karpiak, and J. T. Parsons. 2010. Prevalence and correlates of sexual behavior and risk management among HIV-positive adults over 50. *Sexually Transmitted Diseases* 37(10):615–620.

Gonyea, J. G., A. Curley, K. Melekis, N. Levine, and Y. Lee. 2018. Loneliness and depression among older adults in urban subsidized housing. *Journal of Aging and Health* 30(3):458–474.

Gonzales, L., A. Koci, R. M. Gee, A. Noji, D. Glaser, A. K. Marsh, K. K. Marsh, A. M. Altman, N. Al Salmi, and S. Al Sabei. 2015. Caring for women globally: Psychometric testing of two instruments translated into five languages for use in cardiovascular recovery. *International Journal of Nursing Practice* 21(Suppl 1):27–37.

Gottlieb, L. M., K. Garcia, H. Wing, and R. Manchanda. 2016. Clinical interventions addressing nonmedical health determinants in Medicaid managed care. *American Journal of Managed Care* 22(5):370–376.

Gove, W. R. 1973. Sex, marital status, and mortality. *American Journal of Sociology* 79(1):45–67.

Gow, A. J., A. Pattie, M. C. Whiteman, L. J. Whalley, and I. J. Deary. 2007. Social support and successful aging: Investigating the relationship between lifetime cognitive change and life satisfaction. *Journal of Individual Differences* 28(3):103–115.

Graham, C. L., A. E. Scharlach, and J. Price Wolf. 2014. The impact of the "village" model on health, well-being, service access, and social engagement of older adults. *Health Education & Behavior* 41(1 Suppl):91S–97S.

Graham, J. 2019. *Understanding loneliness in older adults—and tailoring a solution.* https://khn.org/news/understanding-loneliness-in-older-adults-and-tailoring-a-solution (accessed August 13, 2019).

Granbom, M., I. Himmelsbach, M. Haak, C. Lofqvist, F. Oswald, and S. Iwarsson. 2014. Residential normalcy and environmental experiences of very old people: Changes in residential reasoning over time. *Journal of Aging Studies* 29:9–19.

Grant, N., M. Hamer, and A. Steptoe. 2009. Social isolation and stress-related cardiovascular, lipid, and cortisol responses. *Annals of Behavioral Medicine* 37(1):29–37.

Gray, A. 2009. The social capital of older people. *Aging & Society* 29(1):5–31.

Greene, M., N. A. Hessol, C. Perissinotto, R. Zepf, A. Hutton Parrott, C. Foreman, R. Whirry, M. Gandhi, and M. John. 2018. Loneliness in older adults living with HIV. *AIDS and Behavior* 22(5):1475–1484.

Greenhalgh, T., G. Robert, P. Bate, F. Macfarlane, and O. Kyriakidou. 2005. *Diffusion of innovations in health service organisations: A systematic literature review.* Malden, MA: Blackwell Publishing Ltd.

Greiman, L., and C. Ravesloot. 2015. Housing characteristics of households with wheeled mobility device users from the American Housing Survey: Do people live in homes that facilitate community participation? *Community Development* 47(1):63–74.

Gress, J. L., M. G. S. Pedro-Salcedo, T. Kalista, T. F. Kuo, R. Manber, and J. D. Edinger. 2008. Cognitive behavioral therapy for insomnia enhances depression outcome in patients with comorbid major depressive disorder and insomnia. *Sleep* 31(4):489–495.

Greysen, S. R., L. I. Horwitz, K. E. Covinsky, K. Gordon, M. E. Ohl, and A. C. Justice. 2013. Does social isolation predict hospitalization and mortality among HIV+ and uninfected older veterans? *Journal of the American Geriatrics Society* 61(9):1456–1463.

Grieve, R., M. Indian, K. Witteveen, G. A. Tolan, and J. Marrington. 2013. Face-to-face or Facebook: Can social connectedness be derived online? *Computers in Human Behavior* 29(3):604–609.

Griffin, M. L., M. Amodeo, C. Clay, I. Fassler, and M. A. Ellis. 2006. Racial differences in social support: Kin versus friends. *American Journal of Orthopsychiatry* 76(3):374–380.

Griffin, S. O., J. A. Jones, D. Brunson, P. M. Griffin, and W. D. Bailey. 2012. Burden of oral disease among older adults and implications for public health priorities. *American Journal of Public Health* 102(3):411–418.

Grimshaw, J. M., M. P. Eccles, J. N. Lavis, S. J. Hill, and J. E. Squires. 2012. Knowledge translation of research findings. *Implementation Science* 7:50.

Grippo, A. J., D. M. Trahanas, R. R. Zimmerman, II, S. W. Porges, and C. S. Carter. 2009. Oxytocin protects against negative behavioral and autonomic consequences of long-term social isolation. *Psychoneuroendocrinology* 34(10):1542–1553.

Grippo, A. J., H. Pournajafi-Nazarloo, L. Sanzenbacher, D. M. Trahanas, N. McNeal, D. A. Clarke, S. W. Porges, and C. S. Carter. 2012. Peripheral oxytocin administration buffers autonomic but not behavioral responses to environmental stressors in isolated prairie voles. *Stress* 15(2):149–161.

Gum, A. M., S. Shiovitz-Ezra, and L. Ayalon. 2017. Longitudinal associations of hopelessness and loneliness in older adults: Results from the U.S. Health and Retirement Study. *International Psychogeriatrics* 29(9):1451–1459.

Gump, B. B., D. E. Polk, T. W. Kamarck, and S. M. Shiffman. 2001. Partner interactions are associated with reduced blood pressure in the natural environment: Ambulatory monitoring evidence from a healthy, multiethnic adult sample. *Psychosomatic Medicine* 63(3):423–433.

Gustafsson, P. E., U. Janlert, T. Theorell, H. Westerlund, and A. Hammarström. 2012. Social and material adversity from adolescence to adulthood and allostatic load in middle-aged women and men: Results from the Northern Swedish cohort. *Annals of Behavioral Medicine* 43(1):117–128.

Guthrie, D. M., J. G. S. Davidson, N. Williams, J. Campos, K. Hunter, P. Mick, J. B. Orange, M. K. Pichora-Fuller, N. A. Phillips, M. Y. Savundranayagam, and W. Wittich. 2018. Combined impairments in vision, hearing and cognition are associated with greater levels of functional and communication difficulties than cognitive impairment alone: Analysis of interRAI data for home care and long-term care recipients in Ontario. *PLOS ONE* 13(2):e0192971.

Ha, J. H., G. W. Hougham, and D. O. Meltzer. 2019. Risk of social isolation among older patients: What factors affect the availability of family, friends, and neighbors upon hospitalization? *Clinical Gerontology* 42(1):60–69.

Hackett, R. A., M. Hamer, R. Endrighi, L. Brydon, and A. Steptoe. 2012. Loneliness and stress-related inflammatory and neuroendocrine responses in older men and women. *Psychoneuroendocrinology* 37(11):1801–1809.

Hadley Strout, E., L. Fox, A. Castro, P. Haroun, B. Leavitt, C. Ross, M. Sayan, T. Delaney, A. Platzer, J. Hutchins, and J. K. Carney. 2016. Access to transportation for Chittenden County, Vermont, older adults. *Aging Clinical and Experimental Research* 28(4):769–774.

Hafner, K. 2016. Researchers confront an epidemic of loneliness. *The New York Times*. September 5. https://www.nytimes.com/2016/09/06/health/lonliness-aging-health-effects.html (accessed November 20, 2019).

Hagström, E., F. Norlund, A. Stebbins, P. W. Armstrong, K. Chiswell, C. B. Granger, J. López-Sendón, D. Pella, J. Soffer, R. Sy, L. Wallentin, H. D. White, R. A. H. Stewart, and C. Held. 2018. Psychosocial stress and major cardiovascular events in patients with stable coronary heart disease. *Journal of Internal Medicine* 283(1):83–92.

Haines, K. J., T. Quasim, and J. McPeake. 2018. Family and support networks following critical illness. *Critical Care Clinics* 34(4):609–623.

Håkansson, K., S. Rovio, E. L. Helkala, A. R. Vilska, B. Winblad, H. Soininen, A. Nissinen, A. H. Mohammed, and M. Kivipelto. 2009. Association between mid-life marital status and cognitive function in later life: Population based cohort study. *BMJ* 339:b2462.

Hakulinen, C., L. Pulkki-Råback, M. Virtanen, M. Jokela, M. Kivimäki, and M. Elovainio. 2018. Social isolation and loneliness as risk factors for myocardial infarction, stroke and mortality: UK Biobank cohort study of 479,054 men and women. *Heart* 104(18):1536–1542.

Hamilton, B. E., J. A. Martin, M. J. K. Osterman, and L. M. Rossen. 2019. *Births: Provisional data for 2018*. Hyattsville, MD: National Center for Health Statistics.

Hämmig, O. 2019. Health risks associated with social isolation in general and in young, middle and old age. *PLOS ONE* 14(7):e0219663.

Hanratty, B., D. Stow, D. Collingridge Moore, N. K. Valtorta, and F. Matthews. 2018. Loneliness as a risk factor for care home admission in the English Longitudinal Study of Ageing. *Age and Ageing* 47(6):896–900.

Hanson, V. L. 2001. *Web access for elderly citizens.* Paper presented at the Proceedings of the 2001 EC/NSF Workshop on Universal Accessibility of Ubiquitous Computing: Providing for the Elderly. Pp. 14–18.

Harris-Kojetin, L., M. Sengupta, J. P. Lendon, V. Rome, R. Valverde, and C. Caffrey. 2019. *Long-term care providers and services users in the United States, 2015–2016.* Vital Health Statistics, Series 3, Number 43. Hyattsville, MD: National Center for Health Statistics.

Harvath, T. A., and G. L. McKenzie. 2012. *Nursing standard of practice protocol: Depression in older adults.* https://consultgeri.org/geriatric-topics/depression (accessed June 27, 2019).

Haslam, C., T. Cruwys, and S. A. Haslam. 2014. "The we's have it": Evidence for the distinctive benefits of group engagement in enhancing cognitive health in aging. *Social Science and Medicine* 120:57–66.

Hatzenbuehler, M. L., K. M. Keyes, and K. A. McLaughlin. 2011. The protective effects of social/contextual factors on psychiatric morbidity in LGB populations. *International Journal of Epidemiology* 40(4):1071–1080.

Hauck, S., R. P. Winsett, and J. Kuric J. 2012. Leadership facilitation strategies to establish evidence-based practice in an acute care hospital. *Journal of Advanced Nursing* 69(3):664–674.

Havassy, B. E., S. M. Hall, and D. A. Wasserman. 1991. Social support and relapse: Commonalities among alcoholics, opiate users, and cigarette smokers. *Addictive Behaviors* 16(5):235–246.

Hawker, M., and R. Romero-Ortuno. 2016. Social determinants of discharge outcomes in older people admitted to a geriatric medicine ward. *Journal of Frailty & Aging* 5(2):118–120.

Hawkley, L. C., and J. T. Cacioppo. 2010. Loneliness matters: A theoretical and empirical review of consequences and mechanisms. *Annals of Behavioral Medicine* 40(2):218–227.

Hawkley, L. C., and M. Kocherginsky. 2018. Transitions in loneliness among older adults: A 5-year follow-up in the National Social Life, Health, and Aging Project. *Research on Aging* 40(4):365–387.

Hawkley, L. C., C. M. Masi, J. D. Berry, and J. T. Cacioppo. 2006. Loneliness is a unique predictor of age-related differences in systolic blood pressure. *Psychology and Aging* 21(1):152–164.

Hawkley, L. C., K. J. Preacher, and J. T. Cacioppo. 2007. Multilevel modeling of social interactions and mood in lonely and socially connected individuals: The MacArthur social neuroscience studies. In *Oxford handbook of methods in positive psychology.* New York: Oxford University Press. Pp. 559–575.

Hawkley, L. C., M. E. Hughes, L. J. Waite, C. M. Masi, R. A. Thisted, and J. T. Cacioppo. 2008. From social structural factors to perceptions of relationship quality and loneliness: The Chicago Health, Aging, and Social Relations Study. *Journals of Gerontology, Series B: Psychological Sciences and Social Sciences* 63(6):S375–S384.

Hawkley, L. C., R. A. Thisted, and J. T. Cacioppo. 2009. Loneliness predicts reduced physical activity: Cross-sectional & longitudinal analyses. *Health Psychology* 28(3):354–363.

Hawkley, L. C., R. A. Thisted, C. M. Masi, and J. T. Cacioppo. 2010a. Loneliness predicts increased blood pressure: 5-year cross-lagged analyses in middle-aged and older adults. *Psychology and Aging* 25(1):132–141.

Hawkley, L. C., K. J. Preacher, and J. T. Cacioppo. 2010b. Loneliness impairs daytime functioning but not sleep duration. *Health Psychology* 29(2):124–129.

Hawkley, L. C., M. Kozloski, and J. Wong. 2017. A profile of social connectedness in older adults. https://connect2affect.org/wp-content/uploads/2017/03/A-Profile-of-Social-Connectedness.pdf (accessed December 12, 2019).

Hawkley, L. C., K. Wroblewski, T. Kaiser, M. Luhmann, and L. P. Schumm. 2019. Are U.S. older adults getting lonelier? Age, period, and cohort differences. *Psychology and Aging* 34(8): 1144–1157.

Hawton, A., C. Green, A. P. Dickens, S. H. Richards, R. S. Taylor, R. Edwards, C. J. Greaves, and J. L. Campbell. 2011. The impact of social isolation on the health status and health-related quality of life of older people. *Quality of Life Research* 20(1):57–67.

Hay-McCutcheon, M. J., P. E. Reed, and S. Cheimariou. 2018. Positive social interaction and hearing loss in older adults living in rural and urban communities. *Journal of Speech, Language, and Hearing Research* 61(8):2138–2145.

Hayashi, T., H. Umegaki, T. Makino, C. H. Huang, A. Inoue, H. Shimada, and M. Kuzuya. 2020. Combined impact of physical frailty and social isolation on rate of falls in older adults. *Journal of Nutrition, Health & Aging* 24:312–318.

Hayes, M., K. van Stolk-Cooke, and F. Muench. 2015. Understanding Facebook use and the psychological affects of use across generations. *Computers in Human Behavior* 49:507–511.

Hedegaard H., S. C. Curtin, and M. Warner. 2018. *Suicide mortality in the United States, 1999–2017.* NCHS Data Brief, no. 330. Hyattsville, MD: National Center for Health Statistics.

Heimberg, R. G. 2002. Cognitive–behavioral therapy for social anxiety disorder: Current status and future directions. *Biological Psychiatry* 51(1):101–108.

Hennessy, M. B., S. Kaiser, and N. Sachser. 2009. Social buffering of the stress response: Diversity, mechanisms, and functions. *Frontiers in Neuroendocrinology* 30(4):470–482.

Henning-Smith, C., I. Moscovice, and K. Kozhimannil. 2019. Differences in social isolation and its relationship to health by rurality. *Journal of Rural Health* 35(4):540–549.

Hensel, B. K., G. Demiris, and K. L. Courtney. 2006. Defining obtrusiveness in home telehealth technologies: A conceptual framework. *Journal of the American Medical Informatics Association* 13(4):428–431.

Henwood, B. F., J. Lahey, H. Rhoades, D. B. Pitts, J. Pynoos, and R. T. Brown. 2019. Geriatric conditions among formerly homeless older adults living in permanent supportive housing. *Journal of General Internal Medicine* 34(6):802–803.

Heponiemi, T., M. Elovainio, L. Pulkki, S. Puttonen, O. Raitakari, and L. Keltikangas-Jarvinen. 2007. Cardiac autonomic reactivity and recovery in predicting carotid atherosclerosis: The cardiovascular risk in young Finns study. *Health Psychology* 26(1):13–21.

Herbert, C., and J. H. Molinsky. 2019. What can be done to better support older adults to age successfully in their homes and communities? *Health Affairs* 38(5):860–864.

Hernandez, D. C., L. R. Reitzzel, D. W. Wetter, and L. H. McNeill. 2014. Social support and cardiovascular risk factors among black adults. *Ethnicity and Disease* 24(4):444–450.

Heuser, C., and J. Howe. 2019. The relation between social isolation and increasing suicide rates in the elderly. *Quality in Ageing and Older Adults* 20(1):2–9.

HHS (U.S. Department of Health and Human Services). 2001. *The Surgeon General's call to action to prevent and decrease overweight and obesity.* https://www.ncbi.nlm.nih.gov/books/NBK44206 (accessed December 3, 2019).

HHS. 2010. The Surgeon General's vision for a healthy and fit nation. https://www.ncbi.nlm.nih.gov/books/NBK44660 (accessed December 3, 2019).

HHS. 2018. *Dissemination and implementation research in health.* https://grants.nih.gov/grants/guide/pa-files/par-16-238.html (accessed October 1, 2019).

HHS. 2019a. *About Healthy People.* https://www.healthypeople.gov/2020/About-Healthy-People (accessed November 12, 2019).

HHS. 2019b. *2020 topics and objectives: Social determinants of health.* https://www.healthypeople.gov/2020/topics-objectives/topic/social-determinants-of-health (accessed November 12, 2019).

HHS. 2019c. *Healthy People 2030 framework.* https://www.healthypeople.gov/2020/About-Healthy-People/Development-Healthy-People-2030/Framework (accessed November 12, 2019).

HHS. 2019d. *National resource centers.* https://acl.gov/node/2884 (accessed November 13, 2019).

Hinojosa, R., J. Haun, M. S. Hinojosa, and M. Rittman. 2011. Social isolation poststroke: Relationship between race/ethnicity, depression, and functional independence. *Topics in Stroke Rehabilitation* 18(1):79–86.

Hirschman, K. B., E. Shaid, K. McCauley, M. V. Pauly, and M. D. Naylor. 2015. Continuity of care: The transitional care model. *Online Journal of Issues in Nursing* 20(3):1.

Ho, E. C., L. Hawkley, W. Dale, L. Waite, and M. Huisingh-Scheetz. 2018. Social capital predicts accelerometry-measured physical activity among older adults in the U.S.: A cross-sectional study in the National Social Life, Health, and Aging Project. *BMC Public Health* 18(1):804.

Hobbes, T. 1965. Leviathan or the matter, forme, and power of a common-wealth: Ecclesiasticall and civill. In *Laviathon: Reprinted from the edition of 1651 with an essay by the late W. G. Pogson Smith.* London, UK: Oxford University Press.

Hogeboom, D. L., R. J. McDermott, K. M. Perrin, H. Osman, and B. A. Bell-Ellison. 2010. Internet use and social networking among middle aged and older adults. *Educational Gerontology* 36(2):93–111.

Holahan, C. J., R. J. North, C. K. Holahan, R. B. Hayes, D. A. Powers, and J. K. Ockene. 2012. Social influences on smoking in middle-aged and older women. *Psychology of Addictive Behaviors* 26(3):519–526.

Holley, U. A. 2007. Social isolation: A practical guide for nurses assisting clients with chronic illness. *Rehabilitation Nursing* 32(2):51–56.

Holm, A. L., A. K. Berland, and E. Severinsson. 2019. Factors that influence the health of older widows and widowers: A systematic review of quantitative research. *Nursing Open* 6(2):591–611.

Holmbeck, G. N., B. Jandasek, C. Sparks, J. Zukerman, and L. Zurenda. 2008. Theoretical foundations if developmental-behavioral pediatrics. Evidence and practice. In M. L. Wolraich, D. D. Drotar, P. H. Dworkin, and E. C. Perrin (eds.), *Developmental-behavioral pediatrics: Evidence and practice.* Maryland Heights, MO: Mosby. Pp. 13–45.

Holmén, K., K. Ericsson, and B. Winblad. 1999. Quality of life among the elderly. State of mood and loneliness in two selected groups. *Scandinavian Journal of Caring Sciences* 13(2):91–95.

Holmén, K., K. Ericsson, and B. Winblad. 2000. Social and emotional loneliness among non-demented and demented elderly people. *Archives of Gerontology and Geriatrics* 31(3):177–192.

Holt-Lunstad, J. 2018a. Why social relationships are important for physical health: A systems approach to understanding and modifying risk and protection. *Annual Review of Psychology* 69:437–458.

Holt-Lunstad, J. 2018b. The potential public health relevance of social isolation and loneliness: Prevalence, epidemiology, and risk factors. *Public Policy & Aging Report* 27(4):127–130.

Holt-Lunstad, J., and T. B. Smith. 2016. Loneliness and social isolation as risk factors for CVD: Implications for evidence-based patient care and scientific inquiry. *Heart* 102(13):987–989.

Holt-Lunstad, J., and B. N. Uchino. 2019. Social ambivalence and disease (SAD): A theorectical model aimed at understanding the health implications of ambivalent relationships. *Perspectives on Psychological Science* 14(6):941–966.

Holt-Lunstad, J., T. B. Smith, and J. B. Layton. 2010. Social relationships and mortality risk: A meta-analytic review. *PLOS Medicine* 7(7):e1000316.

Holt-Lunstad, J., T. B. Smith, M. Baker, T. Harris, and D. Stephenson. 2015. Loneliness and social isolation as risk factors for mortality: A meta-analytic review. *Perspectives on Psychological Science* 10(2):227–237.

Holt-Lunstad, J., T. F. Robles, and D. A. Sbarra. 2017. Advancing social connection as a public health priority in the United States. *American Psychologist* 72(6):517–530.

Holtslander, L., S. Baxter, K. Mills, S. Bocking, T. Dadgostari, W. Duggleby, V. Duncan, P. Hudson, A. Ogunkorode, and S. Peacock. 2017. Honoring the voices of bereaved caregivers: A metasummary of qualitative research. *BMC Palliative Care* 16(1):48.

Holwerda, T. J., D. J. Deeg, A. T. Beekman, T. G. van Tilburg, M. L. Stek, C. Jonker, and R. A. Schoevers. 2014. Feelings of loneliness, but not social isolation, predict dementia onset: Results from the Amsterdam Study of the Elderly (AMSTEL). *Journal of Neurology, Neurosurgery, and Psychiatry* 85(2):135–142.

Hong, Y. A., and J. Cho. 2017. Has the digital divide widened? Trends of health-related Internet use among older adults from 2003 to 2011. *Journals of Gerontology, Series B: Psychological Sciences and Social Sciences* 72(5):856–863.

Hooker, S. A., M. E. Grigsby, B. Riegel, and D. B. Bekelman. 2015. The impact of relationship quality on health-related outcomes in heart failure patients and informal family caregivers: An integrative review. *Journal of Cardiovascular Nursing* 30(4 Suppl 1):S52–S63.

Hostinar, C. E. 2015. Recent developments in the study of social relationships, stress responses, and physical health. *Current Opinion in Psychology* 5:90–95.

Hostinar, C. E., and M. R. Gunnar. 2015. Social support can buffer against stress and shape brain activity. *American Journal of Bioethics Neuroscience* 6(3):34–42.

Hostinar, C. E., R. M. Sullivan, and M. R. Gunnar. 2014. Psychobiological mechanisms underlying the social buffering of the hypothalamic–pituitary–adrenocortical axis: A review of animal models and human studies across development. *Psychological Bulletin* 140(1):256–282.

House, J. S. 2015. *Beyond Obamacare: Life, death, and social policy.* New York: Russell Sage Foundation.

House, J. S., C. Robbins, and H. L. Metzner. 1982. The association of social relationships and activities with mortality: Prospective evidence from the Tecumseh Community Health Study. *American Journal of Epidemiology* 116(1):123–140.

House, J. S., K. R. Landis, and D. Umberson. 1988. Social relationships and health. *Science* 241(4865): 540–545.

Howick, J., P. Kelly, and M. Kelly. 2019. Establishing a causal link between social relationships and health using the Bradford Hill guidelines. *SSM–Population Health* 8:100402.

HPSM (Health Plan of San Mateo). 2020. Dora's story. https://www.hpsm.org/member-stories/dora (accessed January 2, 2020).

Hripcsak, G., C. B. Forrest, P. F. Brennan, and W. W. Stead. 2015. Informatics to support the IOM social and behavioral domains and measures. *Journal of the American Medical Informatics Association* 22(4):921–924.

HRSA (Health Resources and Services Administration). 2007. *Community health worker national workforce study.* https://bhw.hrsa.gov/sites/default/files/bhw/nchwa/projections/communityhealthworkforce.pdf (accessed October 25, 2019).

Huang, L. B., Y. F. Tsai, C. Y. Liu, and Y. J. Chen. 2017. Influencing and protective factors of suicidal ideation among older adults. *International Journal of Mental Health Nursing* 26(2):191–199.

Hudson, C. G., and N. J. Doogan. 2019. The impact of geographic isolation on mental disability in the United States. *SSM Population Health* 8:100437.

Hughes, M. E., L. J. Waite, L. C. Hawkley, and J. T. Cacioppo. 2004. A short scale for measuring loneliness in large surveys: Results from two population-based studies. *Research on Aging* 26(6):655–672.

Hui Gan, G. Z., A. M. Hill, P. Yeung, S. Keesing, and J. A. Netto. 2019. Pet ownership and its influence on mental health in older adults. *Aging & Mental Health,* June 27 [Epub ahead of print].

Humana. 2018. *Are you feeling lonely? You're not alone. Resources to help fight loneliness & social isolation.* https://populationhealth.humana.com/wp-content/uploads/2019/08/Loneliness-Toolkit.pdf (accessed November 7, 2019).

Humana. 2019. *Talking to your patients about loneliness and social isolation.* https://populationhealth.humana.com/wp-content/uploads/2019/09/quick-guide-to-addressing-loneliness.pdf (accessed November 7, 2019).

Hwang, Y., and G. R. S. Hong. 2018. Predictors of driving cessation in community-dwelling older adults: A 3-year longitudinal study. *Transportation Research Part F: Traffic Psychology and Behaviour* 52:202–209.

Hysong, S. J. 2009. Meta-analysis: Audit and feedback features impact effectiveness on care quality. *Medical Care* 47(3):356–363.

Hysong, S. J., R. G. Best, and J. A. Pugh. 2006. Audit and feedback and clinical practice guideline adherence: Making feedback actionable. *Implementation Science* 1:9.

Hysong, S. J., C. R. Teal, M. J. Khan, and P. Haidet. 2012. Improving quality of care through improved audit and feedback. *Implementation Science* 7:45.

Idler, E., M. Musick, C. Ellison, L. George, N. Krause, M. Ory, K. I. Pargament, L. H. Powell, L. G. Underwood, and D. R. Williams. 2003. Measuring multiple dimensions of religion and spirituality for health research: Conceptual background and findings from the 1998 General Social Survey. *Research on Aging* 25(4):327–365.

Idler, E., J. Blevins, M. Kiser, and C. Hogue. 2017. Religion, a social determinant of mortality? A 10-year follow-up of the health and retirement study. *PLOS ONE* 12(12):e0189134.

Ienca, M., T. Wangmo, F. Jotterand, R. W. Kressig, and B. Elger. 2018. Ethical design of intelligent assistive technologies for dementia: A descriptive review. *Science and Engineering Ethics* 24(4):1035–1055.

IHI (Institute for Healthcare Improvement). 2020. *What is an age-friendly health system?* http://www.ihi.org/Engage/Initiatives/Age-Friendly-Health-Systems/Pages/default.aspx (accessed January 2, 2020).

IOM (Institute of Medicine). 1988. *The future of public health.* Washington, DC: National Academy Press.

IOM. 1992. *The second fifty years: Promoting health and preventing disability.* Washington, DC: National Academy Press.

IOM. 2008. *Retooling for an aging America: Building the health care workforce.* Washington, DC: The National Academies Press.

IOM. 2009. *Initial national priorities for comparative effectiveness research.* Washington, DC: The National Academies Press.

IOM. 2011a. *Clinical practice guidelines we can trust.* Washington, DC: The National Academies Press.

IOM. 2011b. *The future of nursing: Leading change, advancing health.* Washington, DC: The National Academies Press.

IOM. 2012. *Primary care and public health: Exploring integration to improve population health.* Washington, DC: The National Academies Press.

IOM. 2013. *The CTSA program at NIH: Opportunities for advancing clinical and translational research.* Washington, DC: The National Academies Press.

IOM. 2014. *Capturing social and behavioral domains and measures in electronic health records: Phase 2.* Washington, DC: The National Academies Press.

IOM. 2015. *Cognitive aging: Progress in understanding and opportunities for action.* Washington, DC: The National Academies Press.

IPEC (Interprofessional Education Collaborative). 2016. *Core competencies for interprofessional collaborative practice: 2016 update.* https://hsc.unm.edu/ipe/resources/ipec-2016-core-competencies.pdf (accessed June 27, 2019).

Ismail, Z., E. E. Smith, Y. Geda, D. Sultzer, H. Brodaty, G. Smith, L. Agüera-Ortiz, R. Sweet, D. Miller, and C. G. Lyketsos. 2016. Neuropsychiatric symptoms as early manifestations of emergent dementia: Provisional diagnostic criteria for mild behavioral impairment. *Alzheimers & Dementia* 12(2):195–202.

Ivers, N., G. Jamtvedt, S.Flottorp, J. M. Young, J. Odgaard-Jensen, S. D. French, M. A. O'Brien, M. Johansen, J. Grimshaw, and A. D. Oxman. 2012. Audit and feedback: Effects on professional practice and healthcare outcomes. *Cochrane Database of Systematic Reviews* 2012(6):CD000259.

Ivers, N. M., A. Sales, H. Colquhoun, S. Michie, R. Foy, J. J. Francis, and J. M Grimshaw. 2014. No more "business as usual" with audit and feedback interventions: Towards an agenda for a reinvigorated intervention. *Implementation Science* 9:14.

IWH (Institute for Work & Health). 2015. *Primary, secondary and tertiary prevention.* https://www.iwh.on.ca/what-researchers-mean-by/primary-secondary-and-tertiary-prevention (accessed November 10, 2019).

Jackson, S. E., R. A. Hackett, I. Grabovac, L. Smith, and A. Steptoe. 2019. Perceived discrimination, health and wellbeing among middle-aged and older lesbian, gay and bisexual people: A prospective study. *PLOS ONE* 14(5):e0216497.

Jacobs, J. M., A. Cohen, R. Hammerman-Rozenberg, and J. Stessman. 2006. Global sleep satisfaction of older people: The Jerusalem Cohort Study. *Journal of the American Geriatrics Society* 54(2):325–329.

Jacobs, J. M., Y. Rottenberg, A. Cohen, and J. Stessman. 2013. Physical activity and health service utilization among older people. *Journal of the American Medical Directors Association* 14(2):125–129.

Jacobs, S. R., B. J. Weiner, and A. C. Bunger. 2014. Context matters: Measuring implementation climate among individuals and groups. *Implementation Science* 9(1):46.

Jakobsson, U., J. Kristensson, I. R. Hallberg, and P. Midlöv. 2011. Psychosocial perspectives on health care utilization among frail elderly people: An explorative study. *Archives of Gerontology and Geriatrics* 52(3):290–294.

James, B. D., R. S. Wilson, L. L. Barnes, and D. A. Bennett. 2011. Late-life social activity and cognitive decline in old age. *Journal of the International Neuropsychological Society* 17(6):998–1005.

Jamieson, H. A., H. M. Gibson, R. Abey-Nesbit, A. Ahuriri-Driscoll, S. Keeling, and P. J. Schluter. 2018. Profile of ethnicity, living arrangements and loneliness amongst older adults in Aotearoa, New Zealand: A national cross-sectional study. *Australasian Journal on Ageing* 37(1):68–73.

Jaremka, L. M., C. P. Fagundes, J. Peng, J. M. Bennett, R. Glaser, W. B. Malarkey, and J. K. Kiecolt-Glaser. 2013a. Loneliness promotes inflammation during acute stress. *Psychological Science* 24(7):1089–1097.

Jaremka, L. M., M. E. Lindgren, and J. K. Kiecolt-Glaser. 2013b. Synergistic relationships among stress, depression, and troubled relationships: Insights from psychoneuroimmunology. *Depression and Anxiety* 30(4):288–296.

JCHS (Joint Center for Housing Studies). 2018. *Updated household growth projections: 2018–2028 and 2028–2038.* Cambridge, MA: Harvard University. https://www.jchs.harvard.edu/sites/default/files/Harvard_JCHS_McCue_Household_Projections_Rev010319.pdf (accessed July 18, 2019).

Jennings, N. R., and M. Wooldridge. 1998. *Applications of intelligent agents.* Secaucus, NJ: Springer-Verlag.

Jessen, M. A. B., A. V. J. Pallesen, M. Kriegbaum, and M. Kristiansen. 2017. The association between loneliness and health—A survey-based study among middle-aged and older adults in Denmark. *Aging and Mental Health* 22(10):1338–1343.

Jeste, D. V., D. Glorioso, E. E. Lee, R. Daly, S. Graham, J. Liu, A. M. Paredes, C. Nebeker, X. M. Tu, E. W. Twamley, R. Van Patten, Y. Yamada, C. Depp, and H. C. Kim. 2019. Study of independent living residents of a continuing care senior housing community: Sociodemographic and clinical associations of cognitive, physical, and mental health. *American Journal of Geriatric Psychiatry* 27(9):895–907.

Jeuring, H. W., M. L. Stek, M. Huisman, R. C. Oude Voshaar, P. Naarding, R. M. Collard, R. C. van der Mast, R. M. Kok, A. T. F. Beekman, and H. C. Comijs. 2018. A six-year prospective study of the prognosis and predictors in patients with late-life depression. *American Journal of Geriatric Psychiatry* 26(9):985–997.

Johnson, A. M., J. E. Moore, D. A. Chambers, J. Rup, C. Dinyarian, and S. E. Straus. 2019. How do researchers conceptualize and plan for the sustainability of their NIH R01 implementation projects? *Implementation Science* 14(1):50.

Johnson, D., S. Deterding, K. A. Kuhn, A. Staneva, S. Stoyanov, and L. Hides. 2016. Gamification for health and wellbeing: A systematic review of the literature. *Internet Interventions* 6:89–106.

Johnson, J. E. 1999. Urban older adults and the forfeiture of a driver's license. *Journal of Gerontological Nursing* 25(12):12–18.

Johnson, J. E. 2008. Informal social support networks and the maintenance of voluntary driving cessation by older rural women. *Journal of Community Health Nursing* 25(2):65–72.

Johnson, S. R. 2019. *Kaiser to launch social care network.* https://www.modernhealthcare.com/care-delivery/kaiser-launch-social-care-network (accessed November 7, 2019).

Johnston, D., Q. M. Samus, A. Morrison, J. S. Leoutsakos, K. Hicks, S. Handel, R. Rye, B. Robbins, P. V. Rabins, C. G. Lyketsos, and B. S. Black. 2011. Identification of community-residing individuals with dementia and their unmet needs for care. *International Journal of Geriatric Psychiatry* 26(3):292–298.

Jones, D. A., C. R. Victor, and N. J. Vetter. 1985. The problem of loneliness in the elderly in the community: Characteristics of those who are lonely and the factors related to loneliness. *The Journal of the Royal College of General Practitioners* 35(272):136–139.

Jopling, K. 2015. *Promising approaches to reducing loneliness and isolation in later life.* London, UK: AgeUK.

Jøranson, N., I. Pedersen, A. M. Rokstad, and C. Ihlebaek. 2016. Change in quality of life in older people with dementia participating in Paro-activity: A cluster-randomized controlled trial. *Journal of Advanced Nursing* 72(12):3020–3033.

Jowett, B. 2009. *Politics by Aristotle.* http://classics.mit.edu/Aristotle/politics.mb.txt (accessed June 27, 2019).

Jun, J., C. T. Kovner, and A. W. Stimpfel. 2016. Barriers and facilitators of nurses' use of clinical practice guidelines: An integrative review. *International Journal of Nursing Studies* 60:54–68.

Jung, E. H., J. Walden, A. C. Johnson, and S. S. Sundar. 2017. Social networking in the aging context: Why older adults use or avoid Facebook. *Telematics and Informatics* 34(7):1071–1080.

Kaeberlein, M. R., and G. M. Martin. 2015. *Handbook of the biology of aging, 8th edition.* New York: Academic Press.

Kaiser Permanente. 2019. *Kaiser Permanente Northwest launches Thrive Local social health network.* https://about.kaiserpermanente.org/community-health/news/kaiser-permanente-northwest-launches-thrive-local-social-health- (accessed November 4, 2019).

Kanaoka, T., and B. Mutlu. 2015. Designing a motivational agent for behavior change in physical activity. In CHI EA '15: *Proceedings of the 33rd annual ACM Conference extended abstracts on human factors in computing systems.* Pp. 1445–1450.

Kaufman, A. 2016. Beyond Flexner alliance: Social mission in health professions education. *Education for Health* 29(3):277–278.

Kelly, M. E., H. Duff, S. Kelly, J. E. McHugh Power, S. Brennan, B. A. Lawlor, and D. G. Loughrey. 2017. The impact of social activities, social networks, social support and social relationships on the cognitive functioning of healthy older adults: A systematic review. *Systematic Reviews* 6(1):259.

Kemperman, A., P. van den Berg, M. Weijs-Perree, and K. Uijtdewillegen. 2019. Loneliness of older adults: Social network and the living environment. *International Journal of Environmental Research and Public Health* 16(3):406.

Kent de Grey, R. G., B. N. Uchino, R. Trettevik, S. Cronan, and J. N. Hogan. 2018. Social support and sleep: A meta-analysis. *Health Psychology* 37(8):787–798.

Kharicha, K., S. Iliffe, D. Harari, C. Swift, G. Gillmann, and A. E. Stuck. 2007. Health risk appraisal in older people 1: Are older people living alone an "at-risk" group? *British Journal of General Practice* 57(537):271–276.

Kharicha, K., S. Iliffe, J. Manthorpe, C. A. Chew-Graham, M. Cattan, C. Goodman, M. Kirby-Barr, J. H. Whitehouse, and K. Walters. 2017. What do older people experiencing loneliness think about primary care or community based interventions to reduce loneliness? A qualitative study in England. *Health & Social Care in the Community* 25(6):1733–1742.

Khosravi, P., A. Rezvani, and A. Wiewiora. 2016. The impact of technology on older adults' social isolation. *Computers in Human Behavior* 63:594–603.

Khullar, D. 2016. How social isolation is killing us. *The New York Times.* December 22. https://www.nytimes.com/2016/12/22/upshot/how-social-isolation-is-killing-us.html (accessed November 20, 2019).

Kiecolt-Glaser, J. K., and T. L. Newton. 2001. Marriage and health: His and hers. *Psychological Bulletin* 127(4):472–503.

Kim, B. J., C. C. Sangalang, and T. Kihl. 2012. Effects of acculturation and social network support on depression among elderly Korean immigrants. *Aging and Mental Health* 16(6):787–794.

Kim, D. A., E. J. Benjamin, J. H. Fowler, and N. A. Christakis. 2016. Social connectedness is associated with fibrinogen level in a human social network. *Proceedings of the Royal Society B: Biological Sciences* 283(1837):20160958.

Kim, H. J., and K. I. Fredriksen-Goldsen. 2016. Living arrangement and loneliness among lesbian, gay, and bisexual older adults. *Gerontologist* 56(3):548–558.

Kim, H. J., K. Acey, A. Guess, S. Jen, and K. I. Fredriksen-Goldsen. 2016. A collaboration for health and wellness: GROIT Circle and Caring and Aging with Pride. *Generations* 40(2):49–55.

Kimmel, P. L., R. A. Peterson, K. L. Weihs, N. Shidler, S. J. Simmens, S. Alleyne, I. Cruz, J. A. Yanovski, J. H. Veis, and T. M. Phillips. 2000. Dyadic relationship conflict, gender, and mortality in urban hemodialysis patients. *Journal of the American Society of Nephrology* 11(8):1518–1525.

King, K. B., and H. T. Reis. 2012. Marriage and long-term survival after coronary artery bypass grafting. *Health Psychology* 31(1):55–62.

King, S., and H. Dabelko-Schoeny. 2009. "Quite frankly, I have doubts about remaining": Aging-in-place and health care access for rural midlife and older lesbian, gay, and bisexual individuals. *Journal of LGBT Health Research* 5(1–2):10–21.

Kirchner, J., T. Waltz, B. J. Powell, J. L. Smith, and E. K. Proctor. 2018. Implementation strategies. In R. C. Brownson, G. A. Colditz, and E. K. Proctor (eds.), *Dissemination and implementation research in health: Translating science to Practice, 2nd ed.* New York: Oxford University Press. Pp. 245–266.

Kirkpatrick, L. A., D. J. Shillito, and S. L. Kellas. 1999. Loneliness, social support, and perceived relationships with God. *Journal of Social and Personal Relationships* 164(4):513–522.

Kirton, C. 2019. Dissemination. In G. LoBiondo-Wood, J. Haber, and M. G. Titler (eds.), *Evidence-based practice for nursing and healthcare quality improvement.* Philadelphia, PA: Elsevier. Pp. 242–250.

Kline, C. E. 2014. The bidirectional relationship between exercise and sleep: Implications for exercise adherence and sleep improvement. *American Journal of Lifestyle Medicine* 8(6):375–379.

Knowles, M. L., G. M. Lucas, R. F. Baumeister, and W. L. Gardner. 2015. Choking under social pressure: Social monitoring among the lonely. *Personality and Social Psychology Bulletin* 41(6):805–821.

Kobayashi, L. C., and A. Steptoe. 2018. Social isolation, loneliness, and health behaviors at older ages: Longitudinal cohort study. *Annals of Behavioral Medicine* 52(7):582–593.

Kochanek, K. D., S. L. Murphy, J. Q. Xu, and E. Arias. 2019. Deaths: Final data for 2017. *National Vital Statistics Reports* 68(9):1–77. Hyattsville, MD: National Center for Health Statistics. https://www.cdc.gov/nchs/data/nvsr/nvsr68/nvsr68_09-508.pdf (accessed November 21, 2019).

Koenig, H. G., R. E. Westlund, L. K. George, D. G. Blazer, and C. Hybels. 1993. Abbreviating the Duke Social Support Index for use in chronically ill elderly individuals. *Psychosomatics* 34(1):61–69.

Kolodziejczak, K., A. Rosada, J. Drewelies, S. Duzel, P. Eibich, C. Tegeler, G. G. Wagner, K. M. Beier, N. Ram, I. Demuth, E. Steinhagen-Thiessen, and D. Gerstorf. 2019. Sexual activity, sexual thoughts, and intimacy among older adults: Links with physical health and psychosocial resources for successful aging. *Psychology and Aging* 34(3):389–404.

Koszycki, D., M. Benger, J. Shlik, and J. Bradwejn. 2007. Randomized trial of a meditation-based stress reduction program and cognitive behavior therapy in generalized social anxiety disorder. *Behaviour Research and Therapy* 45(10):2518–2526.

Krause-Parello, C. A., and E. E. Gulick. 2013. Situational factors related to loneliness and loss over time among older pet owners. *Western Journal of Nursing Research* 35(7):905–919.

Kroenke, C. H., C. Quesenberry, M. L. Kwan, C. Sweeney, A. Castillo, and B. J. Caan. 2013. Social networks, social support, and burden in relationships, and mortality after breast cancer diagnosis in the Life After Breast Cancer Epidemiology (LACE) study. *Breast Cancer Research and Treatment* 137(1):261–271.

Kueny, A., L. L. Shever, M. Lehan Mackin, and M. G. Titler. 2015. Facilitating the implementation of evidence-based practice through contextual support for nursing leadership. *Journal of Healthcare Leadership* 7:29–39.

Kuiper, J. S., M. Zuidersma, R. C. Oude Voshaar, S. U. Zuidema, E. R. van den Heuvel, R. P. Stolk, and N. Smidt. 2015. Social relationships and risk of dementia: A systematic review and meta-analysis of longitudinal cohort studies. *Ageing Research Reviews* 22:39–57.

Kumar, A., H. Carpenter, R. Morris, S. Iliffe, and D. Kendrick. 2014. Which factors are associated with fear of falling in community-dwelling older people? *Age and Ageing* 43(1):76–84.

Kurina, L. M., K. L. Knutson, L. C. Hawkley, J. T. Cacioppo, D. S. Lauderdale, and C. Ober. 2011. Loneliness is associated with sleep fragmentation in a communal society. *Sleep* 34(11):1519–1526.

Kuyper, L., and T. Fokkema. 2010. Loneliness among older lesbian, gay, and bisexual adults: The role of minority stress. *Archives of Sexual Behavior* 39(5):1171–1180.

Labrum, T., and P. L. Solomon. 2015. Physical elder abuse perpetrated by relatives with serious mental illness: A preliminary conceptual social–ecological model. *Aggression and Violent Behavior* 25:293–303.

Lacey, L. P., C. Manfredi, G. Balch, R. B. Warnecke, K. Allen, and C. Edwards. 1993. Social support in smoking cessation among black women in Chicago public housing. *Public Health Reports* 108(3):387–394.

Lacey, R. E., M. Kumari, and M. Bartley. 2014. Social isolation in childhood and adult inflammation: Evidence from the national child development study. *Psychoneuroendocrinology* 50:85–94.

Lachs, M. S., and K. A. Pillemer. 2015. Elder abuse. *New England Journal of Medicine* 373(20):1947–1956.

Lamb, G., and R. Newhouse. 2018. *Care coordination: A blueprint for action for RNs*. Silver Spring, MD: American Nurses Association.

Lanctôt, K. L., L. Agüera-Ortiz, H. Brodaty, P. T. Francis, Y. E. Geda, Z. Ismail, G. A. Marshall, M. E. Mortby, C. U. Onyike, P. R. Padala, A. M. Politis, P. B. Rosenberg, E. Siegel, D. L. Sultzer, and E. H. Abraham. 2017. Apathy associated with neurocognitive disorders: Recent progress and future directions. *Alzheimers & Dementia* 13(1):84–100.

Lane, K., C. Galambos, L. Phillips, L. Popejoy and M. Rantz. 2019. Aging in place: transitional housing and supported models. In T. Fulmer (ed.), *Handbook of geriatric assessment*. Burlington, MA: Jones & Bartlett. Pp. 365–371.

Laranjo, L., A. G. Dunn, H. L. Tong, A. B. Kocaballi, J. Chen, R. Bashir, D. Surian, B. Gallego, F. Magrabi, A. Y. S. Lau, and E. Coiera. 2018. Conversational agents in healthcare: A systematic review. *Journal of the American Medical Informatics Association* 25(9):1248–1258.

Lauder, W., K. Mummery, M. Jones, and C. Caperchione. 2006a. A comparison of health behaviours in lonely and non-lonely populations. *Psychology, Health & Medicine* 11(2):233–245.

Lauder, W., K. Mummery, and S. Sharkey. 2006b. Social capital, age and religiosity in people who are lonely. *Journal of Clinical Nursing* 15(3):334–340.

LaWall, E., Y. Y. Wu, V. Y. Fan, M. Ashton, and T. Sentell. 2019. Living alone and homelessness as predictors of 30-day potentially preventable hospital readmission. *Preventing Chronic Disease* 16:180189.

Leeming, A., S. A. Murray, and M. Kendall. 2014. The impact of advanced heart failure on social, psychological and existential aspects and personhood. *European Journal of Cardiovascular Nursing* 13(2):162–167.

Leigh-Hunt, N., D. Bagguley, K. Bash, V. Turner, S. Turnbull, N. Valtorta, and W. Caan. 2017. An overview of systematic reviews on the public health consequences of social isolation and loneliness. *Public Health* 152:157–171.

Lennox, L., L. Maher, and J. Reed. 2018. Navigating the sustainability landscape: A systematic review of sustainability approaches in healthcare. *Implementation Science* 13(1):27.

Leoutsakos, J. M., S. N. Forrester, C. D. Corcoran, M. C. Norton, P. V. Rabins, M. I. Steinberg, J. T. Tschanz, and C. G. Lyketsos. 2015. Latent classes of course in Alzheimer's disease and predictors: The Cache County Dementia Progression Study. *International Journal of Geriatric Psychiatry* 30(8):824–832.

Lepore, S. J. 1998. Problems and prospects for the social support-reactivity hypothesis. *Annals of Behavioral Medicine* 20(4):257–269.

LeRoy, A. S., K. W. Murdock, L. M. Jaremka, A. Loya, and C. P. Fagundes. 2017. Loneliness predicts self-reported cold symptoms after a viral challenge. *Health Psychology* 36(5):512–520.

Levin, J. S., and L. M. Chatters. 1998. Religion, health, and psychological well-being in older adults: Findings from three national surveys. *Journal of Aging and Health* 10(4):504–531.

Levine, D. M., B. E. Landon, and J. A. Linder. 2019. Quality and experience of outpatient care in the United States for adults with or without primary care. *JAMA Internal Medicine* 179(3):363–372.

Lewis, G., D. Z. Kounali, K. S. Button, L. Duffy, N. J. Wiles, M. R. Munafò, C. J. Harmer, and G. Lewis. 2017. Variation in the recall of socially rewarding information and depressive symptom severity: A prospective cohort study. *Acta Psychiatrica Scandinavica* 135(5):489–498.

Li, Q., and A. Y. Loke. 2013. A spectrum of hidden morbidities among spousal caregivers for patients with cancer, and differences between the genders: A review of the literature. *European Journal of Oncology Nursing* 17(5):578–587.

Liang, A., I. Piroth, H. Robinson, B. MacDonald, M. Fisher, U. M. Nater, N. Skoluda, and E. Broadbent. 2017. A pilot randomized trial of a companion robot for people with dementia living in the community. *Journal of the American Medical Directors Association* 18(10):871–878.

Lim, L. L., and E. H. Kua. 2011. Living alone, loneliness, and psychological well-being of older persons in Singapore. *Current Gerontology and Geriatrics Research* 2011:673181.

Lim, M. H., T. L. Rodebaugh, M. J. Zyphur, and J. F. Gleeson. 2016. Loneliness over time: The crucial role of social anxiety. *Journal of Abnormal Psychology* 125(5):620–630.

Linden, W., L. Chambers, J. Maurice, and J. W. Lenz. 1993. Sex differences in social support, self-deception, hostility, and ambulatory cardiovascular activity. *Health Psychology* 12(5):376–380.

Lindsay, E. K., S. Young, K. W. Brown, J. M. Smyth, and J. D. Creswell. 2019. Mindfulness training reduces loneliness and increases social contact in a randomized controlled trial. *Proceedings of the National Academy of Sciences* 116(9):3488–3493.

Lisetti, C., R. Amini, U. Yasavur, and N. Rishe. 2013. I can help you change! An empathic virtual agent delivers behavior change health interventions. *ACM Transactions on Management Information Systems* 4(4):1–28.

Locher, J. L., C. S. Ritchie, D. L. Roth, P. S. Baker, E. V. Bodner, and R. M. Allman. 2005. Social isolation, support, and capital and nutritional risk in an older sample: Ethnic and gender differences. *Social Science & Medicine* 60(4):747–761.

Looije, R., M. A. Neerincx, and F. Cnossen. 2010. Persuasive robotic assistant for health self-management of older adults: Design and evaluation of social behaviors. *International Journal of Human–Computer Studies* 68(6):386–397.

Lubben, J. E. 1988. Assessing social networks among elderly populations. *Family and Community Health* 11(3):42–52.

Lubben, J. 2017. Addressing social isolation as a potent killer! *Public Policy & Aging Report* 27(4):136–138.

Lubben, J. E., and M. W. Gironda. 2003. Centrality of social ties to the health and well being of older adults. In B. Berkman and L. K. Harooytan (eds.), *Social work and health care in an aging world.* New York: Springer.

Lubben, J., E. Blozik, G. Gillmann, S. Iliffe, W. von Rentein Kruse, J. C. Beck, and A. E. Stuck. 2006. Performance of an abbreviated version of the Lubben Social Network Scale among three European community-dwelling older adult populations. *The Gerontologist* 46(4):503–513.

Lubben, J., M. Gironda, E. Sabbath, J. Kong, and C. Johnson. 2015. *Social isolation presents a grand challenge for social work.* Grand Challenges for Social Work Initiative working paper no. 7. Cleveland, OH: American Academy of Social Work and Social Welfare.

Lubben, J. E., E. Tracy, S. E. Crewe, E. Sabbath, M. Gironda, C. Johnson, J. Kong, M. Munson, and S. Brown. 2018. Eradicate social isolation. In R. Fong, J. Lubben, and R. P. Barth (eds.), *Grand challenges for social work and society.* New York and Washington, DC: Oxford University Press.

Lubik, A., and T. Kosatsky. 2019. Public health should promote co-operative housing and cohousing. *Canadian Journal of Public Health* 110(2):121–126.

Lukaschek, K., J. Baumert, J. Kruse, C. Meisinger, and K. H. Ladwig. 2017. Sex differences in the association of social network satisfaction and the risk for type 2 diabetes. *BMC Public Health* 17(1):1–8.

Luo, Y., and L. J. Waite. 2014. Loneliness and mortality among older adults in China. *Journals of Gerontology Series B: Psychological Sciences and Social Sciences* 69(4):633–645.

Luo, Y., L. C. Hawkley, L. J. Waite, and J. T. Cacioppo. 2012. Loneliness, health, and mortality in old age: A national longitudinal study. *Social Science & Medicine* 74(6):907–914.

Lykke, S., and C. Handberg. 2019. Experienced loneliness in home-based rehabilitation: Perspectives of older adults with disabilities and their health care professionals. *Global Qualitative Nursing Research* 6:1–12.

Lykken, D. T. 1968. Statistical significance in psychological research. *Psychological Bulletin* 70(3):151–159.

MacKinnon, D. P., and L. J. Luecken. 2008. How and for whom? Mediation and moderation in health psychology. *Health Psychology* 27(2S):S99–S100.

Maes, M., P. Qualter, J. Vanhalst, W. Van den Noortgate, and L. Goossens. 2019. Gender differences in loneliness across the lifespan: A meta-analysis. *European Journal of Personality* 33:642–654.

Magnavita, N., and S. Garbarino. 2017. Sleep, health and wellness at work: A scoping review. *International Journal of Environmental Research and Public Health* 14(11):E1347.

Malani, P., J. Kullgren, J. Piette, E. Solway, D. Singer, and M. Kirch. 2019. *Loneliness and health: National Poll on Healthy Aging.* http://hdl.handle.net/2027.42/148147 (accessed March 28, 2019).

Maloney, S., J. Tunnecliff, P. Morgan, J. E. Gaida, L. Clearihan, S. Sadasivan, D. Davies, S. Ganesh, P. Mohanty, J. Weiner, J. Reynolds, and D. Ilic. 2015. Translating evidence into practice via social media: A mixed-methods study. *Journal of Medical Internet Research* 17(10):e242.

Manatt Health. 2019. *Addressing social factors that affect health: Emerging trends and leading edge practices in Medicaid.* https://www.manatt.com/Manatt/media/Documents/Articles/Social-Factors-That-Affect-Health_Final.pdf (accessed August 13, 2019).

Manemann, S. M., A. M. Chamberlain, V. L. Roger, J. M. Griffin, C. M. Boyd, T. K. M. Cudjoe, D. Jensen, S. A. Weston, M. Fabbri, R. Jiang, and L. J. F. Rutten. 2018. Perceived social isolation and outcomes in patients with heart failure. *Journal of the American Heart Association* 7(11):e008069.

Mann, F., J. K. Bone, B. Lloyd-Evans, J. Frerichs, V. Pinfold, R. Ma, J. Wang, and S. Johnson. 2017. A life less lonely: The state of the art in interventions to reduce loneliness in people with mental health problems. *Social Psychiatry and Psychiatric Epidemiology* 52(6):627–638.

Manzoli, L., P. Villari, G. M. Pirone, and A. Boccia. 2007. Marital status and mortality in the elderly: A systematic review and meta-analysis. *Social Science & Medicine* 64(1):77–94.

Markowitz, J. C., and M. M. Weissman. 2004. Interpersonal psychotherapy: Principles and applications. *World Psychiatry* 3(3):136–139.

Martina, C. M. S., and N. L. Stevens. 2007. Breaking the cycle of loneliness? Psychological effects of a friendship enrichment program for older women. *Aging & Mental Health* 10(5):467–475.

Masi, C. M., H.-Y. Chen, L. C. Hawkley, and J. T. Cacioppo. 2011. A meta-analysis of interventions to reduce loneliness. *Personality and Social Psychology Review* 15(3):219–266.

Matud, M. P. 2004. Gender differences in stress and coping styles. *Personality and Individual Differences* 37(7):1401–1415.

Maxwell, C. J., A. Soo, D. B. Hogan, W. P. Wodchis, E. Gilbart, J. Amuah, M. Eliasziw, B. Hagen, and L. A. Strain. 2013. Predictors of nursing home placement from assisted living settings in Canada. *Canadian Journal of Aging* 32(4):333–348.

May, C. R., M. Johnson, and T. Finch. 2016. Implementation, context and complexity. *Implementation Science* 11(1):141.

Mayo Clinic. 2019. *Cognitive behavioral therapy.* https://www.mayoclinic.org/tests-procedures/cognitive-behavioral-therapy/about/pac-20384610 (accessed April 16, 2019).

Mayo-Wilson, E., S. Dias, I. Mavranezouli, K. Kew, D. M. Clark, A. E. Ades, and S. Pilling. 2014. Psychological and pharmacological interventions for social anxiety disorder in adults: A systematic review and network meta-analysis. *Lancet Psychiatry* 1(5):368–376.

McCormack, B., J. Rycroft-Malone, K. Decorby, A. M. Hutchinson, T. Bucknall, B. Kent, A. Schultz, E. Snelgrove-Clarke, C. Stetler, M. Titler, L. Wallin, and V. Wilson. 2013. A realist review of interventions and strategies to promote evidence-informed healthcare: A focus on change agency. *Implementation Science* 8:107.

McCrory, C., C. Finucane, C. O'Hare, J. Frewen, H. Nolan, R. Layte, P. M. Kearney, and R. A. Kenny. 2016. Social disadvantage and social isolation are associated with a higher resting heart rate: Evidence from the Irish Longitudinal Study on Ageing. *Journals of Gerontology, Series B: Psychological Sciences and Social Sciences* 71(3):463–473.

McGinnis, J. M., P. Williams-Russo, and J. R. Knickman. 2002. The case for more active policy attention to health promotion. *Health Affairs* 21(2):78–93.

McHugh, J. E., and B. A. Lawlor. 2013. Perceived stress mediates the relationship between emotional loneliness and sleep quality over time in older adults. *British Journal of Health Psychology* 18(3):546–555.

McHugh Power, J., C. Hannigan, P. Hyland, S. Brennan, F. Kee, and B. A. Lawlor. 2020. Depressive symptoms predict increased social and emotional loneliness in older adults. *Aging & Mental Health* 24(1):110–118.

McKhann, G. M., D. S. Knopman, H. Chertkow, B. T. Hyman, C. R. Jack, Jr., C. H. Kawas, W. E. Klunk, W. J. Koroshetz, J. J. Manly, R. Mayeux, R. C. Mohs, J. C. Morris, M. N. Rossor, P. Scheltens, M. C. Carrillo, B. Thies, S. Weintraub, and C. H. Phelps. 2011. The diagnosis of dementia due to Alzheimer's disease: Recommendations from the National Institute on Aging–Alzheimer's Association workgroups on diagnostic guidelines for Alzheimer's disease. *Alzheimer's & Dementia* 7(3):263–269.

McKeown, T. 1976. *The rise of population*. New York: Academic Press.

McKeown, T. 1979. *The role of medicine*. Oxford, UK: Blackwell.

McKeown, T. 1988. *The origins of human disease*. Oxford, UK: Blackwell.

McMillen, J. C., and D. R. Adams. 2018. Dissemination and implementation in social service settings. In R. C. Brownson, G. A. Colditz, and E. K. Proctor (eds.), *Dissemination and implementation research in health: Translating science to practice, 2nd ed*. New York: Oxford University Press. Pp. 371–381.

McNicholas, J., and G. M. Collis. 2000. Dogs as catalysts for social interactions: Robustness of the effect. *British Journal of Psychology* 91(Pt 1):61–70.

McWhirter, B. T. 1990. Loneliness: A review of current literature, with implications for counseling and research. *Journal of Counseling and Development* 68(4):417–422.

MDHS (Maine Department of Human Services). 2003. *Introduction to health care and human services: For the personal support specialist (PSS) and certified nurses assistant (CNA) training program*. https://www.maine.gov/dhhs/dlc/licensing/pss/PSS_Student_Manual.pdf (accessed June 27, 2019).

Meals on Wheels America. 2017. *Meals on Wheels America statement on budget blueprint*. https://www.mealsonwheelsamerica.org/learn-more/national/press-room/news/2017/03/16/meals-on-wheels-america-statement-on-budget-blueprint (accessed November 13, 2019).

Melenhorst, A. S., W. A. Rogers, and E. C. Caylor. 2001. The use of communication technologies by older adults: Exploring the benefits from the user's perspective. *Proceedings of the Human Factors and Ergonomics Society 45th Annual Meeting* 45(3):221–225.

Melnyk, B. M., L. Gallagher-Ford, L. E. Long, and E. Fineout-Overholt. 2014. The establishment of evidence-based practice competencies for practicing registered nurses and advanced practice nurses in real-world clinical settings: Proficiencies to improve healthcare quality, reliability, patient outcomes, and costs. *Worldviews on Evidence-Based Nursing* 11(1):5–15.

Merz, E.-M., and J. De Jong Gierveld. 2016. Childhood memories, family ties, sibling support and loneliness in ever-widowed older adults: Quantitative and qualitative results. *Aging & Society* 36:534–561.

Messeri, P., M. Silverstein, and E. Litwak. 1993. Choosing optimal support groups: A review and reformulation. *Journal of Health and Social Behavior* 34(2):122–137.

Meyer, H., and T. R. Johnston. 2014. The national resource center on LGBT aging provides critical training to aging service providers. *Journal of Gerontological Social Work* 57(2–4):407–412.

Mezuk, B., A. Rock, M. C. Lohman, and M. Choi. 2014. Suicide risk in long-term care facilities: A systematic review. *International Journal of Geriatric Psychiatry* 29(12):1198–1211.

Mick, P., and M. K. Pichora-Fuller. 2016. Is hearing loss associated with poorer health in older adults who might benefit from hearing screening? *Ear & Hearing* 37(3):e194–e201.

Mick, P., I. Kawachi, and F. R. Lin. 2014. The association between hearing loss and social isolation in older adults. *Otolaryngology—Head and Neck Surgery* 150(3):378–384.

Mick, P., M. Parfyonov, W. Wittich, N. Phillips, D. Guthrie, and M. K. Pichora-Fuller. 2018. Associations between sensory loss and social networks, participation, support, and loneliness: Analysis of the Canadian Longitudinal Study on Aging. *Canadian Family Physician* 64(1):e33–e41.

Minayo, M. C., and F. G. Cavalcante. 2015. Suicide attempts among the elderly: A review of the literature (2002/2013). *Cien Saude Colet* 20(6):1751–1762.

Mistry, R., J. Rosansky, J. McGuire, C. McDermott, and L. Jarvik. 2001. Social isolation predicts re-hospitalization in a group of older American veterans enrolled in the UPBEAT program: Unified Psychogeriatric Biopsychosocial Evaluation And Treatment. *International Journal of Geriatric Psychiatry* 16(10):950–959.

Mitchell, U. A., P. G. Chebli, L. Ruggiero, and N. Muramatsu. 2019. The digital divide in health-related technology use: The significance of race/ethnicity. *Gerontologist* 59(1):6–14.

Mitchinson, A. R., H. M. Kim, M. Geisser, J. M. Rosenberg, and D. B. Hinshaw. 2008. Social connectedness and patient recovery after major operations. *Journal of the American College of Surgeons* 206(2):292–300.

Miyawaki, C. E. 2015. Association of social isolation and health across different racial and ethnic groups of older Americans. *Ageing and Society* 35(10):2201–2228.

Moffatt, S., M. Steer, S. Lawson, L. Penn, and N. O'Brien. 2017. Link Worker social prescribing to improve health and well-being for people with long-term conditions: Qualitative study of service user perceptions. *BMJ Open* 7(7):e015203.

Moon, H., S. Rote, and W. E. Haley. 2018. Factors that contribute to remaining in the community among older adults. *Aging & Mental Health* 22(11):1502–1509.

Moore, S., A. Teixeira, and S. Stewart. 2014. Effect of network social capital on the chances of smoking relapse: A two-year follow-up study of urban-dwelling adults. *American Journal of Public Health* 104(12):e72–e76.

Morris, J. C. 1993. The clinical dementia rating (CDR): Current version and scoring rules. *Neurology* 43(11):2412–2414.

Morris, Z. A. 2019. Loneliness as a predictor of work disability onset among nondisabled, working older adults in 14 countries. *Journal of Aging and Health*, April 9 [Epub ahead of print].

Moukouta, C. S., K. Kokou-Kpolou, D. Mbassa Menick, H. Deligne, M. Dailly, and F. Soltani. 2017. Difficulties in the management of elderly migrants. *Geriatrie et Psychologie Neuropsychiatrie du Vieillissement* 15(4):409–416.

Moyle, W., U. Kellett, A. Ballantyne, and N. Gracia. 2011. Dementia and loneliness: An Australian perspective. *Journal of Clinical Nursing* 20(9-10):1445–1453.

Msowoya, A. L., and S. M. Gephart. 2019. Patient-centered evidence-based practices. In G. LoBiondo-Wood, J. Haber, and M. G. Titler (eds.), *Evidence-based practice for nursing and healthcare quality improvement.* Philadelphia, PA: Elsevier. Pp. 219–230.

Mueller, M. K., N. R. Gee, and R. M. Bures. 2018. Human–animal interaction as a social determinant of health: Descriptive findings from the health and retirement study. *BMC Public Health* 18(1):305.

Mullen, F. 2017. Social mission in health professions education: Beyond Flexner. *JAMA* 318(2):122–123.

Mullen, R. A., S. Tong, R. T. Sabo, W. R. Liaw, J. Marshall, D. E. Nease, Jr., A. H. Krist, and J. J. Frey, III. 2019. Loneliness in primary care patients: A prevalence study. *Annals of Family Medicine* 17(2):108–115.

Muraco, A., J. Putney, C. Shiu, and K. I. Fredriksen-Goldsen. 2018. Lifesaving in every way: The role of companion animals in the lives of older lesbian, gay, bisexual, and transgender adults age 50 and over. *Research on Aging* 40(9):859–882.

Murray, D. R., M. G. Haselton, M. Fales, and S. W. Cole. 2019. Subjective social status and inflammatory gene expression. *Health Psychology* 38(2):182–186.

Musich, S., S. S. Wang, K. Hawkins, and C. S. Yeh. 2015. The impact of loneliness on quality of life and patient satisfaction among older, sicker adults. *Gerontology and Geriatric Medicine* 1:2333721415582119.

Nachega, J. B., C. Morroni, J. M. Zuniga, R. Sherer, C. Beyrer, S. Solomon, M. Schechter, and J. Rockstroh. 2012. HIV-related stigma, isolation, discrimination, and serostatus disclosure: A global survey of 2035 HIV-infected adults. *Journal of the International Association of Physicians in AIDS Care* 11(3):172–178.

NADSP (National Alliance for Direct Support Professionals). 2016. *Direct support professional competency areas: The foundation of direct support practice.* https://nadsp.org/wp-content/uploads/2017/07/National-Direct-Support-Professional-Competency-Areas-Brochure-FINAL.pdf (accessed June 27, 2019).

NASEM (National Academies of Sciences, Engineering, and Medicine). 2016a. *A framework for educating health professionals to address the social determinants of health.* Washington, DC: The National Academies Press.

NASEM. 2016b. *Families caring for an aging America*. Washington, DC: The National Academies Press.

NASEM. 2016c. *Assessing progress on the Institute of Medicine report* The Future of Nursing. Washington, DC: The National Academies Press.

NASEM. 2017. *Accounting for social risk factors in Medicare payment*. Washington, DC: The National Academies Press.

NASEM. 2019. *Integrating social care into the delivery of health care: Moving upstream to improve the nation's health*. Washington, DC: The National Academies Press.

Naylor, M. D., K. H. Bowles, K. M. McCauley, M. C. Maccoy, G. Maislin, M. V. Pauly, and R. Krakauer. 2013. High-value transitional care: Translation of research into practice. *Journal of Evaluation in Clinical Practice* 19(5):727–733.

Naylor, M. D., K. B. Hirschman, M. P. Toles, O. F. Jarrin, E. Shaid, and M. V. Pauly. 2018. Adaptations of the evidence-based Transitional Care Model in the U.S. *Social Science & Medicine* 213:28–36.

NCBDE (National Certification Board for Diabetes Educators). 2019. *National Certification Board for Diabetes Educators*. www.ncbde.org (accessed September 24, 2019).

NCDHHS (North Carolina Department of Health and Human Services). 2018. *Healthy opportunities pilots fact sheet*. https://files.nc.gov/ncdhhs/SDOH-HealthyOpptys-FactSheet-FINAL-20181114.pdf (accessed November 10, 2019).

NCI (National Cancer Institute). 2011. *NCI dictionary of cancer terms*. https://www.cancer.gov/publications/dictionaries/cancer-terms (accessed October 25, 2019).

NCOA (National Council on Aging). 2019. *Healthy aging facts: Chronic disease*. https://www.ncoa.org/news/resources-for-reporters/get-the-facts/healthy-aging-facts (accessed July 26, 2019).

NCSL (National Conference of State Legislatures). 2019. *Medicaid 1115 waivers by state*. http://www.ncsl.org/research/health/medicaid-1115-waivers-by-state.aspx (accessed November 13, 2019).

Needell, N. J., and N. Mehta-Naik. 2016. Is pet ownership helpful in reducing the risk and severity of geriatric depression? *Geriatrics* 1(4):PMC6371194.

Neill, O. 2003. Some limits of informed consent. *Journal of Medical Ethics* 29(1):4–7.

Nersesian, P. V., H. R. Han, G. Yenokyan, R. S. Blumenthal, M. T. Nolan, M. D. Hladek, and S. L. Szanton. 2018. Loneliness in middle age and biomarkers of systemic inflammation: Findings from Midlife in the United States. *Social Science and Medicine* 209:174–181.

Newman, S. D., C. Li, and J. S. Krause. 2016. Social isolation after spinal cord injury: Indicators from the Longitudinal Aging Study. *Rehabilitation Psychology* 61(4):408–416.

Ng, D. M., and R. W. Jeffery. 2003. Relationships between perceived stress and health behaviors in a sample of working adults. *Health Psychology* 22(6):638–642.

Nicolaisen, M., and K. Thorsen. 2017. What are friends for? Friendships and loneliness over the lifespan—From 18 to 79 years. *International Journal of Aging and Human Development* 84(2):126–158.

NIH (National Institutes of Health). 2014. *Role of community health workers*. https://www.nhlbi.nih.gov/health/educational/healthdisp/role-of-community-health-workers.htm (accessed October 25, 2019).

NIH. 2016. *Effects of pregnenolone on perceived social isolation*. https://clinicaltrials.gov/ct2/show/NCT02826577 (accessed March 28, 2019).

NIH. 2017. *To screen or not to screen? The benefits and harms of screening tests*. https://newsinhealth.nih.gov/2017/03/screen-or-not-screen (accessed July 27, 2019).

NIH. 2019. *NIH public health campaigns*. https://prevention.nih.gov/research-priorities/dissemination-implementation/nih-public-health-campaigns (accessed October 25, 2019).

Nocon, A., and M. G. Pearson. 2000. The roles of friends and neighbors in providing support for older people. *Ageing and Society* 20(3):341–367.

Noel, L., F. Phillips, K. Tossas-Milligan, K. Spear, M. L. Vanderford, R. A. Winn, R. C. Vanderpool, and S. G. Eckhardt. 2019. Community–academic partnerships: Approaches to engagement. *American Society for Clinical Oncology Educational Book* 39:88–95.

Northcott, S., B. Moss, K. Harrison, and K. Hilari. 2016. A systematic review of the impact of stroke on social support and social networks: Associated factors and patterns of change. *Clinical Rehabilitation* 30(8):811–831.

Norton, S., F. E. Matthews, D. E. Barnes, K. Yaffe, and C. Brayne. 2014. Potential for primary prevention of Alzheimer's disease: An analysis of population-based data. *Lancet Neurology* 13(8):788–794.

Nuffield Council on Bioethics. 2009. *Dementia: Ethical issues.* London, UK: Nuffield Council on Bioethics.

NYSDOH (New York State Department of Health). 2002. *Home care curriculum.* https://www.health.ny.gov/professionals/home_care/curriculum/docs/home_care_curriculum.pdf (accessed June 27, 2019).

NYSDOH. 2017. VBP social determinants of health (SDH) and community based organizations (CBOs) informational webinar. https://www.health.ny.gov/health_care/medicaid/redesign/dsrip/vbp_library/docs/2017-08-25_sdh_cbo_slides.pdf (accessed December 19, 2019).

NYSDOH. 2019. Social determinants of health (SDH) and community based organizations (CBOs). https://www.health.ny.gov/health_care/medicaid/redesign/sdh/index.htm (accessed December 19, 2019).

O'Brien, M. A., S. Rogers, G. Jamtvedt, A. D. Oxman, J. Odgaard-Jensen, D. T. Kristoffersen, L. Forsetlund, D. Bainbridge, N. Freemantle, D. A. Davis, R. B. Haynes, and E. L. Harvey. 2007. Educational outreach visits: Effects on professional practice and health care outcomes. *Cochrane Database of Systematic Reviews* 2007(4):CD000409.

Oliveira, V. C., M. L. Ferreira, L. Morso, H. B. Albert, K. M. Refshauge, and P. H. Ferreira. 2015. Patients' perceived level of social isolation affects the prognosis of low back pain. *European Journal of Pain* 19(4):538–545.

Ollonqvist, K., H. Palkeinen, T. Aaltonen, T. Pohjolainen, P. Puukka, K. Hinkka, and S. Pontinen. 2012. Alleviating loneliness among frail older people: Findings from a randomized controlled trial. *International Journal of Mental Health Promotion* 10(2):26–34.

O'Malley, A. S., E. C. Rich, L. Shang, T. Rose, A. Ghosh, D. Poznyak, and D. Peikes. 2019. New approaches to measuring the comprehensiveness of primary care physicians. *Health Services Research* 54(2):356–366.

Omran, A. R. 1971. The epidemiological transition: A theory of the epidemiology of population change. *Millbank Memorial Fund Quarterly* 49(4):509–538.

Ong, A. D., and J. C. Allaire. 2005. Cardiovascular intraindividual variability in later life: The influence of social connectedness and positive emotions. *Psychology and Aging* 20(3):476–485.

Ong, A. D., B. N. Uchino, and E.Wethington. 2016. Loneliness and health in older adults: A mini-review and synthesis. *Gerontology* 62(4):443–449.

Orth-Gomer, K. and J. V. Johnson. 1987. Social network interaction and mortality: A six year follow-up study of a random sample of the Swedish population. *Journal of Chronic Diseases* 40(10):949–957.

Ortman, J. M., V. A. Velkoff, and H. Hogan. 2014. *An aging nation: The older population in the United States.* Current Population Reports, P25-1140. Washington, DC: U.S. Census Bureau.

Pacala, J. T., and B. Yueh. 2012. Hearing deficits in the older patient: "I didn't notice anything." *JAMA* 307(11):1185–1194.

Palmer, A. D., J. T. Newsom, and K. S. Rook. 2016. How does difficulty communicating affect the social relationships of older adults? An exploration using data from a national survey. *Journal of Communication Disorders* 62:131–146.

Pantoja, T., J. M. Grimshaw, N. Colomer, C. Castañon, and J. Leniz Martelli. 2019. Manually-generated reminders delivered on paper: Effects on professional practice and health care outcomes. *Cochrane Database of Systematic Reviews* 2019(12):CD001174.

Pappas, G., S. Queen, W. Hadden, and G. Fisher. 1993. The increasing disparity in mortality between socioeconomic groups in the United States, 1960 and 1986. *New England Journal of Medicine* 329(2):103–109.

Park, S., B. Kim, and Y. Han. 2018. Differential aging in place and depressive symptoms: Interplay among time, income, and senior housing. *Research on Aging* 40(3):207–231.

Park, Y.-J., and I.-H. Park. 2010. Effect of tai chi exercise on loneliness, sleep pattern, and instrumental activities of daily living in elderly women. *Journal of Muscle and Joint Health* 17(2):151–161.

Parry, S. W., C. Bamford, V. Deary, T. L. Finch, J. Gray, C. MacDonald, P. McMeekin, N. J. Sabin, I. N. Steen, S. L. Whitney, and E. M. McColl. 2016. Cognitive–behavioural therapy–based intervention to reduce fear of falling in older people: Therapy development and randomised controlled trial—The Strategies for Increasing InDependence, Confidence and Energy (STRIDE) Study. *Health Technology Assessment* 20(56):1–206.

Parsons, P. L., B. Mezuk, S. Ratliff, and K. L. Lapane. 2011. Subsidized housing, not subsidized health: Health status and fatigue among elders in public housing and other community settings. *Ethnicity & Disease* 21(1):85–90.

Paúl, C., and O. Ribeiro. 2009. Predicting loneliness in old people living in the community. *Reviews in Clinical Gerontology* 19(1):53–60.

Pearl, R. 2014. Kaiser Permanente Northern California: Current experiences with Internet, mobile, and video technologies. *Health Affairs* 33(2):251–257.

Pearson, C. F., C. C. Quinn, S. Loganathan, A. R. Datta, B. B. Mace, and D. C. Grabowski. 2019. The forgotten middle: Many middle-income seniors will have insufficient resources for housing and health care. *Health Affairs* 38(5):851–859.

Peerenboom, L., R. M. Collard, P. Naarding, and H. C. Comijs. 2015. The association between depression and emotional and social loneliness in older persons and the influence of social support, cognitive functioning and personality: A cross-sectional study. *Journal of Affective Disorders* 182:26–31.

Penninkilampi, R., A. N. Casey, M. F. Singh, and H. Brodaty. 2018. The association between social engagement, loneliness, and risk of dementia: A systematic review and meta-analysis. *Journal of Alzheimer's Disease* 66(4):1619–1633.

Perissinotto, C. M., and K. E. Covinsky. 2014. Living alone, socially isolated or lonely—What are we measuring? *Journal of General Internal Medicine* 29(11):1429–1431.

Perissinotto, C. M., I. S. Cenzer, and K. E. Covinsky. 2012. Loneliness in older persons: A predictor of functional decline and death. *Archives of Internal Medicine* 172(14):1078–1083.

Perlman, D., and L. Peplau. 1998. Loneliness. In H. S. Friedman (ed.), *Encyclopedia of Mental Health*, Vol. 2. San Diego, CA: Academic Press. Pp. 571–581.

Perren, K., S. Arber, and K. Davidson. 2003. Men's organisational affiliations in later life: The influence of social class and marital status on informal group membership. *Aging and Society* 23:69–82.

Pescheny, J. V., Y. Pappas, and G. Randhawa. 2018. Facilitators and barriers of implementing and delivering social prescribing services: A systematic review. *BMC Health Services Research* 18(1):86.

Petersen, J., S. Thielke, D. Austin, and J. Kaye. 2016. Phone behaviour and its relationship to loneliness in older adults. *Aging and Mental Health* 20(10):1084–1091.

Pew Research Center. 2017. *Tech adoption climbs among older adults.* http://assets.pewresearch.org/wp-content/uploads/sites/14/2017/05/16170850/PI_2017.05.17_Older-Americans-Tech_FINAL.pdf (accessed June 27, 2019).

Pew Research Center. 2018. *Social media fact sheet.* https://www.pewinternet.org/fact-sheet/social-media (accessed June 27, 2019).

Pew Research Center. 2019a. *Baby boomers retire.* https://www.pewresearch.org/fact-tank/2010/12/29/baby-boomers-retire (accessed July 31, 2019).

Pew Research Center. 2019b. *Mobile fact sheet.* https://www.pewinternet.org/fact-sheet/mobile (accessed October 18, 2019).

PHI. 2018a. *The direct care workforce: 2018 in review.* https://phinational.org/wp-content/uploads/2018/12/Direct-Care-Workforce-Year-in-Review-2018-PHI.pdf (accessed September 27, 2019).

PHI. 2018b. *Savvy social media: 6 lessons from Minnesota and Wisconsin.* https://phinational.org/savvy-social-media-6-lessons-from-minnesota-and-wisconsin (accessed June 27, 2019).

PHI. 2019a. *60 caregiver issues.* https://60caregiverissues.org (accessed June 27, 2019).

PHI. 2019b. *Home health aide nursing assistant training requirements by state.* https://phinational.org/advocacy/home-health-aide-training-requirements-state-2016 (accessed June 27, 2019).

PHI. 2019c. *Nursing assistant training requirements by state.* https://phinational.org/advocacy/nurse-aide-training-requirements-state-2016 (accessed June 27, 2019).

PHI. 2019d. *Personal care aide training requirements.* https://phinational.org/advocacy/personal-care-aide-training-requirements (accessed June 27, 2019).

Pinna, G. 2010. In a mouse model relevant for post-traumatic stress disorder, selective brain steroidogenic stimulants (SBSS) improve behavioral deficits by normalizing allopregnanolone biosynthesis. *Behavioral Pharmacology* 21(5–6):438–450.

Pinquart, M., and S. Sörensen. 2000. Influences of socioeconomic status, social network, and competence on subjective well-being in later life: A meta-analysis. *Psychology and Aging* 15(2):187–224.

Pinquart, M., and S. Sörensen. 2001. Influences on loneliness in older adults: A meta-analysis. *Basic and Applied Social Psychology* 23(4):245–266.

Ploeg, J., M. Markle-Reid, B. Davies, K. Higuchi, W. Gifford, I. Bajnok, H. McConnell, J. Plenderleith, S. Foster, and S. Bookey-Bassett. 2014. Spreading and sustaining best practices for home care of older adults: A grounded theory study. *Implementation Science* 9:162.

Podsakoff, P. M., S. B. MacKenzie, J. Y. Lee, and N. P. Podsakoff. 2003. Common method biases in behavioral research: A critical review of the literature and recommended remedies. *Journal of Applied Psychology* 88(5):879–903.

Polley, M., M. Dixon, K. Pilkington, D. Ridge, N. Herbert, C. Drinkwater, J. Fleming, A. McGregor, M. Bertotti, C. Frostick, D. Hopewell, R. Kimberlee, and L. Pedro. 2016. *Report of the Annual Social Prescribing Network Conference.* London, UK: University of Westminster.

Portacolone, E. 2018. Structural factors of elders' isolation in a high-crime neighborhood: An in-depth perspective. *Public Policy & Aging Report* 27(4):152–155.

Portacolone, E., C. Perissinotto, J. C. Yeh, and S. R. Greysen. 2018. "I feel trapped": The tension between personal and structural factors of social isolation and the desire for social integration among older residents of a high-crime neighborhood. *Gerontologist* 58(1):79–88.

Powell, J., and U. Deetjen. 2019. Characterizing the digital health citizen: Mixed-methods study deriving a new typology. *Journal of Medical Internet Research* 21(3):e11279.

Price, E. L., S. Bereknyei, A. Kuby, W. Levinson, and C. H. Braddock, III. 2012. New elements for informed decision making: A qualitative study of older adults' views. *Patient Education and Counseling* 86(3):335–341.

Price, J., R. Repetti, T. Robles, and J. E. Carroll. 2018. Self-disclosure interacts with positive and negative features of romantic social relationships on telomere length. *Psychosomatic Medicine* 80(3):A146–A147.

Pronk, M., D. J. Deeg, C. Smits, T. G. van Tilburg, D. J. Kuik, J. M. Festen, and S. E. Kramer. 2011. Prospective effects of hearing status on loneliness and depression in older persons: Identification of subgroups. *International Journal of Audiology* 50(12):887–896.

Pronk, M., D. J. Deeg, and S. E. Kramer. 2013. Hearing status in older persons: A significant determinant of depression and loneliness? Results from the Longitudinal Aging Study Amsterdam. *American Journal of Audiology* 22(2):316–320.

Provoost, S., H. M. Lau, J. Ruwaard, and H. Riper. 2017. Embodied conversational agents in clinical psychology: A scoping review. *Journal of Medical Internet Research* 19(5):e151.

Pu, L., W. Moyle, C, Jones, and M. Todorovic. 2019. The effectiveness of social robots for older adults: A systematic review and meta-analysis of randomized controlled studies. *Gerontologist* 59(1):e37–e51.

Public Health England. 2019. *NHS population screening explained.* https://www.gov.uk/guidance/nhs-population-screening-explained (accessed August 13, 2019).

Puljak, L. 2016. Using social media for knowledge translation, promotion of evidence-based medicine and high-quality information on health. *Journal of Evidence-Based Medicine* 9(1):4–7.

Putnam, R. D. 2001. *Bowling alone: The collapse and revival of American community.* New York: Simon & Schuster.

Puvill, T., S. Kusumastuti, R. Lund, E. L. Mortensen, J. Slaets, J. Lindenberg, and R. G. J. Westendorp. 2019. Do psychosocial factors modify the negative association between disability and life satisfaction in old age? *PLOS ONE* 14(10):e0224421.

Qualter, P., J. Vanhalst, R. Harris, E. Van Roekel, G. Lodder, M. Bangee, M. Maes, and M. Verhagen. 2015. Loneliness across the life span. *Perspectives on Psychological Science* 10(2):250–264.

Quine, S., Y. Wells, D. de Vaus, and H. Kendig. 2007. When choice in retirement decisions is missing: Qualitative and quantitative findings of impact on well-being. *Australasian Journal on Ageing* 26(4):173–179.

Quirke, E., H. H. Konig, and A. Hajek. 2019. Association between caring for grandchildren and feelings of loneliness, social isolation and social network size: A cross-sectional study of community dwelling adults in Germany. *BMJ Open* 9(12):e029605.

Rabin, B. A., and R. C. Brownson. 2018. Terminology for dissemination and implementation research. In R. C. Brownson, G. A. Colditz, and E. K. Proctor (eds.), *Dissemination and implementation research in health: Translating science to practice*. New York: Oxford University Press. Pp. 20–45.

Raina, P., D. Waltner-Toews, B. Bonnett, C. Woodward, and T. Abernathy. 1999. Influence of companion animals on the physical and psychological health of older people: An analysis of a one-year longitudinal study. *Journal of the American Geriatrics Society* 47(3):323–329.

Ramage-Morin, P. L. 2016. Hearing difficulties and feelings of social isolation among Canadians aged 45 or older. *Health Reports* 27(11):3–12.

Ramage-Morin, P. L., and H. Gilmour. 2013. Urinary incontinence and loneliness in Canadian seniors. *Health Reports* 24(10):3–10.

Ramos, A. K., D. Su, L. Lander, and R. Rivera. 2015. Stress factors contributing to depression among Latino migrant farmworkers in Nebraska. *Journal of Immigrant & Minority Health* 17(6):1627–1634.

Ratnapradipa, K. L., J. Wang, M. Berg-Weger, and M. Schootman. 2018. Coming out of "retirement"—Predictors of driving resumption among older drivers. *Innovation in Aging* 2(3):1–10.

Redfoot, D. L., and A. Kochera. 2005. Targeting services to those most at risk: Characteristics of residents in federally subsidized housing. *Journal of Housing for the Elderly* 18(3-4):137–163.

Redfoot, D., L. Feinberg, and A. Houser. 2013. *The aging of the baby boom and the growing care gap: A look at future declines in the availability of family caregivers*. Washington, DC: AARP Public Policy Institute.

Reid, L., W. Lahey, B. Livingstone, and M. McNally. 2018. Ethical and legal implications of frailty screening. *Journal of Frailty and Aging* 7(4):224–232.

Reiners, F., J. Sturm, L. J. W. Bouw, and E. J. M. Wouters. 2019. Sociodemographic factors influencing the use of eHealth in people with chronic diseases. *International Journal of Environmental Research and Public Health* 16(4):E645.

Reisberg, B., S. H. Ferris, M. J. de Leon, and T. Crook. 1982. The global deterioration scale for assessment of primary degenerative dementia. *American Journal of Psychiatry* 139(9):1136–1139.

Rejeski, W. J., A. Thompson, P. H. Brubaker, and H. S. Miller. 1992. Acute exercise: Buffering psychosocial stress responses in women. *Health Psychology* 11(6):355–362.

Rendall, M. S., M. M. Weden, M. M. Favreault, and H. Waldron. 2011. The protective effect of marriage for survival: A review and update. *Demography* 48(2):481–506.

Repke, M. A., and C. Ipsen. 2020. Differences in social connectedness and perceived isolation among rural and urban adults with disabilities. *Disability and Health Journal* 13(1):100829.

Ribu, L., and A. Wahl. 2004. Living with diabetic foot ulcers: A life of fear, restrictions, and pain. *Ostomy Wound Management* 50(2):57–67.

Richard, A., S. Rohrmann, C. L. Vandeleur, M. Schmid, J. Barth, and M. Eichholzer. 2017. Loneliness is adversely associated with physical and mental health and lifestyle factors: Results from a Swiss national survey. *PLOS ONE* 12(7):e0181442.

Richter, A., U. von Thiele Schwarz, C. Lornudd, R. Lundmark, R. Mosson, and H. Hasson. 2016. iLead—A transformational leadership intervention to train healthcare managers' implementation leadership. *Implementation Science* 11(1):108.

Rico-Uribe, L. A., F. F. Caballero, N. Martin-Maria, M. Cabello, J. L. Ayuso-Mateos, and M. Miret. 2018. Association of loneliness with all-cause mortality: A meta-analysis. *PLOS ONE* 13(1):e0190033.

Riffin, C., P. H. Van Ness, J. L. Wolff, and T. Fried. 2019. Multifactorial examination of caregiver burden in a national sample of family and unpaid caregivers. *Journal of the American Geriatric Society* 67(2):277–283.

Rijnaard, M. D., J. van Hoof, B. M. Janssen, H. Verbeek, W. Pocornie, A. Eijkelenboom, H. C. Beerens, S. L. Molony, and E. J. Wouters. 2016. The factors influencing the sense of home in nursing homes: A systematic review from the perspective of residents. *Journal of Aging Research* 2016:6143645.

Riley, B. L., C. D. Willis, B. Holmes, D. T. Finegood, A. Best, and J. D. McIsaac. 2018. Systems thinking and dissemination and implementation research. In R. C. Brownson, G. A. Colditz, and E. K. Proctor (eds.), *Dissemination and implementation research in health: Translating science to practice, 2nd ed.* New York: Oxford University Press. Pp. 143–155.

Rim, T. H., A. W. J. Teo, H. H. S. Yang, C. Y. Cheung, and T. Y. Wong. 2020. Retinal vascular signs and cerebrovascular diseases. *Journal of Neuro-Ophthalmology* 40(1):44–59.

Ris, I., W. Schnepp, and R. Mahrer Imhof. 2019. An integrative review on family caregivers' involvement in care of home-dwelling elderly. *Health & Social Care in the Community* 27(3):e95–e111.

Rizvi, M. A. K., and M. Z. Hossain. 2017. Relationship between religious belief and happiness: A systematic literature review. *Journal of Religion and Health* 56(5):1561–1582.

Robinaugh, D. J., N. J. LeBlanc, H. A. Vuletich, and R. J. McNally. 2014. Network analysis of persistent complex bereavement disorder in conjugally bereaved adults. *Journal of Abnormal Psychology* 123(3):510–522.

Robins, L. M., K. D. Hill, C. F. Finch, L. Clemson, and T. Haines. 2018. The association between physical activity and social isolation in community-dwelling older adults. *Aging and Mental Health* 22(2):175–182.

Robinson, H., B. MacDonald, N. Kerse, and E. Broadbent. 2013. The psychosocial effects of a companion robot: A randomized controlled trial. *Journal of the American Medical Directors Association* 14(9):661–667.

Robles, T. F. 2014. Marital quality and health: Implications for marriage in the 21st century. *Current Directions in Psychological Science* 23(6):427–432.

Robles, T. F., and J. K. Kiecolt-Glaser. 2003. The physiology of marriage: Pathways to health. *Physiology & Behavior* 79(3):409–416.

Robles, T. F., R. B. Slatcher, J. M. Trombello, and M. M. McGinn. 2014. Marital quality and health: A meta-analytic review. *Psychological Bulletin* 140(1):140–187.

Roelfs, D. J., E. Shor, M. Curreli, L. Clemow, M. M. Burg, and J. E. Schwartz. 2012. Widowhood and mortality: A meta-analysis and meta-regression. *Demography* 49(2):575–606.

Rogers, E. M. 2003. *Diffusion of innovations, 5th ed.* New York: The Free Press.

Rokach, A. 1996. The subjectivity of loneliness and coping with it. *Psychological Reports* 79(2):475–481.

Roland, D. 2018. Social media, health policy, and knowledge translation. *Journal of the American College of Radiology* 15(1 Pt B):149–152.

Rook, K. S., and S. T. Charles. 2017. Close social ties and health in later life: Strengths and vulnerabilities. *American Psychologist* 72(6):567–577.

Rosenberg, P. B., M. A. Nowrangi, and C. G. Lyketsos. 2015. Neuropsychiatric symptoms in Alzheimer's disease: What might be associated brain circuits? *Molecular Aspects of Medicine* 43-44:25–37.

Rosenquist, J. N., J. Murabito, J. H. Fowler, and N. A. Christakis. 2010. The spread of alcohol consumption behavior in a large social network. *Annals of Internal Medicine* 152(7):426–433.

Rote, S., T. D. Hill, and C. G. Ellison. 2013. Religious attendance and loneliness in later life. *Gerontologist* 53(1):39–50.

Rouxel, P., A. Heilmann, P. Demakakos, J. Aida, G. Tsakos, and R. G. Watt. 2017. Oral health–related quality of life and loneliness among older adults. *European Journal of Ageing* 14(2):101–109.

Rueda, S., S. Law, and S. B. Rourke. 2014. Psychosocial, mental health, and behavioral issues of aging with HIV. *Current Opinion in HIV and AIDS* 9(4):325–331.

Russell, C., A. Campbell, and I. Hughes. 2008. Ageing, social capital and the Internet: Findings from an exploratory study of Australian "silver surfers." *Australasian Journal on Ageing* 27(2):78–82.

Russell, D. W. 1996. UCLA Loneliness Scale (version 3): Reliability, validity, and factor structure. *Journal of Personality Assessment* 66(1):20–40.

Russell, D., L. A. Peplau, and C. E. Cutrona. 1980. The revised UCLA Loneliness Scale: Concurrent and discriminant validity evidence. *Journal of Personality and Social Psychology* 39(3):472–480.

Ruwanpathirana, T., A. Owen, and C. M. Reid. 2015. Review on cardiovascular risk prediction. *Cardiovascular Therapeutics* 33(2):62–70.

RWJF (Robert Wood Johnson Foundation). 2010. *A new way to talk about the social determinants of health.* https://www.rwjf.org/en/library/research/2010/01/a-new-way-to-talk-about-the-social-determinants-of-health.html (accessed September 27, 2019).

Saczynski, J. S., L. A. Pfeifer, K. Masaki, E. S. Korf, D. Laurin, L. White, and L. J. Launer. 2006. The effect of social engagement on incident dementia: The Honolulu–Asia Aging Study. *American Journal of Epidemiology* 163(5):433–440.

Sakai, Y., Y. Nonaka, Y. I. Nakano, and K. Yasuda. 2012. Listener agent for elderly people with dementia. In *Proceedings of the Seventh Annual ACM/IEEE International Conference on Human–Robot Interaction.* Pp. 199–200.

Salari, S. M., and M. Rich. 2001. Social and environmental infantilization of aged persons: Observations in two adult day care centers. *International Journal of Aging & Human Development* 52(2):115–134.

Salinas, J., A. Beiser, J. J. Himali, C. L. Satizabal, H. J. Aparicio, G. Weinstein, F. J. Mateen, L. F. Berkman, J. Rosand, and S. Seshadri. 2017. Associations between social relationship measures, serum brain-derived neurotrophic factor, and risk of stroke and dementia. *Alzheimer's and Dementia* 3(2):229–237.

Sanders, A. E., J. Nininger, J. Absher, A. Bennett, S. Shugarman, and R. Roca. 2017. Quality improvement in neurology: Dementia management quality measurement set update. *American Journal of Psychiatry* 174(5):493–498.

Santini, S., G. Andersson, and G. Lamura. 2016. Impact of incontinence on the quality of life of caregivers of older persons with incontinence: A qualitative study in four European countries. *Archives of Gerontology and Geriatrics* 63:92–101.

Saulsberry, A., M. Marko-Holguin, K. Blomeke, C. Hinkle, J. Fogel, T. Gladstone, C. Bell, M. Reinecke, M. Corden, and B. W. Van Voorhees. 2013. Randomized clinical trial of a primary care internet-based intervention to prevent adolescent depression: One-year outcomes. *Journal of the Canadian Academy of Child and Adolescent Psychiatry* 22(2):106–117.

Saxon, S. V., M. J. Etten, and E. A. Perkins. 2015. *Physical change and aging, sixth edition:A guide for the helping professions.* New York: Springer.

Schaap, R., A. de Wind, P. Coenen, K. Proper, and C. Boot. 2018. The effects of exit from work on health across different socioeconomic groups: A systematic literature review. *Social Science & Medicine* 198:36–45.

Schiaffino, S., and A. Amandi. 2009. Building an expert travel agent as a software agent. *Expert Systems With Applications* 36(2):1291–1299.

Schneider, J. M., B. Gopinath, C. M. McMahon, S. R. Leeder, P. Mitchell, and J. J. Wang. 2011. Dual sensory impairment in older age. *Journal of Aging & Health* 23(8):1309–1324.

Schoenbach, V. J., B. H. Kaplan, L. Fredman, and D. G. Kleinbaum. 1986. Social ties and mortality in Evans County, Georgia. *American Journal of Epidemiology* 123(4):577–591.

Schrempft, S., M. Jackowska, M. Hamer, and A. Steptoe. 2019. Associations between social isolation, loneliness, and objective physical activity in older men and women. *BMC Public Health* 19(1):74.

Schutter, N., T. J. Holwerda, M. L. Stek, J. J. Dekker, D. Rhebergen, and H. C. Comijs. 2017. Loneliness in older adults is associated with diminished cortisol output. *Journal of Psychosomatic Research* 95:19–25.

Schwarzbach, M., M. Luppa, S. Forstmeier, H.-H. König, and S. G. Riedel-Heller. 2014. Social relations and depression in late life—A systematic review. *International Journal of Geriatric Psychiatry* 29(1):1–21.

Scott, J. 1988. Trend report: Social network analysis. *Sociology* 22(1):109–127.

Seeman, M., and C. S. Anderson. 1983. Alienation and alcohol: The role of work, mastery, and community in drinking behavior. *American Sociological Review* 48(1):60–77.

Segel-Karpas, D., L. Ayalon, and M. E. Lachman. 2018. Loneliness and depressive symptoms: The moderating role of the transition into retirement. *Aging & Mental Health* 22(1):135–140.

Serra, M., M. G. Pisu, M. Littera, G. Papi, E. Sanna, F. Tuveri, L. Usala, R. H. Purdy, and G. Biggio. 2000. Social isolation-induced decreases in both the abundance of neuroactive steroids and GABA(A) receptor function in rat brain. *Journal of Neurochemistry* 75(2):732–740.

Shankar, A., A. McMunn, J. Banks, and A. Steptoe. 2011. Loneliness, social isolation, and behavioral and biological health indicators in older adults. *Health Psychology* 30(4):377–385.

Shankar, A., M. Hamer, A. McMunn, and A. Steptoe. 2013. Social isolation and loneliness: Relationships with cognitive function during 4 years of follow-up in the English Longitudinal Study of Ageing. *Psychosomatic Medicine* 75(2):161–170.

Sharkey, A., and N. Sharkey. 2012. Granny and the robots: Ethical issues in robot care for the elderly. *Ethics and Information Technology* 14(1):27–40.

Shaw, J. G., M. Farid, C. Noel-Miller, N. Joseph, A. Houser, S. M. Asch, J. Bhattacharya, and L. Flowers. 2017. Social isolation and Medicare spending: Among older adults, objective isolation increases expenditures while loneliness does not. *Journal of Aging and Health* 29(7):1119–1143.

Shelton, R. C., R. E. Goldman, K. M. Emmons, G. Sorensen, and J. D. Allen. 2011. An investigation into the social context of low-income, urban black and Latina women: Implications for adherence to recommended health behaviors. *Health Education & Behavior* 38(5):471–481.

Shever, L. L., M. G. Titler, M. L. Mackin, and A. Kueny. 2011. Fall prevention practices in adult medical–surgical nursing units described by nurse managers. *Western Journal of Nursing Research* 33(3):385–397.

Shiells, K., L. Pivodic, I. Holmerová, and L. Van den Block. 2019. Self-reported needs and experiences of people with dementia living in nursing homes: A scoping review. *Aging and Mental Health* June 4:1–16 [Epub ahead of print].

Shiovitz-Ezra, S., and S. A. Leitsch. 2010. The role of social relationships in predicting loneliness: The National Social Life, Health, and Aging Project. *Social Work Research* 34(3):157–167.

Shiu, C., A. Muraco, and K. Fredriksen-Goldsen. 2016. Invisible care: Friend and partner care among older lesbian, gay, bisexual, and transgender (LGBT) adults. *Journal for the Society for Social Work and Research* 7(3):527–546.

Shor, E., and D. J. Roelfs. 2015. Social contact frequency and all-cause mortality: A meta-analysis and meta-regression. *Social Science & Medicine* 128:76–86.

Shuman, C. J., X. Liu, M. L. Aebersold, D. Tschannen, J. Banaszak-Holl, and M. G. Titler. 2018a. Associations among unit leadership and unit climates for implementation in acute care: A cross-sectional study. *Implementation Science* 13(1):62–72.

Shuman, C. J., X. J. Xie, K. A. Herr, and M. G. Titler. 2018b. Sustainability of evidence-based acute pain management practices for hospitalized older adults. *Western Journal of Nursing Research* 40(12):1749–1764.

Shuman, C. J., K. Powers, J. Banaszak-Holl, and M. G. Titler. 2019. Unit leadership and climates for evidence-based practice implementation in acute care: A cross-sectional descriptive study. *Journal of Nursing Scholarship* 51(1):114–124.

Sibbald, B., and J. M. Holroyd-Leduc. 2012. Protecting our most vulnerable elders from abuse. *Canadian Medical Association Journal* 184(16):1763.

Sivam, A., K. E. Wroblewski, G. Alkorta-Aranburu, L. L. Barnes, R. S. Wilson, D. A. Bennett, and J. M. Pinto. 2016. Olfactory dysfunction in older adults is associated with feelings of depression and loneliness. *Chemical Senses* 41(4):293–299.

Slavich, G. M., and S. W. Cole. 2013. The emerging field of human social genomics. *Clinical Psychological Science* 1(3):331–348.

Smith, S. G., R. O'Conor, W. Aitken, L. M. Curtis, M. S. Wolf, and M. S. Goel. 2015. Disparities in registration and use of an online patient portal among older adults: Findings from the LitCog cohort. *Journal of the American Medical Informatics Association* 22(4):888–895.

Smith, T. W., and K. D. Jordan. 2015. Interpersonal motives and social-evaluative threat: Effects of acceptance and status stressors on cardiovascular reactivity and salivary cortisol response. *Psychophysiology* 52(2):269–276.

Snelling, S. 2019. *Can public awareness campaigns convince people to care about aging?* https://strianews.com/can-public-awareness-campaigns-convince-people-to-care-about-aging (accessed September 27, 2019).

Soler, M. V., L. Agüera-Ortiz, J. O. Rodríguez, C. M. Rebolledo, A. P. Muñoz, I. R. Pérez, E. O. Ruiz, A. B. Sánchez, V. H. Cano, L. C. Chillón, S. F. Ruiz, J. L. Alvarez, B. L. Salas, J. M. C. Plaza, F. M. Rico, G. A. Dago, and P. M. Martín. 2015. Social robots in advanced dementia. *Frontiers in Aging Neuroscience* 7:133.

Soper, M. H. 2017. *Providing value-added services for Medicare–Medicaid enrollees: Considerations for integrated health plans.* https://www.chcs.org/media/PRIDE-Value-Added-Services_012617.pdf (accessed November 10, 2019).

Sorell, T., and H. Draper. 2014. Robot carers, ethics, and older people. *Ethics and Information Technology* 16(3):183–195.

South, J., T. J. Higgins, J. Woodall, and S. M. White. 2008. Can social prescribing provide the missing link? *Primary Health Care Research & Development* 9(4):310–318.

Spahni, S., D. Morselli, P. Perrig-Chiello, and K. M. Bennett. 2015. Patterns of psychological adaptation to spousal bereavement in old age. *Gerontology* 61(5):456–468.

Sparrow, R., and L. Sparrow. 2006. In the hands of machines? The future of aged care. *Minds and Machines* 16(2):141–161.

Spitzer, S. B., M. M. Llabre, G. H. Ironson, M. D. Gellman, and N. Schneiderman. 1992. The influence of social situations on ambulatory blood pressure. *Psychosomatic Medicine* 54(1):79–86.

Squires, J. E., I. D. Graham, A. M. Hutchinson, S. Michie, J. J. Francis, A. Sales, J. Brehaut, J. Curran, N. Ivers, J. Lavis, S. Linklater, S. Fenton, T. Noseworthy, J. Vine, and J. M. Grimshaw. 2015. Identifying the domains of context important to implementation science: A study protocol. *Implementation Science* 10(1):135.

Stacey, D., F. Légaré, K. Lewis, M. J. Barry, C. L. Bennett, K. B. Eden, M. Holmes-Rovner, H. Llewellyn-Thomas, A. Lyddiatt, R. Thomson, and L. Trevena. 2017. Decision aids for people facing health treatment or screening decisions. *Cochrane Database of Systematic Reviews* 2017(4):CD001431.

Stack, S. 1998. Marriage, family and loneliness: A cross-national study. *Sociological Perspectives* 41(2):415–432.

Stahl, S. T., A. M. Arnold, J. Y. Chen, S. Anderson, and R. Schulz. 2016. Mortality after bereavement: The role of cardiovascular disease and depression. *Psychosomatic Medicine* 78(6):697–703.

Stanley, I. H., Y. Conwell, C. Bowen, and K. A. Van Orden. 2014. Pet ownership may attenuate loneliness among older adult primary care patients who live alone. *Aging & Mental Health* 18(3):394–399.

Statista. 2020. *Share of adults in the United States who use the Internet in 2019, by age group.* https://www.statista.com/statistics/266587/percentage-of-internet-users-by-age-groups-in-the-us (accessed January 2, 2020).

Steele, I. H., N. Thrower, P. Noroian, and F. M. Saleh. 2018. Understanding suicide across the lifespan: A United States perspective of suicide risk factors, assessment and management. *Journal of Forensic Sciences* 63(1):162–171.

Steensma, J. T., M. W. Kreuter, C. M. Casey, and J. M. Bernhardt. 2018. Enhancing dissemination through marketing and distribution systems: A vision for public health. In R. C. Brownson, G. A. Colditz, and E. K. Proctor (eds.), *Dissemination and implementation research in health: Translating science to practice, 2nd ed.* New York: Oxford University Press. Pp. 191–200.

Steptoe, A., K. Lundwall, and M. Cropley. 2000. Gender, family structure and cardiovascular activity during the working day and evening. *Social Science & Medicine* 50(4):531–539.

Steptoe, A., N. Owen, S. R. Kunz-Ebrecht, and L. Brydon. 2004. Loneliness and neuroendocrine, cardiovascular, and inflammatory stress responses in middle-aged men and women. *Psychoneuroendocrinology* 29(5):593–611.

Steptoe, A., A. Shankar, P. Demakakos, and J. Wardle. 2013. Social isolation, loneliness, and all-cause mortality in older men and women. *Proceedings of the National Academy of Sciences* 110(15):5797–5801.

Stern, Y. 2012. Cognitive reserve in ageing and Alzheimer's disease. *Lancet Neurology* 11(11):1006–1012.

Stetler, C. B., J. A. Ritchie, J. Rycroft-Malone, A. A. Schultz, and M. P. Charns. 2009. Institutionalizing evidence-based practice: An organizational case study using a model of strategic change. *Implementation Science* 4(1):78.

Stewart, M., D. Craig, K. MacPherson, and S. Alexander. 2001. Promoting positive affect and diminishing loneliness of widowed seniors through a support intervention. *Public Health Nursing* 18(1):54–63.

Stickley, A., A. Koyanagi, B. Roberts, E. Richardson, P. Abbott, S. Tumanov, and M. McKee. 2013. Loneliness: Its correlates and association with health behaviours and outcomes in nine countries of the former Soviet Union. *PLOS ONE* 8(7):e67978.

Stickley, A., Z. I. Santini, and A. Koyanagi. 2017. Urinary incontinence, mental health and loneliness among community-dwelling older adults in Ireland. *BMC Urology* 17(1):29.

Stimson, R. J., and R. McCrea. 2004. A push–pull framework for modelling the relocation of retirees to a retirement village: The Australian experience. *Environment and Planning A* 36(8): 1451–1470.

Stirman, S. W., and J. W. Dearing. 2019. Sustainability of cancer practices and programs. In D. A. Chambers, C. A. Vinson, and W. E. Norton (eds.), *Advancing the science of implementation across the cancer continuum*. New York: Oxford University Press. Pp. 312–329.

Stokes, J. P. 1985. The relation of social network and individual difference variables to loneliness. *Journal of Personality and Social Psychology* 48(4):981–990.

Stover, S. 2018. *Reaching rural America with broadband internet service.* https://theconversation.com/reaching-rural-america-with-broadband-internet-service-82488 (accessed June 27, 2019).

Strassner, C., E. Frick, G. Stotz-Ingenlath, N. Buhlinger-Göpfarth, J. Scezcsenyi, J. Krisam, F. Schalhorn, J. Valentini, R. Stolz, and S. Joos. 2019. Holistic care program for elderly patients to integrate spiritual needs, social activity, self-care into disease management in primary care (HoPES3): Study protocol for a cluster-randomized trial. *Trials* 20(1):364.

Straus, S. E., W. S. Richardson, P. Glasziou, and R. B. Haynes. 2010. *Evidence-based medicine: How to practice and teach it, 4th ed.* New York: Elsevier.

Strawbridge, W. J., M. I. Wallhagen, S. J. Shema, and G. A. Kaplan. 2000. Negative consequences of hearing impairment in old age: A longitudinal analysis. *Gerontologist* 40(3):320–326.

Strawbridge, W. J., S. J. Shema, R. D. Cohen, and G. A. Kaplan. 2001. Religious attendance increases survival by improving and maintaining good health behaviors, mental health, and social relationships. *Annals of Behavioral Medicine* 23(1):68–74.

Strawbridge, W. J., M. I. Wallhagen, and S. J. Shema. 2007. Impact of spouse vision impairment on partner health and well-being: A longitudinal analysis of couples. *Journals of Gerontology, Series B: Psychological Sciences and Social Sciences* 62(5):S315–S322.

Sum, S., R. M. Mathews, I. Hughes, and A. Campbell. 2008. Internet use and loneliness in older adults. *CyberPsychology and Behavior* 11(2):208–211.

Sung, Y. K., L. Li, C. Blake, J. Betz, and F. R. Lin. 2016. Association of hearing loss and loneliness in older adults. *Journal of Aging and Health* 28(6):979–994.

Sutherland Shire Council. 2018. *Council combats loneliness.* http://www.sutherlandshire.nsw.gov.au/Council/News-and-Publications/News/Council-Combats-Loneliness (accessed November 10, 2019).

Sving, E., L. Gunningberg, M. Högman, and A. G. Mamhidir. 2012. Registered nurses' attention to and perceptions of pressure ulcer prevention in hospital settings. *Journal of Clinical Nursing* 21(9–10):1293–1303.

Syme, S. L. 1974. Behavioral factors associated with the etiology of physical disease: A social epidemiological approach. *American Journal of Public Health* 64(11):1043–1045.

Szanton, S. L., Q. L. Xue, B. Leff, J. Guralnik, J. L. Wolff, E. K. Tanner, C. Boyd, R. J. Thorpe, Jr., D. Bishai, and L. N. Gitlin. 2019. Effect of a biobehavioral environmental approach on disability among low-income older adults: A randomized clinical trial. *JAMA Internal Medicine* 179(2):204–211.

Szreter, S. 1988. The importance of social intervention in Britain's mortality decline c.1850–1914: A re-interpretation of the role of public health. *Social History of Medicine* 1:1–37.

Szreter, S. 1997. Economic growth, disruption, deprivation, disease, and death: On the importance of the politics of public health for development. *Population and Development Review* 23(4):693–728.

Szreter, S. 2000. Social capital, the economy, and education in historical perspective. In *Social capital: Critical perspectives*. New York: Oxford University Press.

Taipale, S., J. Vincent, B. Sapio, G. Lugano, and L. Fortunati. 2015. Introduction: Situating the human in social robots. In J. Vincent, S. Taipale, B. Sapio, G. Lugano, and L. Fortunati (eds.), *Social robots from a human perspective*. Dordrecht, Netherlands: Springer. Pp. 1–7.

Takagi, E., and Y. Saito. 2019. Japanese older adults' loneliness, family relationships and mortality: Does one's living arrangement make a difference? *Geriatrics & Gerontology International* 20(2):156–160.

Tanaka, M., A. Ishii, E. Yamano, H. Ogikubo, M. Okazaki, K. Kamimura, Y. Konishi, S. Emoto, and Y. Watanabe. 2012. Effect of a human-type communication robot on cognitive function in elderly women living alone. *Medical Science Monitor* 18(9):CR550–CR557.

Tanne, D., U. Goldbourt, and J. H. Medalie. 2004. Perceived family difficulties and prediction of 23-year stroke mortality among middle-aged men. *Cerebrovascular Disease* 18(4):277–282.

Tanskanen, J., and T. Anttila. 2016. A prospective study of social isolation, loneliness, and mortality in Finland. *American Journal of Public Health* 106(11):2042–2048.

Taylor, H. O., R. J. Taylor, A. W. Nguyen, and L. Chatters. 2018a. Social isolation, depression, and psychological distress among older adults. *Journal of Aging and Health* 30(2):229–246.

Taylor, H. O., Y. Wang, and N. Morrow-Howell. 2018b. Loneliness in senior housing communities. *Journal of Gerontological Social Work* 61(6):623–639.

Taylor, J. L., L. Roberts, M. D. Hladek, M. Liu, M. Nkimbeng, C. M. Boyd, and S. L. Szanton. 2019. Achieving self-management goals among low income older adults with functional limitations. *Geriatric Nursing* 40(4):424–430.

Taylor, R. J., L. M. Chatters, A. T. Woodward, and E. Brown. 2013. Racial and ethnic differences in extended family, friendship, fictive kin and congregational informal support networks. *Family Relations* 62(4):609–624.

Teerawichitchainan, B., W. Pothisiri, and G. T. Long. 2015. How do living arrangements and intergenerational support matter for psychological health of elderly parents? Evidence from Myanmar, Vietnam, and Thailand. *Social Science & Medicine* (136–137):106–116.

Teo, A. R., R. Lerrigo, and M. A. M. Rogers. 2013a. The role of social isolation in social anxiety disorder: A systematic review and meta-analysis. *Journal of Anxiety Disorders* 27(4):353–364.

Teo, A. R., H. Choi, and M. Valenstein. 2013b. Social relationships and depression; Ten-year follow-up from a nationally representative study. *PLOS ONE* 8(4):e62396.

Teo, A. R., H. Choi, S. B. Andrea, M. Valenstein, J. T. Newsom, S. K. Dobscha, and K. Zivin. 2015. Does mode of contact with different types of social relationships predict depression in older adults? Evidence from a nationally representative survey. *Journal of the American Geriatrics Society* 63(10):2014–2022.

TFAH (Trust for America's Health). 2020. *Age-friendly public health studies*. https://www.tfah.org/story/age-friendly-case-studies (accessed January 2, 2020).

Theeke, L. A. 2009. Predictors of loneliness in U.S. adults over age sixty-five. *Archives of Psychiatric Nursing* 23(5):387–396.

Theeke, L. A. 2010. Sociodemographic and health-related risks for loneliness and outcome differences by loneliness status in a sample of U.S. older adults. *Research in Gerontological Nursing* 3(2):113–125.

Thoits, P. A. 1995. Stress, coping, and social support processes: Where are we? What next? *Journal of Health and Social Behavior* (extra issue):53–79.

Tian, Q. 2016. Intergeneration social support affects the subjective well-being of the elderly: Mediator roles of self-esteem and loneliness. *Journal of Health Psychology* 21(6):1137–1144.

Tibblin, G., K. Svardsudd, L. Welin, and B. Larsson. 1986. The theory of general susceptibility. In S. O. Isacsson and L. Janzon (eds.), *Social support: Health and disease*. Stockholm, Sweden: Almqvist and Wiksell. Pp. 11–19.

Tilvis, R. S., M. H. Kähönen-Vare, J. Jolkkonen, J. Valvanne, K. H. Pitkala, and T. E. Strandberg. 2004. Predictors of cognitive decline and mortality of aged people over a 10-year period. *Journals of Gerontology, Series A: Biological Sciences and Medical Sciences* 59(3):268–274.

Tisminetzky, M., J. Gurwitz, D. D. McManus, J. S. Saczynski, N. Erskine, M. E. Waring, M. Anatchkova, H. Awad, D. C. Parish, D. Lessard, C. Kiefe, and R. Goldberg. 2016. Multiple chronic conditions and psychosocial limitations in patients hospitalized with an acute coronary syndrome. *American Journal of Medicine* 129(6):608–614.

Titler, M. G. 2010. Translation science and context. *Research and Theory for Nursing Practice* 24(1):35–55.

Titler, M. G. 2014. Overview of evidence-based practice and translation science. *Nursing Clinics of North America* 49(3):269–274.

Titler, M. G. 2018. Developing an evidence-based practice. In G. LoBiondo-Wood and J. Haber (eds.), *Nursing research: Methods and critical appraisal for evidence-based practice, 9th ed.* Philadelphia, PA: Elsevier. Pp. 383–405.

Titler, M. G., and C. Anderson. 2019. Implementation strategies for stakeholders. In G. LoBiondo-Wood, J. Haber, and M. G. Titler (eds.), *Evidence-based practice for nursing and healthcare quality improvement.* Philadelphia, PA: Elsevier. Pp. 206–218.

Titler, M. G., and L. Q. Everett. 2001. Translating research into practice: Considerations for critical care investigators. *Critical Care Nursing Clinics of North America* 13(4):587–604.

Titler, M. G., K. Herr, J. M. Brooks, X. J. Xie, G. Ardery, M. L. Schilling, J. L. Marsh, L. Q. Everett, and W. R. Clarke. 2009. Translating research into practice intervention improves management of acute pain in older hip fracture patients. *Health Services Research* 44(1):264–287.

Titler, M. G., P. Conlon, M. A. Reynolds, R. Ripley, A. Tsodikov, D. S. Wilson, and M. Montie. 2016. The effect of a translating research into practice intervention to promote use of evidence-based fall prevention interventions in hospitalized adults: A prospective pre–post implementation study in the U.S. *Applied Nursing Research* 31:52–59.

Tonetti, M. S., P. Bottenberg, G. Conrads, P. Eickholz, P. Heasman, M. C. Huysmans, R. Lopez, P. Madianos, F. Muller, I. Needleman, B. Nyvad, P. M. Preshaw, I. Pretty, S. Renvert, F. Schwendicke, L. Trombelli, G. J. van der Putten, J. Vanobbergen, N. West, A. Young, and S. Paris. 2017. Dental caries and periodontal diseases in the ageing population: Call to action to protect and enhance oral health and well-being as an essential component of healthy ageing—Consensus report of group 4 of the joint EFP/ORCA workshop on the boundaries between caries and periodontal diseases. *Journal of Clinical Periodontology* 44(Suppl 18):S135–S144.

Tong, S. T., W. R. Liaw, P. L. Kashiri, J. Pecsok, J. Rozman, A. W. Bazemore, and A. H. Krist. 2018. Clinician experiences with screening for social needs in primary care. *Journal of the American Board of Family Medicine* 31(3):351–363.

Toohey, A. M., G. R. McCormack, P. K. Doyle-Baker, C. L. Adams, and M. J. Rock. 2013. Dog-walking and sense of community in neighborhoods: Implications for promoting regular physical activity in adults 50 years and older. *Health Place* 22:75–81.

Tricco, A. C., H. M. Ashoor, R. Cardoso, H. MacDonald, E. Cogo, M. Kastner, L. Perrier, A. McKibbon, J. M. Grimshaw, and S. E. Straus. 2016. Sustainability of knowledge translation interventions in healthcare decision-making: A scoping review. *Implementation Science* 11:55.

Troya, M. I., O. Babatunde, K. Polidano, B. Bartlam, E. McCloskey, L. Dikomitis, and C. A. Chew-Graham. 2019. Self-harm in older adults: Systematic review. *British Journal of Psychiatry* 214(4):186–200.

Trybusińska, D., and A. Saracen. 2019. Loneliness in the context of quality of life of nursing home residents. *Open Medicine* 14:354–361.

Tsai, H. H., and Y. F. Tsai. 2011. Changes in depressive symptoms, social support, and loneliness over 1 year after a minimum 3-month videoconference program for older nursing home residents. *Journal of Medical Internet Research* 13(4):e93.

Tse, M. M., S. K. Tang, V. T. Wan, and S. K. Vong. 2014. The effectiveness of physical exercise training in pain, mobility, and psychological well-being of older persons living in nursing homes. *Pain Management Nursing* 15(4):778–788.

Tseng, Y. C., S. H. Y. Liu, M. F. Lou, and G. S. Huang. 2018. Quality of life in older adults with sensory impairments: A systematic review. *Quality of Life Research* 27(8):1957–1971.

Tsiourti, C., E. Joly, C. Wings, M. B. Moussa, and K. Wac. 2014. Virtual assistive companions for older adults: Qualitative field study and design implications. In *Proceedings of the 8th International Conference on Pervasive Computing Technologies for Healthcare.* Brussels: ICST. Pp. 57–64.

Tucker, J. S., H. S. Friedman, D. L. Wingard, and J. E. Schwartz. 1996. Marital history at midlife as a predictor of longevity: Alternative explanations to the protective effect of marriage. *Health Psychology* 15(2):94–101.

Tung, E. L., L. C. Hawkley, K. A. Cagney, and M. E. Peek. 2019. Social isolation, loneliness, and violence exposure in urban adults. *Health Affairs* 38(10):1670–1678.

Tung, J., and Y. Gilad. 2013. Social environmental effects on gene regulation. *Cellular and Molecular Life Sciences* 70(22):4323–4339.

Tunnecliff, J., J. Weiner, J. E. Gaida, J. L. Keating, P. Morgan, D. Ilic, L. Clearihan, D. Davies, S. Sadasivan, P. Mohanty, S. Ganesh, J. Reynolds, and S. Maloney. 2017. Translating evidence to practice in the health professions: A randomized trial of Twitter vs Facebook. *Journal of the Medical Informatics Association* 24(2):403–408.

Uchino, B. N. 2006. Social support and health: A review of physiological processes potentially underlying links to disease outcomes. *Journal of Behavioral Medicine* 29(4):377–387.

Uchino, B. N. 2009a. What a lifespan approach might tell us about why distinct measures of social support have differential links to physical health. *Journal of Social and Personal Relationships* 26(1):53–62.

Uchino, B. N. 2009b. Understanding the links between social support and physical health: A lifespan perspective with emphasis on the separability of perceived and received support. *Perspectives on Psychological Science* 4(3):236–255.

Uchino, B. N., J. T. Cacioppo, W. Malarkey, and R. Glaser. 1995. Individual differences in cardiac sympathetic control predict endocrine and immune responses to acute psychological stress. *Journal of Personality and Social Psychology* 69(4):736–743.

Uchino, B. N., J. T. Cacioppo, and J. K. Kiecolt-Glaser. 1996. The relationship between social support and physiological processes: A review with emphasis on underlying mechanisms and implications for health. *Psychological Bulletin* 119(3):488–531.

Uchino, B. N., J. Holt-Lunstad, D. Uno, R. Betancourt, and T. S. Garvey. 1999. Social support and age-related differences in cardiovascular function: An examination of potential mediators. *Annals of Behavioral Medicine* 21(2):135–142.

Uchino, B. N., M. Carlisle, W. Birmingham, and A. A. Vaughn. 2011. Social support and the reactivity hypothesis: Conceptual issues in examining the efficacy of received support during acute psychological stress. *Biological Psychology* 86(2):137–142.

Uchino, B. N., R. Trettevik, R. G. Kent de Grey, S. Cronan, J. Hogan, and B. R. W. Baucom. 2018. Social support, social integration, and inflammatory cytokines: A meta-analysis. *Health Psychology* 37(5):462–471.

Uehara, E., M. Flynn, R. Fong, J. Brekke, R. P. Barth, C. Coulton, K. Davis, D. DiNitto, J. D. Hawkins, J. Lubben, R. Manderscheid, Y. Padilla, M. Sherraden, and K. Walters. 2013. Grand challenges for social work. *Journal of the Society for Social Work and Research* 4(3):165–170.

Umberson, D. 1987. Family status and health behaviors: Social control as a dimension of social integration. *Journal of Health and Social Behavior* 28(3):306–319.

Umberson, D., K. Williams, D. A. Powers, H. Liu, and B. Needham. 2006. You make me sick: Marital quality and health over the life course. *Journal of Health and Social Behavior 47*(1):1–16.

UnitedHealth Group. 2018. *UnitedHealthcare expands Navigate4Me to bring personalized, holistic care to more people.* https://www.unitedhealthgroup.com/newsroom/2018/2018-12-09-uhc-expands-navigate4me-program.html (accessed November 4, 2019).

U.S. Census Bureau. 2018. *Households by age of the householder: 1960–present* (Table HH-3). https://www.census.gov/data/tables/time-series/demo/families/households.html (accessed November 12, 2019).

Utz, R. L., K. L. Swenson, M. Caserta, D. Lund, and B. deVries. 2014. Feeling lonely versus being alone: Loneliness and social support among recently bereaved persons. *Journals of Gerontology Series B: Psychological Sciences and Social Sciences* 69(1):85–94.

Vagelatos, N. T., and G. D. Eslick. 2013. Type 2 diabetes as a risk factor for Alzheimer's disease: The confounders, interactions, and neuropathology associated with this relationship. *Epidemiologic Reviews* 35:152–160.

Vallée, M., W. Mayo, and M. Le Moal. 2001. Role of pregnenolone, dehydroepiandrosterone and their sulfate esters on learning and memory in cognitive aging. *Brain Research Reviews* 37(1–3):301–312.

Valtorta, N. K., M. Kanaan, S. Gilbody, S. Ronzi, and B. Hanratty. 2016a. Loneliness and social isolation as risk factors for coronary heart disease and stroke: Systematic review and meta-analysis of longitudinal observational studies. *Heart* 102(13):1009–1016.

Valtorta, N. K., M. Kanaan, S. Gilbody, and B. Hanratty. 2016b. Loneliness, social isolation and social relationships: What are we measuring? A novel framework for classifying and comparing tools. *BMJ Open* 6(4):e010799.

Valtorta, N. K., M. Kanaan, S. Gilbody, and B. Hanratty. 2018a. Loneliness, social isolation and risk of cardiovascular disease in the English Longitudinal Study of Ageing. *European Journal of Preventive Cardiology* 25(13):1387–1396.

Valtorta, N. K., D. C. Moore, L. Barron, D. Stow, and B. Hanratty. 2018b. Older adults' social relationships and health care utilization: A systematic review. *American Journal of Public Health* 108(4):e1–e10.

van Deursen, A. J. A. M., and J. A. G. M. van Dijk. 2019. The first-level digital divide shifts from inequalities in physical access to inequalities in material access. *New Media & Society* 21(2):354–375.

Van Eerd, D., K. Newman, R. DeForge, R. Urquhart, E. Cornelissen, and K. N. Dainty. 2016. Knowledge brokering for healthy aging: A scoping review of potential approaches. *Implementation Science* 11(1):140.

van Wijngaarden, E., C. Leget, and A. Goossensen. 2015. Ready to give up on life: The lived experience of elderly people who feel life is completed and no longer worth living. *Social Science & Medicine* 138:257–264.

Vardoulakis L.P., L. Ring, B. Barry, C. L. Sidner, and T. Bickmore. 2012. Designing relational agents as long term social companions for older adults. In Y. Nakano, M. Neff, A. Paiva, and M. Walker (eds.), *Intelligent Virtual Agents*. IVA 2012. Lecture Notes in Computer Science, vol. 7502. Berlin, Heidelberg, Germany: Springer.

Vázquez, A., C. Jenaro, N. Flores, M. J. Bagnato, M. C. Pérez, and M. Cruz. 2018. eHealth interventions for adult and aging population with intellectual disability: A review. *Frontiers in Physiology* 9:2323.

VDMAS (Virginia Department of Medical Assistance Services). 2003. *Personal care aide training curriculum*. Richmond, VA: Virginia Department of Medical Assistance Services.

Veazie, S., J. Gilbert, K. Winchell, R. Paynter, and J.-M. Guise. 2019. *Addressing social isolation to improve the health of older adults: A rapid review*. Rockville, MD: Agency for Healthcare Research and Quality.

Ventola, C. L. 2014. Social media and health care professionals: Benefits, risks, and best practices. *Pharmacy and Therapeutics* 39(7):491–520.

Verdery, A. M., and R. Margolis. 2017. Projections of white and black older adults without living kin in the United States, 2015 to 2060. *Proceedings of the National Academy of Sciences* 114(42):11109–11114.

Verduyn, P., O. Ybarra, M. Résibois, J. Jonides, and E. Kross. 2017. Do social network sites enhance or undermine subjective well-being? A critical review. *Social Issues and Policy Review* 11(1):274–302.

Verma, S. 2018. CMS approves North Carolina's innovative Medicaid demonstration to help improve health outcomes. *Health Affairs Blog*, October 24. https://www.healthaffairs.org/do/10.1377/hblog20181024.406020/full (accessed December 2, 2019).

Versloot, J., A. Grudniewicz, A. Chatterjee, L. Hayden, M. Kastner, and O. Bhattacharyya. 2015. Format guidelines to make them vivid, intuitive, and visual: Use simple formatting rules to optimize usability and accessibility of clinical practice guidelines. *International Journal of Evidence-Based Healthcare* 13(2):52–57.

Victor, C. R., and A. Bowling. 2012. A longitudinal analysis of loneliness among older people in Great Britain. *Journal of Psychology* 146(3):313–331.

Victor, C. R., V. Burholt, and W. Martin. 2012. Loneliness and ethnic minority elders in Great Britain: An exploratory study. *Journal of Cross-Cultural Gerontology* 27(1):65–78.

Viruell-Fuentes, E. A., J. D. Morenoff, D. R. Williams, and J. S. House. 2013. Contextualizing nativity status, Latino social ties, and ethnic enclaves: An examination of the "immigrant social ties hypothesis." *Ethnicity & Health* 18(6):586–609.

Visser, M. A., and F. El Fakiri. 2016. The prevalence and impact of risk factors for ethnic differences in loneliness. *European Journal of Public Health* 26(6):977–983.

Vitak, J., N. Proferes, K. Shilton, and Z. Ashktorab. 2017. Ethics regulation in social computing research: Examining the role of institutional review boards. *Journal of Empirical Research on Human Research Ethics* 12(5):372–382.

von Soest, T., M. Luhmann, T. Hansen, and D. Gerstorf. 2020. Development of loneliness in midlife and old age: Its nature and correlates. *Journal of Personality and Social Psychology* 118(2):388–406.

Vozikaki, M., M. Linardakis, and A. Philalithis. 2017. Preventive health services utilization in relation to social isolation in older adults. *Journal of Public Health* 25(5):545–556.

Wagner, J., N. Ram, J. Smith, and D. Gerstorf. 2016. Personality trait development at the end of life: Antecedents and correlates of mean-level trajectories. *Journal of Personality & Social Psychology* 111(3):411–429.

Wallace, R., C. Lees, M. Minou, D. Singleton, and G. Stratton. 2014. Effects of a 12-week community exercise programme on older people. *Nursing Older People* 26(1):20–26.

Wallhagen, M. I., W. J. Strawbridge, and G. A. Kaplan. 1996. 6-year impact of hearing impairment on psychosocial and physiologic functioning. *Nurse Practitioner* 21(9):11–14.

Walsh, C. G., J. D. Ribeiro, and J. C. Franklin. 2018. Predicting suicide attempts in adolescents with longitudinal clinical data and machine learning. *Journal of Child Psychology and Psychiatry* 59(12):1261–1270.

Walters, K., K. Kharicha, C. Goodman, M. Handley, J. Manthorpe, M. Cattan, S. Morris, C. S. Clarke, J. Round, and S. Iliffe. 2017. Promoting independence, health and well-being for older people: A feasibility study of computer-aided health and social risk appraisal system in primary care. *BMC Family Practice* 18(1):47.

Wand, A. P. F., C. Peisah, B. Draper, and H. Brodaty. 2018. Why do the very old self-harm? A qualitative study. *American Journal of Geriatric Psychiatry* 26(8):862–871.

Wang, X. M., S. Brisbin, T. Loo, and S. Straus. 2015. Elder abuse: An approach to identification, assessment and intervention. *Canadian Medical Association Journal* 187(8):575–581.

Wang, Y., L. Kung, and T. A. Byrd. 2018. Big data analytics: Understanding its capabilities and potential benefits for healthcare organizations. *Technological Forecasting and Social Change* 126:3–13.

Warner, C. B., A. R. Roberts, A. B. Jeanblanc, and K. B. Adams. 2017. Coping resources, loneliness, and depressive symptoms of older women with chronic illness. *Journal of Applied Gerontology* 38(3):295–322.

Warner, D. F., S. A. Adams, and R. K. Anderson. 2019. The good, the bad, and the indifferent: Physical disability, social role configurations, and changes in loneliness among married and unmarried older adults. *Journal of Aging Health* 31(8):1423–1453.

Warner, L. M., B. Schuz, L. Aiken, J. P. Ziegelmann, S. Wurm, C. Tesch-Romer, and R. Schwarzer. 2013. Interactive effects of social support and social conflict on medication adherence in multimorbid older adults. *Social Science & Medicine* 87:23–30.

Weinstein, B. E., and I. M. Ventry. 1982. Hearing impairment and social isolation in the elderly. *Journal of Speech and Hearing Research* 25(4):593–599.

Weinstein, B. E., L. W. Sirow, and S. Moser. 2016. Relating hearing aid use to social and emotional loneliness in older adults. *American Journal of Audiology* 25(1):54–61.

Weiss, R. S. 1974. *Loneliness: The experience of emotional and social isolation.* Cambridge, MA: MIT Press.

Weissman, M. M., J. Pathak, and A. Talati. 2020. Personal life events—A promising dimension for psychiatry in electronic health records. *JAMA Psychiatry* 77(20):115–116.

Welin, L., K. Svärdsudd, S. Ander-Peciva, G. Tibblin, B. Tibblin, B. Larsson, and L. Wilhelmsen. 1985. Prospective study of social influences on mortality: The study of men born in 1913 and 1923. *Lancet* 325(8434):915–918.

Whisman, M. A. 2010. Loneliness and the metabolic syndrome in a population-based sample of middle-aged and older adults. *Health Psychology* 29(5):550–554.

White, H., E. McConnell, E. Clipp, L. G. Branch, R. Sloane, C. Pieper, and T. L. Box. 2002. A randomized controlled trial of the psychosocial impact of providing internet training and access to older adults. *Aging & Mental Health* 6(3):213–221.

WHO (World Health Organization). 2018. *Elder abuse: Key facts*. https://www.who.int/news-room/fact-sheets/detail/elder-abuse (accessed January 29, 2019).

WHO. 2019a. *Early detection of cancer*. https://www.who.int/cancer/detection/en (accessed November 26, 2019).

WHO. 2019b. *Health promotion and disease prevention through population-based interventions, including action to address social determinants and health inequity*. http://www.emro.who.int/about-who/public-health-functions/health-promotion-disease-prevention.html (accessed November 10, 2019).

Wick, J. Y. 2017. Aging in place: Our house is a very, very, very fine house. *Consultant Pharmacist* 32(10):566–574.

Wiktorsson, S., B. Runeson, I. Skoog, S. Ostling, and M. Waern. 2010. Attempted suicide in the elderly: Characteristics of suicide attempters 70 years and older and a general population comparison group. *American Journal of Geriatric Psychiatry* 18(1):57–67.

Wiles, J. L., A. Leibing, N. Guberman, J. Reeve, and R. E. Allen. 2012. The meaning of "aging in place" to older people. *Gerontologist* 52(3):357–366.

Wilkins, R., O. Adams, and A. Brancker. 1989. Changes in mortality by income in urban Canada from 1971 to 1986. *Health Reports* 1(2):137–174.

Williams, N. J., M. A. Grandner, D. M. Wallace, Y. Cuffee, C. Airhihenbuwa, K. Okuyemi, G. Ogedegbe, and G. Jean-Louis. 2016. Social and behavioral predictors of insufficient sleep among African Americans and Caucasians. *Sleep Medicine* 18:103–107.

Wilson, D. S., M. Montie, P. Conlon, M. Reynolds, R. Ripley, and M. G. Titler. 2016. Nurses' perceptions of implementing fall prevention interventions to mitigate patient-specific fall risk factors. *Western Journal of Nursing Research* 38(8):1012–1034.

Wilson, J. M. G., and G. Jungner. 1968. *Principles and practice of screening for disease*. Geneva, Switzerland: World Health Organization.

Wilson, R. S., K. R. Krueger, S. E. Arnold, J. A. Schneider, J. F. Kelly, L. L. Barnes, Y. Tang, and D. A. Bennett. 2007. Loneliness and risk of Alzheimer disease. *Archives of General Psychiatry* 64(2):234–240.

Winningham, R. G., and N. L. Pike. 2007. A cognitive intervention to enhance institutionalized older adults' social support networks and decrease loneliness. *Aging & Mental Health* 11(6):716–721.

Wong, C. A., and L. M. Giallonardo. 2013. Authentic leadership and nurse-assessed adverse patient outcomes. *Journal of Nursing Management* 21(5):740–752.

Wong, J. S. M., and L. J. P. Waite. 2017. Elder mistreatment predicts later physical and psychological health: Results from a national longitudinal study. *Journal of Elder Abuse & Neglect* 29(1):15–42.

Woods, J. A., K. R. Wilund, S. A. Martin, and B. M. Kistler. 2012. Exercise, inflammation and aging. *Aging and Disease* 3(1):130–140.

Wormald, A. D., P. McCallion, and M. McCarron. 2019. The antecedents of loneliness in older people with an intellectual disability. *Research in Developmental Disabilities* 85:116–130.

WSDSHS (Washington State Department of Social and Health Services). 2009. *Revised fundamentals of caregiving: Facilitator's guide*. https://www.dshs.wa.gov/sites/default/files/ALTSA/hcs/documents/Facilitators%20Guide%20RFOC.pdf (accessed June 27, 2019).

Wu, Y., S. Damnée, H. Kerhervé, C. Ware, and A. Rigaud. 2015. Bridging the digital divide in older adults: A study from an initiative to inform older adults about new technologies. *Clinical Interventions in Aging* 10:193–201.

Xia, N., and H. Li. 2018. Loneliness, social isolation, and cardiovascular health. *Antioxidants and Redox Signaling* 28(9):837–851.

Xu, M., P. A. Thomas, and D. Umberson. 2016. Marital quality and cognitive limitations in late life. *Journals of Gerontology, Series B: Psychological Sciences and Social Sciences* 71(1):165–176.

Yaghoubzadeh, R., M. Kramer, K. Pitsch, and S. Kopp. 2013. Virtual agents as daily assistants for elderly or cognitively impaired people: Studies on acceptance and interaction feasibility. In R. Aylett, B. Krenn, C. Pelachaud, and H. Shimodaira (eds.), *Intelligent virtual agents*. IVA 2013. Lecture Notes in Computer Science, vol. 8108. Berlin: Springer. Pp. 79–91.

Yamada, J., J. E. Squires, C. A. Estabrooks, C. Vicotor, and B. Stevens. 2017. The role of organizational context in moderating the effect of research use on pain outcomes in hospitalized children: A cross-sectional study. *BMC Health Services Research* 17(1):68.

Yang, Y. C., C. Boen, K. Gerken, T. Li, K. Schorpp, and K. M. Harris. 2016. Social relationships and physiological determinants of longevity across the human life span. *Proceedings of the National Academy of Sciences* 113(3):578–583.

Yeginsu, C. 2018. U.K. appoints a minister for loneliness. *The New York Times*. January 17. https://www.nytimes.com/2018/01/17/world/europe/uk-britain-loneliness.html (accessed August 11, 2019)

Yildirim, Y., and S. Kocabiyik. 2010. The relationship between social support and loneliness in Turkish patients with cancer. *Journal of Clinical Nursing* 19(5–6):832–839.

Yip, S. O., M. A. Dick, A. M. McPencow, D. K. Martin, M. M. Ciarleglio, and E. A. Erekson. 2013. The association between urinary and fecal incontinence and social isolation in older women. *American Journal of Obstetrics and Gynecology* 208(2):e141–e146.

Young, K. A., Y. Liu, K. L. Gobrogge, H. Wang, and Z. Wang. 2014. Oxytocin reverses amphetamine-induced deficits in social bonding: Evidence for an interaction with nucleus accumbens dopamine. *Journal of Neuroscience* 34(25):8499–8506.

Yousefi Nooraie, R., A. Marin, R. Hanneman, L. Lohfeld, and M. Dobbins. 2017. Implementation of evidence-informed practice through central network actors; A case study of three public health units in Canada. *BMC Health Services Research* 17(1):208.

Yu, L., P. A. Boyle, E. Segawa, S. Leurgans, J. A. Schneider, R. S. Wilson, and D. A. Bennett. 2015. Residual decline in cognition after adjustment for common neuropathologic conditions. *Neuropsychology* 29(3):335–343.

Yusif, S., J. Soar, and A. Hafeez-Baig. 2016. Older people, assistive technologies, and the barriers to adoption: A systematic review. *International Journal of Medical Informatics.* 94:112–116.

Zebhauser, A., L. Hofmann-Xu, J. Baumert, S. Hafner, M. E. Lacruz, R. T. Emeny, A. Doring, E. Grill, D. Huber, A. Peters, and K. H. Ladwig. 2014. How much does it hurt to be lonely? Mental and physical differences between older men and women in the KORA-Age study. *International Journal of Geriatric Psychiatry* 29(3):245–252.

Zhu, V. J., L. A. Lenert, B. E. Bunnell, J. S. Obeid, M. Jefferson, and C. H. Halbert. 2019. Automatically identifying social isolation from clinical narratives for patients with prostate cancer. *BMC Medical Informatics and Decision Making* 19(1):43.

Zickuhr, K., and M. Madden. 2012. *Older adults and internet use.* https://www.pewresearch.org/internet/2012/06/06/older-adults-and-internet-use (accessed June 27, 2019).

Zijlstra, G. A. R, J. C. Van Haastregt, T. Ambergen, E. Van Rossum, J. T. Van Eijk, S. L. Tennstedt, and G. I. Kempen. 2009. Effects of a multicomponent cognitive behavioral group intervention on fear of falling and activity avoidance in community-dwelling older adults: Results of a randomized controlled trial. *Journal of the American Geriatrics Society* 57(11):2020–2028.

Zivin, K., and N. A. Christakis. 2007. The emotional toll of spousal morbidity and mortality. *American Journal of Geriatric Psychiatry* 15(9):772–779.

Zuboff, S. 2019. *The age of surveillance capitalism: The fight for a human future at the new frontier of power.* New York: PublicAffairs.

Zwijsen, S. A., A. R. Niemeijer, and C. M. P. M. Hertogh. 2011. Ethics of using assistive technology in the care for community-dwelling elderly people: An overview of the literature. *Aging & Mental Health* 15(4):419–427.

A

Public Meeting Agendas

Committee on the Health and Medical Dimensions of
Social Isolation and Loneliness in Older Adults

FIRST COMMITTEE MEETING

DECEMBER 10, 2018

National Academy of Sciences Building
2101 Constitution Avenue
Washington, DC 20418

Open Session

11:15 a.m.	**Welcome Study Sponsors and Introductory Remarks** *Dan Blazer II, Committee Chair* *Lisa Marsh Ryerson, AARP Foundation*
	Discussion and Q&A *Committee Members*
12:30 p.m.	**Adjournment of Public Session**

SECOND COMMITTEE MEETING

FEBRUARY 27, 2019

Keck Center of the National Academies
500 Fifth Street, NW
Washington, DC 20001

Open Session

9:00 a.m.	**Welcome and Opening Remarks** *Dan Blazer II, Committee Chair*
9:15 a.m.	**PANEL: Interventions** *Jeanne-Marie Guise, Agency for Healthcare Research and Quality Evidence-Based Practice Centers* *Jessica Retrum, Metropolitan State University of Denver (via Zoom)* *Lucy Savitz, Kaiser Permanente Center for Health Research* *Speaker Q&A with Audience*
10:45 a.m.	**PANEL: Technology** *Colin Walsh, Vanderbilt University Medical Center (via Zoom)* *Steve Ewell, Consumer Technology Association Foundation* *Speaker Q&A with Audience*
11:45 a.m.	**Lunch**
12:30 p.m.	**PANEL: State of the Science** *James Coan, University of Virginia* *Bert Uchino, University of Utah (via Zoom)* *Speaker Q&A with Audience*
1:30 p.m.	**Break**

1:45 p.m. **PANEL: Public Health Considerations**
Martha Bruce, The Dartmouth Institute
Linda Fried, Columbia University
Speaker Q&A with Audience

2:45 p.m. **Open Public Comment Period**

3:30 p.m. **Adjournment of Public Session**

THIRD COMMITTEE MEETING – DAY ONE

APRIL 24, 2019

Beckman Center of the National Academies of Sciences,
Engineering, and Medicine
100 Academy Way
Irvine, CA 92617

Open Session

12:45 p.m. **Welcome and Opening Remarks**
Dan Blazer II, Committee Chair

12:50 p.m. **The Role of Technology**
Sara Czaja, Weill Cornell Medicine (via Zoom)

1:20 p.m. **Addressing Social Determinants of Health**
Michael Monson, Centene Corporation (via Zoom)

2:00 p.m. **Coalitions to Address Social Isolation and Loneliness**
Maureen Feldman, Social Isolation Impact Project
Jeanne-Marie Guise, Agency for Healthcare Research and Quality Evidence-Based Practice Centers

3:15 p.m. **Adjournment of Public Session**

THIRD COMMITTEE MEETING – DAY TWO

APRIL 25, 2019

Beckman Center of the National Academies of
Sciences, Engineering, and Medicine
100 Academy Way
Irvine, CA 92617

Open Session

8:00 a.m.	**Welcome and Opening Remarks** *Dan Blazer II, Committee Chair*
8:05 a.m.	**Addressing Social Determinants of Health** *Sachin Jain, CareMore (via Zoom)*
8:45 a.m.	**Adjournment of Public Session**

B

Committee and Staff Biographies

Dan G. Blazer II, M.D., M.P.H., Ph.D. (*Chair*), is the J.P. Gibbons Professor of Psychiatry Emeritus and a professor of community and family medicine at Duke University as well as an adjunct professor in the Department of Epidemiology, School of Public Health, University of North Carolina. He is the author or co-author of more than 180 book chapters, more than 220 published abstracts, and nearly 500 peer-reviewed articles. He is also the editor or author of 40 books. Many of the book chapters and scientific articles are on the topics of late life depression, epidemiology, consultation liaison psychiatry, the interface between religion and psychiatry, and the epidemiology of substance use disorders. Most of his research projects have focused on the prevalence of physical and mental illness in the elderly. He has served as the principal investigator (PI) of the Duke University Established Populations for Epidemiologic Studies of the Elderly, the Piedmont Health Survey of the Elderly, and the MacArthur Field Studies of Successful Aging. He also was the original PI of the Duke Clinical Research Center for Late Life Depression. Dr. Blazer is an elected member of the National Academy of Medicine from which he received the Walsh McDermott Award for Distinguished Lifetime Service to the Academy.

Susan Beane, M.D., joined Healthfirst in 2009, bringing with her extensive professional experience in managed care. As the executive medical director at Healthfirst, Dr. Beane focuses on care management and clinical provider partnerships, programs especially designed to improve the delivery of vital, evidence-based health care to members. Dr. Beane, a dedicated primary care physician and board-certified internist, is a strong proponent of collaborating with and engaging providers to improve health outcomes. Dr. Beane leads Healthfirst in collaborating with major health care delivery systems and local and national policy experts on the design, implementation, and dissemination of innovative, outcomes-focused models of care. Her research contributions span the health of caregivers, obesity, and maternal health. Prior to joining Healthfirst, Dr. Beane served as the chief medical officer for Affinity Health Plan for 5 years—during which time she helped Affinity Health Plan become a top performer in quality and member satisfaction. Before that, she worked at AmeriChoice and HIP USA as a medical director. Dr. Beane is a graduate of Princeton University and the Columbia University College of Physicians and Surgeons.

Cynthia M. Boyd, M.D., M.P.H., is a professor at the Johns Hopkins University School of Medicine in the Department of Medicine, Division of Geriatric Medicine and Gerontology, and is a core faculty member at the Johns Hopkins Center on Aging and Health and the Roger C. Lipitz Center for Integrated Health Care. Dr. Boyd is jointly appointed in the Department of Health Policy and Management and Epidemiology at the Johns Hopkins Bloomberg School of Public Health. She is trained in internal medicine, geriatric medicine, and epidemiology. Her work has focused on person- and family-centered care for people with multiple chronic conditions in order to improve health and well-being, and it includes epidemiological research, health services, research, systematic reviews, guidelines, and clinical trials. Dr. Boyd has focused on interventions to improve outcomes for older adults with multiple chronic conditions through community-based and health care interventions.

Linda Burnes Bolton, Dr.P.H., R.N., FAAN, is the senior vice president for nursing and the chief nursing executive at Cedars-Sinai Medical Center. Her research, teaching, and clinical expertise include nursing and patient care outcomes, improving organization performance, quality care, and cultural diversity within the health professions. Dr. Burnes Bolton is a past president of the American Organization of Nurse Executives, the American Academy of Nursing, and the National Black Nurses Association. She has provided leadership for several state and national programs, including service as chair of the national advisory committee of Transforming Care at the Bedside, Veterans Affairs Commission on Nursing, and the vice chair of the Robert Wood Johnson Foundation Initiative on the Future of Nursing at the Institute of Medicine. Dr. Burnes Bolton earned her bachelor of science degree in nursing from Arizona State University. She completed her master of science degree in nursing, master's in public health, and doctorate in public health at the University of California, Los Angeles.

George Demiris, Ph.D., FACMI, is a PIK (Penn Integrates Knowledge) University Professor at the University of Pennsylvania with joint appointments in the School of Nursing and the Perelman School of Medicine. He focuses his research on the use of information technology to support older adults and their family caregivers and to explore innovative solutions to promote independent aging and patient and family engagement. One area of his research includes the use of behavioral sensing, "smart home," and "Internet of Things" technologies to promote independence for community-dwelling older adults and their families. Such emerging technologies introduce challenges and opportunities in terms of engaging older adults in decision making, making sense of vast amounts of data, and promoting effective data visualizations as well as addressing ethical considerations. Dr. Demiris is also an elected member of the National Academy of Medicine.

Nancy J. Donovan, M.D., is the director of the Division of Geriatric Psychiatry at Brigham and Women's Hospital and an associate researcher at Massachusetts General Hospital. She is an investigator in observational neuroimaging studies of aging at Massachusetts General Hospital and in clinical trials research at the Center for Alzheimer Research and Treatment. Dr. Donovan's research examines late life neuropsychiatric symptoms and their underlying biological substrates, including the association between a number of emotional and behavioral symptoms (such as loneliness) and preclinical Alzheimer's disease. In her clinical work, she provides care for older adults with psychiatric and cognitive disorders. She received her medical degree from the Columbia University Vagelos College of Physicians and Surgeons and completed psychiatric residency training at the Stanford University Medical Center. She is an assistant professor of psychiatry at the Harvard Medical School.

Robert Espinoza, M.P.A., is the vice president of policy at PHI, an organization focused on the direct care workforce, where he oversees its national policy advocacy, research, and strategic communications division. For more than 20 years Mr. Espinoza has spearheaded high-profile advocacy campaigns and written landmark reports on aging and long-term care; lesbian, gay, bisexual, and transgender (LGBT) rights; racial justice; and immigration, among other topics. Prior to PHI, he served as the senior director for public policy and communications at SAGE, the country's premier organization for LGBT older adults. In 2010 he co-founded the Diverse Elders Coalition, a historic federal coalition focused on improving aging supports for communities of color and LGBT communities. Mr. Espinoza received his M.P.A., with honors, from New York University, and his B.A. in English and B.S. in journalism from the University of Colorado Boulder.

Colleen Galambos, Ph.D., ACSW, LCSW, LCSW-C, FGSA, is the Helen Bader Endowed Chair in Applied Gerontology at the University of Wisconsin–Milwaukee and an adjunct professor at the Medical College of Wisconsin. She is a center scientist with the Center for Aging and Translational Research, Center for Urban Population Health, and a member of the Clinical and Translational Science Institute of Southeast Wisconsin. She currently serves as the secretary general of the North American Chapter of the International Society of Gerontechnology and is past chair of the National Association of Social Workers Aging Practice Section. Dr. Galambos's practice experience includes clinical, administrative, policy, and research positions in a variety of health and long-term care organizations. She is a fellow of the Gerontological Society of America and a National Association of Social Workers Pioneer. She is the author of 3 books and more than 140 peer-reviewed publications. Dr. Galambos's research interests include care transitions and advance care planning, aging in place, abuse in later life, health and long-term care, systems quality improvement, gerontechnology, and interprofessional practice.

Julianne Holt-Lunstad, Ph.D., is a professor of psychology and neuroscience at Brigham Young University. She focuses her research on the long-term health effects of social connection. Her work has been seminal in the recognition of social isolation and loneliness as risk factors for early mortality. Dr. Holt-Lunstad has worked with government organizations aimed at addressing this issue. She has provided expert testimony in a U.S. congressional hearing, provided expert recommendations for the U.S. Surgeon General Emotional Well-Being in America Initiative, and is currently a member of the technical working group for the UK Cross Departmental Loneliness Team. She also serves as a scientific advisor for the Australian Coalition to End Loneliness, the Foundation for Art & Healing, and research advisory panel for AARP Services, Inc., United Healthcare, and Rural Aging.

James S. House, Ph.D., is the Angus Campbell Distinguished University Professor Emeritus of Survey Research, Public Policy, and Sociology at the University of Michigan Institute for Social Research and an elected member of the American Academy of Arts & Sciences, the National Academy of Medicine, and the National Academy of Sciences. He received his B.A. in history (minor in psychology) from Haverford College and his Ph.D. in social psychology from the University of Michigan. His research career has focused on the role of social and psychological factors in the etiology and course of health and illness, initially on occupational stress and health, then social relationships and support in relation to health, and currently on the role of psychosocial factors in understanding and alleviating social disparities in health and the way health changes with age. Professor House has been the founding principal investigator or co-principal investigator of the Americans' Changing Lives study, the Changing Lives of Older Couples study, and the Chicago Community Adult Health Study.

Kathleen McGarry, Ph.D., is a professor of economics at the University of California, Los Angeles, and a research associate at the National Bureau of Economic Research. She was previously a professor of economics at Dartmouth College and served as a senior economist at the White House Council of Economic Advisers. Dr. McGarry's research focuses on the well-being of the elderly with particular attention paid to public and private transfers, including the Medicare and Supplemental Security Income programs, and the transfer of resources within families. Her research combines work on the financial aspects of aging with issues related to health economics to examine insurance coverage among the elderly. Dr. McGarry's current work analyzes the importance of end-of-life medical expenses, particularly expenses associated with nursing homes and home health care, and the effect of caregiving on the well-being of family care providers. She is a co-investigator for the Health and Retirement Study.

Jeanne Miranda, Ph.D., is a professor in the Department of Psychiatry and Biobehavioral Sciences at the University of California, Los Angeles (UCLA). She is a mental health services researcher who has focused her work on providing mental health care to low-income and minority communities. She holds a Ph.D. in clinical psychology from University of Kansas and completed postdoctoral training at the University of California, San Francisco. Dr. Miranda's major research contributions have been in evaluating the impact of mental health care for ethnic minority communities. She is an investigator in two UCLA centers focusing on improving disparities in health care for ethnic minorities. She was the senior scientific editor of *Mental Health: Culture, Race and Ethnicity, a Supplement to Mental Health: A Report of the Surgeon General* (2001). She became a member of the National Academy of Medicine in 2005 and was the 2008 recipient of the Emily Mumford Award for Contributions to Social Medicine from Columbia University.

Laurie Lovett Novak, Ph.D., M.H.S.A., is an assistant professor of biomedical informatics at the Vanderbilt University Medical Center. In the Department of Biomedical Informatics, she serves as the director of the Center of Excellence in Applied Artificial Intelligence. Dr. Novak conducts ethnographic research to advance theory and contribute to the development of technology and social interventions in several domains. These include the everyday management of chronic illness among the elderly and in other populations, the implementation of artificial intelligence into everyday work practices in health care, and the social and ethical dimensions of new forms of population health management. She received a B.A. in finance from Murray State University, an M.H.S.A. in health management and policy from the University of Michigan, and a Ph.D. in medical and organizational anthropology from Wayne State University.

Carla M. Perissinotto, M.D., M.H.S., is an associate professor in the Division of Geriatrics, Department of Medicine at the University of California, San Francisco (UCSF), and is board certified in internal medicine, geriatrics, and palliative medicine. Since 2017, she has served as the associate chief for geriatrics clinical programs at UCSF. In this role she oversees and develops new clinical programs serving older adults across care settings. Her main work is in UCSF

Care at Home, which provides medical care to home-bound older adults, and in embedded geriatrics consulting practices. From 2008 to 2017, Dr. Perissinotto spent a portion of her clinical time at the Over 60 Health Center, a federally qualified health center, serving adults over age 55 in Alameda County. At Over 60, Dr. Perissinotto directed the educational programs for UCSF learners and focused on practice change by establishing a team-based model for community-based geriatrics seeing adults across a continuum of care. Dr. Perissinotto gained national and international recognition for her research on the effects of loneliness on the health of older adults. Most recently, her research has focused on integration of loneliness assessments in health care, and evaluation and implementation of community-based programs focused on ameliorating loneliness and isolation in adults.

Juliann G. Sebastian, Ph.D., R.N., FAAN, is the dean of the College of Nursing at the University of Nebraska Medical Center and a professor of nursing. Her areas of expertise are the organization of care delivery systems, care for underserved populations, academic nursing practice, nurse-managed health centers, and doctor of nursing practice program curricula. Dr. Sebastian earned her bachelor's and master's degrees in nursing from the University of Kentucky (UK) College of Nursing and a doctorate in business administration from UK's College of Business and Economics. She served as chair of the board of directors for the American Association of Colleges of Nursing (2016–2018) and has served on the boards of directors of several nonprofit organizations. She has presented at numerous national and international conferences and has published numerous papers, book chapters, and abstracts and three books related to community nursing. In 1999 Dr. Sebastian was inducted as a fellow in the American Academy of Nursing.

NATIONAL ACADEMIES OF SCIENCES, ENGINEERING, AND MEDICINE STAFF

Tracy A. Lustig, D.P.M., M.P.H., is a senior program officer in the Health and Medicine Division of the National Academies of Sciences, Engineering, and Medicine. Dr. Lustig was trained in podiatric medicine and surgery and spent several years in private practice. In 1999 she was awarded a congressional fellowship with the American Association for the Advancement of Science and spent 1 year working in the office of Ron Wyden of the U.S. Senate. Dr. Lustig joined the National Academies in 2004. Much of her work has focused on the health care workforce and the aging of the U.S. population. She was the study director for consensus studies on the geriatrics workforce, oral health, and ovarian cancer research. She also directed workshops on the oral health workforce, the allied health workforce, telehealth, assistive technologies, home health care, hearing loss, and stereotypes in aging and disability. In 2009 she staffed a National Academies–wide initiative on the Grand Challenges of an Aging Society and subsequently helped to launch the Forum on Aging, Disability, and Independence, which she currently directs. Dr. Lustig has a doctor of podiatric medicine degree from Temple University and a master of public health degree with a concentration in health policy from The George Washington University.

Jennifer A. Cohen, M.P.H., is a program officer in the Health and Medicine Division of the National Academies. She received her undergraduate degree and her M.P.H. from the University of Maryland, College Park. She has worked on a number of projects at the National Academies, including *Organ Procurement and Transplantation*, *Clearing the Air: Asthma and Indoor Air Exposures*, *Veterans and Agent Orange: Update 2000 . . . Update 2014*, *Post-Vietnam Exposure in Agent Orange-Contaminated C-123 Aircraft*, *The Health Effects of Cannabis and Cannabinoids*, and *Getting to Zero Alcohol-Impaired Driving Fatalities*. She was also the rapporteur for the workshop summary *Challenges and Successes in Reducing Health Disparities*.

Caroline M. Cilio, M.B.E., until October 2019, was an associate program officer in the Health and Medicine Division of the National Academies. Ms. Cilio joined the National Academies in 2016 and worked on the Forum on Aging, Disability, and Independence; a consensus study on returning individual research results to participants; a workshop on physician-assisted death; and the Forum on Medical and Public Health Preparedness for Disasters and Emergencies. Ms. Cilio holds a master of bioethics degree and a B.A. in health and societies, an interdisciplinary study focused on medical sociology and health policy, from the University of Pennsylvania.

Kendall Logan, is a senior program assistant in the Health and Medicine Division of the National Academies. She received her bachelor of arts in anthropology with a public health minor from Haverford College. Ms. Logan joined the National Academies in 2018 and has also worked on the standing committee on Medical and Epidemiological Aspects of Air Pollution on U.S. Government Employees and Their Families and the consensus study on temporomandibular disorders.

Andrew M. Pope, Ph.D., is the director of the Board on Health Sciences Policy. He has a Ph.D. in physiology and biochemistry from the University of Maryland and has been a member of the National Academies staff since 1982 and of the Health and Medicine Division staff since 1989. His primary interests are science policy, biomedical ethics, and environmental and occupational influences on human health. During his tenure at the National Academies, Dr. Pope has directed numerous studies on topics that range from injury control, disability prevention, and biologic markers to the protection of human subjects of research, National Institutes of Health priority-setting processes, organ procurement and transplantation policy, and the role of science and technology in countering terrorism. Since 1998 Dr. Pope has served as the director of the Board on Health Sciences Policy, which oversees and guides a program of activities that is intended to encourage and sustain the continuous vigor of the basic biomedical and clinical research enterprises needed to ensure and improve the health and resilience of the public. Ongoing activities include forums on neuroscience, genomics, drug discovery and development, and medical and public health preparedness for catastrophic events. Dr. Pope is the recipient of the Health and Medicine Division's Cecil Award and the National Academy of Sciences' President's Special Achievement Award.